PSYCHOTHERAPY
A DYNAMIC APPROACH

Psychotherapy
a dynamic approach

PAUL A. DEWALD M.D.

Training and Supervising Analyst (Geographic),
Chicago Institute for Psychoanalysis

Clinical Professor of Psychiatry,
St Louis University School of Medicine

Director of Treatment Service,
Psychoanalytic Foundation of St Louis

Consultant, St Louis State Hospital

SECOND EDITION

Blackwell Scientific Publications
Oxford and Edinburgh

SEN 632 06160 X

FIRST PUBLISHED 1964
SECOND EDITION 1969

Printed in Great Britain by
ADLARD AND SON LTD, DORKING
and bound by
THE KEMP HALL BINDERY, OXFORD

TO NELL

'It is very probable, too, that the large-scale application of our therapy will compel us to alloy the pure gold of analysis freely with the copper of direct suggestion; and hypnotic influence, too, might find a place in it again, as it has in the treatment of war neuroses. But, whatever form this psychotherapy for the people may take, whatever the elements out of which it is compounded, its most effective and most important ingredients will assuredly remain those borrowed from strict and untendentious psychoanalysis.'

SIGMUND FREUD (1919)
Lines of Advance in
Psychoanalytic Therapy

Contents

Acknowledgements to First Edition

I want to express my debt to all of the various people who have been my patients during the past 15 years, each of whom has given me the opportunity to learn something different. I am also deeply grateful to the various students I have had the pleasure of teaching in a number of different settings. Their questions, uncertainties and desire for understanding have forced me to conceptualize my own ideas more carefully, and to put them into communicable form.

In the preparation of this volume, I wish to thank Doctors Joan Fleming, John W. Higgins and Alex H. Kaplan, and Mrs Janet Golden for their helpful criticisms of the manuscript. I am indebted to Mrs Ann Mounts for her dedicated secretarial work.

My wife helped in assembling the references, and her encouragement and support were vital throughout the whole project.

Introduction to Second Edition

In the years since the first edition of this volume was published, psychoanalysis has come under increasing attack from a large number of sources, both inside and outside the field of psychiatry. Most of this criticism and depreciation is directed toward psychoanalysis as a specific treatment-method, and involves such things as the occurrence of therapeutic limitations, issues of statistical cure rates, and its lack of applicability as a general therapeutic instrument for the treatment of the majority of psychiatrically ill patients.

In the area of the general understanding of human behaviour, and in the further development of psychoanalytic theory, there have likewise been continuing pressures for modification and change. Generally speaking these criticisms have been more temperate, and focused at the substance of elaborations or modifications of basic theory, and of continuing attempts to derive methods for verification or validation of psychoanalytic observations and postulates. Many of these criticisms and suggested modifications arise from scientific work using both the psychoanalytic method and experimental or observational approaches other than psychoanalysis *per se*. These issues generally represent the applications of the scientific method and a progressive evolution of concepts which occur as part of any scientific discipline that seeks to advance human knowledge and understanding.

However, most of the basic concepts with which this book deals (such as the existence of unconscious motivational forces within the mind, the dynamic steady state, homeostasis and psychic equilibrium, the structural model of mental functioning, concepts of transference and counter-transference, the genetic and dynamic approaches to understanding of human behaviour, the interrelationships between the individual's intra-psychic experience and his external environment, etc.) remain as corner stones of present-day psychiatric understanding. Although the vocabulary and semantics may differ somewhat, such conceptualizations from psychoanalytic experience and understanding are deeply imbedded in the current stream of thinking in modern psychiatry. Whether the focus of therapeutic interest and intent is the individual, the family, or the community, the basic data and conceptual extrapolations remain meaningful and pertinent to the understanding of behaviour, whether seen individually or in the setting of larger groups. Indeed, psychoanalytic observations and theory aid in understanding the group process itself.

With the changing patterns in the delivery of health care and in the expectations of the population at large, and with successful efforts at community education in regard to mental health and mental illness, ever larger numbers of individuals are presenting themselves for psychiatric evaluation and treatment. Psychiatry is being asked to contribute its understanding, as well as its therapeutic efforts, into much broader and more inclusive areas of human behaviour and interaction than ever before. The pressures of therapeutic need are increasing, and there is likewise an increased interest in developing methods of preventive psychiatry. The growing emphasis on psychiatric services for the poor, the shift of psychiatric interest away from the traditional middle- or upper-class patient, and the extension of psychiatric services into the community are illustrated by the rapid development of the community mental health movement in the United States. There are pressing needs to develop new therapeutic methods applicable to a variety of different social classes and types of patients, and applicable in a more effective and generally economical fashion than have been available heretofore.

However, such pressures for service, and the increasing awareness of the impact of social and cultural forces on the individual, do not in any way negate the existence or importance of internal intra-psychic factors, and the complexity of interrelationship between the individual and his environment. The needs for the development of new approaches to therapy should not lead us to discard or minimize the knowledge or lessons painstakingly acquired and learned through years of clinical observation and research. The needs for the development of brief forms of therapy do not offset or wipe out the technical and theoretical advances achieved from the long-term and intensive study of patients. Instead, these latter experiences and the conceptualizations derived from them can provide the theoretical principles from which more practical and immediate therapeutic experimentation and development can occur. Random, non-conceptualized, impulsive, or anti-theoretical attempts at therapy, no matter how well intentioned, may prove uneconomical in the long run.

Psychoanalysis as a generalized theory of behaviour can shed conceptual light and understanding upon the multiple varieties of human behaviour and interrelationships, including all forms of therapeutic interchange, whether conducted with individual patients or with larger groups of people. Its lessons and its understanding should not be overlooked in the search for new therapeutic modalities, even though extensive modifications of technique may occur as therapeutic applications are broadened. The rationale and effects of such treatment modalities as Behaviour Therapy, Learning Theory, Conditioning, Reciprocal Innervation, etc., can be effectively understood within the framework of general psychoanalytic theory. Psychoanalytic theory can offer significant insights for the further development of effective therapeutic techniques applicable to larger numbers and types of patients.

It is for these reasons that the decision was made to publish a second edition of this book. This book remains the only systematic and definitive attempt to apply the insights of psychoanalytic theory to supportive, active, or non-analytic psychotherapies. It is an attempt to develop a rational, consistent, and communicable theory of supportive treatment, and to delineate and compare such forms of therapy from more traditionally insight-directed analytic approaches to the treatment of mental disability. Supportive treatment as developed here includes treatments of long or brief duration, treatments aimed at suppression of symptoms or modification of behaviour, and treatments applicable to the total social class spectrum. It is the thesis of this book that if the basic understanding of human motivation and behaviour supplied by psychoanalysis are systematically applied to non-analytic therapeutic methods, a theoretical structure for such methods can be developed and they can be carried out with increased effectiveness.

Introduction to First Edition

Proficiency in psychotherapy is a clinical skill which is acquired only gradually, and in large measure is the result of continuing and varied experience in the therapeutic setting with patients. As with any clinical skill, the more intensive and varied is the young therapist's experience, the greater are the opportunities for learning and for improving himself in his therapeutic capacity. The technique of psychotherapy cannot be taught or learned in purely didactic fashion. However, in the process of obtaining the clinical experience necessary to develop these skills, the young therapist is faced with difficulties and problems which may interfere with his learning progress, or may impair his ability to make constructive use of his contacts with patients. Most people starting in this field have only a vague or incomplete theoretical orientation, and generally a minimum of clinical experience as a background. In spite of careful or frequent supervision, the young therapist is on his own in most of his contacts with patients.

Although the use of a clinical trial-and-error method can provide valuable learning experiences, this is not the most efficient or economical way of developing a skill. Different from other clinical specialities, psychotherapy is for the most part a private process between patient and therapist, and the introduction of a third person as an observer (either the trainee observing the supervisor, or the supervisor observing the trainee), drastically changes the total therapeutic situation. The use of closed circuit TV, one-way mirrors and tape recordings has helped in the teaching and learning of this technique, but there are still many limitations.

During his training and early experience, the young psychiatrist is usually reading or hearing from people who are much his senior in experience about problems or techniques with which he has had little personal contact. Not infrequently, he becomes discouraged that in his own work with patients he cannot demonstrate or find the same things mentioned by others, or at times he may take things out of context and attempt to apply them somewhat inappropriately to his own case material and experience.

Furthermore, the structure of most training programmes results in the relatively inexperienced therapist often being assigned patients who represent the most advanced degrees of psychopathology and who therefore often have the poorest therapeutic prognosis, and create some of the most difficult therapeutic problems. This is frequently accompanied with the recommendation, 'Just give this patient supportive treatment', but little attention is paid in an organized way as to what constitutes support and how this is to be accomplished. This is also at times accompanied by a directly or indirectly expressed depreciation of supportive treatment. Pushed by his own therapeutic ambition, and comparing himself with somewhat more advanced colleagues, the young therapist may at times be bewildered, unclear and unsure of himself in the therapeutic situation.

In the face of these problems and stresses on the developing therapist, a number of responses are common. Some people lose interest in therapy, and instead turn to research. While this may offer hope for the future, it does not meet the therapeutic needs and challenges of today. Others come to rely exclusively on drug chemistry or somatic therapies. Some develop a 'defeatist attitude' which borders on therapeutic nihilism, with the feeling that it doesn't make any difference what is done in psychotherapy, since the patient will either get well or not get well regardless. Still others respond to the patient on the basis of intuition or common sense, and in a trial-and-error fashion, and gradually evolve a technique based partly on their own personal experiences and partly on those of their supervisors. Their concepts of treatment are often vague or unstructured, and in essence they must acquire in their own individual learning much of the cumulative knowledge obtained in other settings by other people.

Other therapists deal with their uncertainties by asking a variety of highly specific questions, such as: 'What does the therapist do when the patient says thus', or, 'How do you handle this situation?' This leads to a type of 'cook-book' psychotherapy, in which the young therapist is essentially looking for a recipe which he can apply in specific quantities and at specified times in hopes thereby of bringing some order to his thinking and treatment. The problem here is that such questions are not readily answered by simple responses since they vary in accordance with a number of factors in the specific situation, and an answer which does not take account of these factors can only be partially helpful at best. If the therapist attempts to apply in a rote or memorized fashion specific interactions or interventions without a general understanding of why they are being made, he becomes more of a mechanical technician, and much of the skill and effectiveness in psychotherapy is lost.

The inexperienced psychotherapist is in need of a theoretical frame of reference and orientation to the problems and technique of psychotherapy. This can provide him with a background on which to make observations in his own clinical experience, and against which to weigh and judge the particular therapeutic interventions or interactions that he makes. Such a background can also provide a number of unifying concepts, whereby he can begin to appreciate some of the similarities and differences in therapeutic technique as applied to various patients and settings.

It is in this connection that a book such as this on the *theory and technique of psychotherapy* can serve a useful function. And psychoanalysis can serve effectively as a theoretical and unifying framework within which the various clinical observations can be organized and conceptualized.

Psychoanalysis as a specific method of therapy is an extremely intense, long-term and difficult type of treatment. In proportion to the total number of people with emotional and mental disturbances and disorders, only a relatively small number have thus far been treated in formal psychoanalysis. As a specific method of treatment, psychoanalysis cannot fulfil the therapeutic needs of the majority of psychiatric patients. The investment of time, effort and money are too great, and the number of qualified psychoanalysts (and the rate at which new ones are trained) is too small for this method of treatment to be applied on a mass scale. Furthermore, for a variety of reasons to be considered later, formal psychoanalysis would not be the treatment of choice for the majority of psychiatric patients, even if an analyst and the necessary time and money were available. Although many of the patients who have successfully completed a full psychoanalysis consider the required investments to have been worth while, it remains a form of treatment applicable to a relatively small number of patients.

Psychoanalysis, however, is also a general theory of behaviour, apart from its specific therapeutic application. Based on the intensive and 'microscopic' study of relatively normal as well as pathological phenomena, psychoanalytic theory offers a comprehensive conceptualization of the functioning of the human mind in states of health and of psychopathology. It provides an internally consistent theory of total behaviour based on clinical observation and the conceptualization derived from it. One of the areas of human interaction which can be conveniently and systematically understood within the psychoanalytic theoretical framework is the process and technique of other forms of psychotherapy.

This book is an attempt to apply the unifying concepts of psychoanalysis to the broad spectrum of interactions of the psychotherapeutic process. The main focus is on individual psychotherapy, although some of the concepts elaborated will have applicability to other variations of treatment such as group therapy, family treatment, or the milieu therapy of a hospital setting.

The book is based on material presented by the author in seminar form to groups of psychiatric residents and fellows at the University of Rochester Medical Center, at Washington University School of Medicine, and at St Louis University School of Medicine.

Section I of the book may be considered as a presentation of the general problem of psychodynamics. It is a highly condensed summary of some of the aspects of general psychoanalytic theory which have a particular pertinence to the theory and technique of psychotherapy. Section II is likewise a condensation of the psychoanalytic theory of psychopathology, as formulated within the more general theory of human behaviour. Neither of these sections should be construed as a complete exposition of their respective areas, but rather they should be considered as a summarized general background and basis for the theory and technique of psychotherapy which is developed in Section III.

Since the book is primarily addressed to the relatively inexperienced psychiatrist in training, there has been a deliberate omission of the more highly theoretical, abstract and controversial aspects of basic theory. The greater the reader's familiarity with the basic concepts of psychoanalytic theory, the more useful will be the condensations presented here. The suggested references at the end of each chapter are designed to help the reader expand his understanding of the basic general theoretical framework. However, in none of the chapters has there been an attempt systematically to survey the literature, or to present a complete bibliography on the particular subject.

In Section III on psychotherapy, the material is deliberately presented in the form of a somewhat artificial dichotomy of supportive versus insight-directed psychotherapy. This is being done for pedagogic reasons, with full recognition that in the usual clinical situation such sharp dichotomies do not always exist or persist. However, the emphasis is on providing the relatively inexperienced therapist with a framework of orientation in which the similarities and differences of therapeutic approaches can become more readily apparent. Once the general framework and structure of psychotherapy have been grasped and understood, the therapist can avoid random or contradictory responses or interventions and instead he can integrate his behaviour in keeping with an internally consistent overall theory of therapeutic technique.

Supportive and brief forms of psychotherapy offer a considerable challenge to the skill of the therapist. The patient population is frequently severely and seriously disabled, time is often a pressing factor and decisions must frequently be made on the basis of incomplete evidence, data or understanding. However, if the therapist has a clear understanding of the basic principles of psychopathology and behaviour, as well as the theory of therapy, he can begin to develop rational and consistent therapeutic techniques which will permit the broadest possible application to the various clinical problems that he faces.

SECTION I
Psychodynamics

CHAPTER I

The Mental Apparatus

Psychoanalytic theory began as an attempt by Freud to organize and conceptualize the data derived from his clinical observations of patients. His study of the phenomena of hypnosis, neurotic symptoms and dreams suggested to him that large components of mental life were unconscious, and occurred without the individual's awareness of their existence.

His own introspective self-analysis, and the detailed study of his own dreams further supported this finding, as did his studies on the psychology of slips and errors, and the psychology of wit and humour.

In these early studies, he was particularly struck by the many and varied manifestations of the sexual instincts, and by the significance and con tinuing importance of early life experiences and ideas. He became increasingly interested in the existence of various manifestations of infantile and childhood sexuality, and their persistence in a variety of forms in the conscious and unconscious mental life of the adult.

He proposed the theory that neuroses arose from a disturbance in the function and discharge of these sexual instincts, resulting from internal conflicts between them and the rest of the individual's personality. The infantile and childhood sexual instincts and memories were thought of as comprising one area of mental function, designated the System Unconscious. Essentially all other mental functions were thought to comprise the Ego-instincts, and were designated as occurring in the Systems Preconscious and Conscious.

Anxiety was thought to result from dammed-up sexual instincts or libido being inadequately or incorrectly discharged, and thus directly converted to anxiety.

Freud developed and presented these ideas as the *topographical hypothesis* in his monumental book, *The Interpretation of Dreams*. This theory served as the early basis of attempts to understand the aetiology and persistence of neurotic phenomena.

The early technique of psychoanalysis as a method of treatment followed logically from these theoretical formulations, and was the first systematic attempt at psychotherapy based on a rational and internally consistent theory of psychopathology.

Further details of these early theoretical formulations will not be developed here, but the interested reader is referred to the literature on the subject. The topographical hypothesis formed a useful framework for the initial collection of analytic material, but continuing clinical experience indicated that these formulations did not permit a ready understanding of some of the newer data derived from clinical observation. In particular, clinical observation showed that a large number of mental functions which were *not* related to the instincts were nevertheless unconscious to the patient, and many manifestations of aggression in mental life had the other characteristics of instincts. Furthermore, anxiety could not always be understood as the result of dammed-up libido.

These were among the factors which forced Freud to modify his theoretical formulations in a group of papers published in 1920–27, and led him to develop the *structural hypothesis*. This theory and the second theory of anxiety (to be described), have served as the subsequent basic theoretical conceptualization of analytic observations, although there have been significant modifications and extensions, particularly since the elaboration of ego psychology initiated by Anna Freud in 1936, and carried on by many workers since that time.

Conscious, Preconscious and Unconscious

The earlier topographical hypothesis had divided mental phenomena into the Systems Unconscious, Preconscious and Conscious. In the later structural hypothesis, mental processes are still conceived of in terms of unconscious, preconscious and conscious phenomena, but these terms now have an adjectival quality and are descriptive, rather than attempts to localize an area of function.

Conscious is defined as those aspects of mental function which at the time of observation are within the current awareness of the individual. This may include a large variety of thoughts, sensations and feelings, but the critical point is that the individual at that moment is aware of their existence and has focused some part of his current attention on them.

The quality of *preconscious* is related to those mental processes which are not currently within the conscious awareness of the individual, but which are readily available to his conscious mind, and can be brought to consciousness with a minimal expenditure of psychic energy.

By *unconscious* is meant those mental functions or processes which are not currently in the consciousness of the individual, and which require a significant expenditure of psychic energy to be made conscious.

This distinction can be illustrated as follows. If an individual is thinking about and aware of the name of a popular song, this song would be currently conscious. If the individual is not thinking about this song, but is asked the name of it by someone else who directs his attention to the song and he is able correctly and immediately to give the name, the song would have been preconscious prior to the time that the individual focused his attention upon it and brought it to consciousness. Everybody has had the experience, however, of knowing very well that he has not forgotten the name of a particular song, and of feeling that it is 'on the tip of my tongue', and yet in spite of considerable effort, energy and various attempts to do so, is unable, for the moment, to remember the correct name. At this particular moment, the song and its name would be unconscious since in spite of considerable effort, it cannot be brought to consciousness. The fact that it is still present in the mind is attested to by the individual's own awareness that he 'knows it', and by the fact that if someone else mentions it, there is an instantaneous recognition and awareness of the correct name. And frequently at a later time the correct name may return to the individual's consciousness without the necessity for the investment of energy that was attempted previously.

This illustration is meant only to demonstrate the quality of unconsciousness, and does not illustrate many of the other aspects of unconscious mental phenomena to be considered later.

The qualities conscious, preconscious or unconscious as applied to mental phenomena may be considered to exist on a continuum. Each may be seen as zonal, with gradations within the zone, and with no sharp dividing line between them.

Psychic Energy

The concept of *psychic energy* is an obscure and unclarified one. However, subjective as well as objective observations of human behaviour permit the postulation of its existence, even though the mechanisms are unknown by which the metabolic functioning of brain cells is converted into various types of thought processes. And as yet there is no accurate way of measuring the quanta of energy involved. Therefore, the differentiation between unconscious, preconscious and conscious on the basis of the expenditure of psychic energy required to bring a mental process into conscious awareness is based only on rough approximations and relationships.

However, the concept of psychic energy refers to repeated observations that there are various forces operative in mental life; that these appear to have different intensities; that the intensity of these forces varies among different individuals; that the strength of these forces within a given individual may shift or change; and that these observed forces are related to factors of motivation. As will be developed later, this concept of psychic energy has heuristic value in understanding the dynamics of the human mind.

The act of directing mental or psychic energy and investing it in any mental process within the mind itself is known as the act of *cathecting*. The quantity of psychic energy which is so invested in such a mental process, although undefined in terms of a precise measurement, is known as a *cathexis*.

Id, Ego and Super-ego

In the structural hypothesis, the mental apparatus is divided by definition into three major functional groupings, namely, the *id*, *ego* and *super-ego*. As will be seen in the following definitions and descriptions, all mental processes can be conceptualized as belonging in one of these three groups of functions.

It must be explicitly understood that the structural hypothesis and the grouping of mental processes as id, ego and super-ego is a theoretical abstraction based on a series of arbitrary definitions. These abstractions and groupings have a particular usefulness in understanding psychic and mental function, but although they are referred to as 'psychic structures' they do not correspond to any type of central nervous system structure, organization or group of physiological or neurological functions.

There is considerable misunderstanding about this because in much of the literature these structures are described in an anthropomorphic fashion as if they had a separate existence of their own. They represent groupings of mental functions and phenomena based on an agreed-upon definition of terms, but divided in such a way that they prove eventually to have usefulness for the understanding and conceptualization of psychodynamics and psychopathology. The idea of a 'structure' is based on the repeated observation that once established, the various functions included in any one of the groups tend to be organized in a characteristic way, to become automatic in operation, to be repetitive and persistent, and to have a slow rate of change.

Therefore, although they are not 'real' structures in the sense of having any type of separate existence, there is nevertheless an internal consistency within these groupings and an interrelatedness between them which therefore permit us to *think* of them as psychic structures, recognizing, however, that they are purely arbitrary groups of functions.

The *id* is that portion of the mental apparatus whose function it is to give psychic representation in the mind to the energic, instinctual forces originating in the biological organization of the organism. The term 'instinct' has been the source of much confusion, since in psychoanalytic theory it has been used differently than in general biological theory, resulting from the problem of translating Freud's original term 'trieb' into English. 'Instinct' in psychoanalysis refers to the general, driving biological forces more closely related to the biology than to the psychology of the human organism, and *not* to the highly complex, organized, inborn patterns of behaviour seen in lower species.

By mechanisms that are as yet unknown, some of these biological forces eventually achieve a psychic representation within the mind at which time they are known in psychoanalytic theory as *drives*. In brief, the drive is the psychic representation in the mental apparatus of the biological instinct. There are multiple drives present in the id, but these can be grouped as relating either to the sexual drives in the broadest sense of the term, or to the aggressive drives.

The id is totally unconscious, and its functions are organized in accordance with the pleasure principle and the primary process. *The pleasure principle* involves the concept that drives seek direct and immediate gratification regardless of any other factors or forces which impinge on the situation. The drives will vary in their intensity from time to time, and the stronger the drive, the greater will be the pressure for immediate discharge gratification and thus for reduction of drive tension. In and of themselves, the drives take no cognisance of such things as the impact or effect of the reality situation, the presence or absence of an appropriate object, or the overall effects of drive discharge.

The primary process is a mode of thought characteristic of the early thinking processes in the infant and child, and is contrasted with the *secondary process*, which is a later mode of thought acquired through learning, experience, trial and error, and education by the environment. This primary process mode of thought of the infant and the very young child is characterized chiefly by the concept of mobility of cathexis. This means that the representation of objects or other mental processes may be rapidly cathected with drive energy, either sexual, or aggressive, and may also be rapidly decathected of this drive energy. As a result, there may be sharp changes and shifts in the investment of psychic representations of objects and other mental processes within the id, depending on the nature and intensity of the drives at any one particular moment, and the various mental representations which present themselves as objects for these drives.

Descriptively, this results in the phenomena of condensation and displacement, which are likewise characteristic of primary process thought. In the case of *displacement*, mental representations of objects or other processes may be cathected by drives which are only indirectly related to these objects. In the case of *condensation*, one mental process or object representation within the mind may be the target of a number of different drives simultaneously.

Mobility of cathexis, condensation and displacement also mean that the usual learned laws and concepts of rationality and logic do not exist in the primary process mode of thinking, and that instead there is a disregard for compatibility, sequence, time-relations and cause and effect. Opposites may co-exist simultaneously and there is no conception of negative. This mode of thought persists in a timeless fashion since id functions are totally unconscious and therefore are not directly influenced by learning or experience.

The mode of thought of the primary process is best exemplified by the manifest content of a dream during sleep. A variety of distortions and disturbances in logical sequence, cause and effect, time and spatial arrangement, contradiction and the existence of opposites, may occur. One figure or place in the dream may be a composite made up of many figures or places. People and memories from one era in the person's life may interact with those from an entirely different era. Allusions and small fragments of experiences may occur without being completed. And feelings or thoughts which are associated with one person may be displaced and experienced towards someone else.

Usually during the dream itself, the dreamer has a sense of active participation and involvement, and the dream has the quality of reality. It is only as the dreamer wakes, or after he has woken up, that these irrational and illogical connections and distortions lose their realistic quality and the person becomes aware of the incongruity of the events or people in the dream as it occurred.

Another characteristic of the id and the primary process is the existence of symbolism and symbol formation. This is a form of displacement by which an object, because of a specific quality or attribute which can be associated with some other object or some aspect of a drive comes to stand for (and in this sense to symbolize) a drive which may or may not be directly related to it originally.

The universality of certain types of symbols arises from the fact that a number of drives, and conflicts over these drives, occur in all children by virtue of the human condition and the prolonged period required for human development, learning and maturation. In the course of development, as the child perceives more and more things in the world about him, certain objects present themselves as available for drive cathexes in the child's attempted solution of these universal conflicts. Thus the object, by virtue of its parts or qualities, eventually becomes symbolic of that which is unconscious and for other reasons cannot be expressed consciously. Examples of such universal childhood conflicts and problems include the issues of sexuality, death, birth, the body and its parts. The child will seek symbols for these in its interactions and experiences within its own specific environment and culture, so that the specific symbols chosen will differ with cultural experience and availability.

An example of this might be the percept of a coca-cola bottle, which may be realistically perceived and remain undistorted. However, drives which are seeking discharge will cathect whatever internal images or external percepts will permit a displacement of drive energy in accordance with the primary process mode of thought. Therefore, because of its neck and elongated shape, the bottle could represent a phallic symbol, and as such be invested with a variety of drives relating to masculine or phallic activity. At the same time, it is also a hollow vessel with a cavity, and hence it may be used to represent a feminine symbol and be invested with drives relating to feminine, receptive sexuality. It is also filled with a liquid which may be drunk, and hence might be cathected with drives relating to nutrition, sucking and the taking-in of various substances. Because of its consistency, shape and the fact that it is made of glass, it might also serve as a weapon, and hence be cathected with drives relating to aggression, and the expression of aggressive impulses. Whether or not such a percept will be cathected with drive energy through primary process displacement will be a function of the nature and intensity of the particular drives at the moment, and of the nature and qualities of the available objects or percepts. As there are shifts in drive intensity, there may be a de-cathexis of one object, and a re-cathexis of some other object more suitable to the expression of the particular predominating drive at that moment.

Although earlier psychoanalytic theory postulated that the drives originate entirely in the biological functions of the organism, this has been challenged by more recent data. This is particularly true for the theory of aggression, and there is on-going debate as to whether aggression is a primary inborn drive, or whether it develops very early in life as the result of frustration. And subsequently aggressive drive manifestations can be observed as at least partly a response to external stimulation. Even the vicissitudes of the sexual drives have been demonstrated to be influenced by non-biological factors and stimulation.

However these issues are ultimately settled, in the clinical and behavioural situation the id processes are totally unconscious and cannot be directly observed. However, by virtue of their drive quality, they produce derivatives, the effects of which are closer to consciousness and may be observed in the individual's conscious and preconscious thought, behaviour and feeling. It is through observation and study of these drive-derivatives that the existence of the underlying unconscious drives is inferred.

Although the id drives seek direct and immediate discharge as described before, other mental processes (such as perception, judgment, motor activity, etc.) which are defined as part of ego function, are required to effect such drive discharge. In other words, id drives do not have a direct access to motility or to the external environment, but must be mediated by ego functions to be described shortly.

The *super-ego* is that portion of the mental apparatus whose function it is to judge the other mental functions critically, in terms of moral standards of right and wrong, good and bad, punishment and reward. The super-ego is partly conscious and preconscious, this element corresponding to what ordinarily is called the conscience. But it is also largely unconscious, and this unconscious aspect of super-ego function relates to more primitive and archaic considerations of punishment and reward.

Super-ego formation involves the internalization to varying degrees of the parental standards and attitudes of right and wrong, and of reward and punishment. These are experienced by the child from infancy onwards, but are particularly influenced by the child's attempts to identify with the parents in the conflicts over the resolution of the oedipus complex.

These incorporated early parental images, which form the nucleus of unconscious super-ego function, do not necessarily reflect parental attitudes and standards as they actually occurred, but rather are an internalization of the child's perception, anticipation and interpretation of the parents' attitudes. The child will also tend to project on to the parents his own hostile or aggressive impulses and then to anticipate the parents' reaction in kind. In this way the ultimate super-ego threat and demands include the child's projections and distortions of the parents and their attitudes occurring at the time that the incorporation and identification took place.

In addition to concepts of punishment, the super-ego also includes the representation in the mind of the ideals to which the individual strives, known as the *ego-ideal*. These ideals likewise are partly preconscious and partly unconscious and they are based on childhood fantasy and conceptions of the parental images. These are later incorporated, and hence the individual's ideals for himself may be permanently influenced by the primary process and early fantasied distortions.

Although the major impetus to super-ego development has been the internalization of the parental images as individuals, the parents and their attitudes and concepts are also representative of society generally. Hence there is an impact on super-ego formation from social and cultural forces as represented first by the parents, and later by other objects with whom the developing child comes in contact. And, in turn, super-ego functions play an important role in the continuity of social and cultural forces from one generation to the next.

The conscious and preconscious super-ego functions are capable of continuous modification as influenced by relationships and identifications with people other than the parents, and particularly with the peer group in adolescence. However, the unconscious infantile and early childhood parental images that have been incorporated as super-ego functions persist essentially unchanged since they are not accessible to conscious learning.

The *ego* is defined as that group of mental processes whose function it is to perceive and recognize the various forces impinging on the organism both from the internal and the external environments, to synthesize and integrate these, and to execute those functions and activities necessary to maintain a state of internal and external adaptation. This group of functions includes such things as perception, memory, thought, intelligence, the motor-functions, judgment and the assessment of reality. It also includes those efforts that the organism makes to alter the internal or external environments, or to adapt itself to either of these.

The ego operates in accordance with the reality principle, as opposed to the pleasure principle of the id. The *reality principle* involves the assessment of the total situation, including all of the various forces impinging on the individual, with an ultimate selection or judgment for the choice of response made on the basis of the greatest good and long-term benefit for the total organism. The reality principle may involve a blocking of drive gratification or a change in the object of a drive, or the substitution of a future pleasure for a present one, with the ultimate aim of achieving the greatest amount of satisfaction and pleasure and the least amount of pain or danger. Since the individual is ultimately seeking the greatest possible gain and satisfaction within the limitations of the internal and external reality situation, it may be said that the reality principle is a further functioning of the pleasure principle, but taking account of other factors than the immediacy of the drives.

The ego also functions in accordance with the *secondary process* mode of thought, in which concepts of logic, sequence, cause and effect, contradiction and negative are recognized. This means also that in comparison to the mobility of cathexis operative in the primary process, in the secondary process there is a relative stability of cathexis and the maintenance of a more constant set of investments of psychic energy.

The ego functions are partly on a conscious and preconscious level, but there are also a significant number of ego functions which occur unconsciously. Among the latter are the psychological mechanisms of defence which will be considered separately in a later chapter.

A full description and elaboration of the development of ego functions and their ultimate integration into an internally consistent, cohesive pattern of functioning and interrelationship is beyond the scope of this discussion. This is a highly complex and, in some areas, still unclarified subject and interested readers are referred to various discussions of this in the psychoanalytic literature.

For the purposes of this presentation it will be sufficient to point out that ego development involves the interaction of two main developmental streams. The first of these are the innate, inborn and constitutional ego apparatuses, some of which (i.e. perception) exist in varying degrees of maturity at the time of birth, and others of which unfold in a developmentally predetermined, chronological pattern specific to the species. For example, in motor-behaviour, which is by definition an ego-function, there are initially only undifferentiated motor responses, usually involving a total response of the organism. With the subsequent development of the central nervous system, myelinization of nerve tracts, and further growth and maturation of the organism generally, there is a progressive refinement and capacity to control motor activity as the child develops within certain species-specific time intervals. The capacity to sit, to crawl, to walk, for dexterous movements of the hands and arms, etc., develops sequentially and at roughly the same age for most children. Similarly, the capacity for speech, for memory, for abstract thinking and conceptualization, etc., are also dependent on the biological maturation of the specific apparatus involved in the carrying out of these functions.

The other main developmental stream is the psychological impact on ego development initiated and sustained by the interaction of the developing organism with what has been called the 'average expected or anticipated environment'. The impact of this environment, from the psychological and experiential standpoint, will significantly influence ego-development, depending on the nature and types of interaction which occur.

The various sub-groups of ego functions may develop at different rates, depending on the nature of the biological and constitutional apparatuses and their subsequent development, as well as the nature and effects of the various psychological processes and experiences. In some instances there may be general disturbances or distortions of ego development, while at other times specific ego functions may be enhanced or inhibited while general ego development is not completely affected.

The major portion of ego development occurs in the first five or six years of life. But there is continuous further development of the ego as the organism matures, and as the development of the various apparatuses and the increasing interaction between the organism and psychological environment proceeds.

In considering ego-development, it is necessary to take into account what is the expected and appropriate capacity of the organism in relationship to its chronological age, as well as in relationship to the specific life experiences that have been undergone.

For example, in comparing a child of 1 year with a child of 3, significant ego difference would be anticipated, not only in terms of intellect, perception, motor and other physical capacities, but also in terms of psychological capacities, such as the ability to tolerate frustration. A child of 1 will have very little capacity for this, and if frustrated will quickly have a massive or generalized discharge, whereas in a child of 3 it would be anticipated that he should now be in a position psychologically to master some of the tension related to frustration, at least up to a certain point. Whereas a child of 1 year may not be psychologically capable of comfortably separating himself physically from the mother, in a child of 3 there should be sufficient ego development to permit such separation without undue anxiety, at least for short intervals. In each instance, the response would be normal for the respective chronological age.

On the other hand, if the 1-year-old child is capable of separating from the mother without apparent anxiety, it would suggest that there may have been a failure in development of a relationship with her, since normally one would not anticipate that the ego would be well enough developed to permit this separation without conflict. Similarly, if a child of 3 cannot separate from the mother without manifest disturbance, there has been a failure in ego development which by this time should have been sufficient to master the conflict situation.

Similarly, if both of these children are compared to a child of 6 or an adolescent of 16, one would anticipate significant differences as ego functions have developed and unfolded. This would be related to physical and underlying biological development as well as to psychological maturation and integration. These differences would be illustrated by the capacity for increasingly complicated physical and mechanical activity, as well as the capacity for the use of the mind in increasingly complex functions involving memory, intelligence, abstract thinking and judgment.

At the other end of the biological scale, there also occur significant ego changes but in the reverse direction. During the process of ageing there may be a significant and progressive deterioration of previously established ego functions. These may include the loss or reduction of motor, sensory and intellectual ego capacities, as well as the loss or change in complex psychological ego integrations or patterns of behaviour. The rate of such losses may vary among the different ego functions, and such losses may at times be limited to specific ego functions, or at other times be more generalized. Such involutional and senescent ego changes may occur as a result of the combination of biological and psychological processes.

Although once they are developed the functions which make up the ego have a general internal consistency for the individual, it must be recognized that this is not a static, once-and-for-all type of organization. There are significant and continuously modifying changes within the ego generally, as well as within specific sub-groups of functions in response to various influences. For example, such factors as fatigue, sleep, delirium, illness, sensory deprivation, trauma, prolonged stress, or conflict of various types will all exert an influence on ego functions which may at times be highly specific and at other times be more generalized.

It should again be emphasized that this conception of the mental apparatus remains a theoretical abstraction, based upon an accepted set of definitions. The id, ego and super-ego have no separate existence of their own, and represent convenient groupings of the various types of mental processes and functions.

What becomes apparent, however, is that the nature of these groupings takes into account the possibility of contradictory, and hence of conflict-producing, processes within the mind, or between these functional groups. It also takes into account the possibility of conflict between the total organism and the external environment. The usefulness of this frame of reference is that it provides a way of conceptualizing and understanding both the subjective and the objective aspects of human behaviour, and thus can provide the framework for a general dynamic theory of behaviour and of mental functioning, both normal and pathological. These concepts will be further developed in the next chapter on psychodynamics.

SUGGESTED READING

ARLOW, JACOB A. & BRENNER, CHARLES (1964) *Psychoanalytic Concepts and the Structural Theory*. International Universities Press Inc, New York

BRENNER, CHARLES (1955) *An Elementary Textbook of Psychoanalysis*. International Universities Press Inc, New York

FREUD, SIGMUND (1923) *The Ego and the Id*. Standard Edition of Complete Psychological Works, Vol. 19. The Hogarth Press, London

FREUD, SIGMUND (1933) *New Introductory Lectures on Psychoanalysis*. W.W.Norton & Co Inc, New York; or Standard Edition of Complete Psychological Works, Vol. 22, The Hogarth Press, London

GILL, MERTON M. (1963) *Topography and Systems in Psychoanalytic Theory*. Psychological Issues, Monograph 10. International Universities Press Inc, New York

HARTMAN, HEINZ (1956) The development of the ego concept in Freud's work. *Int. J. Psycho-Anal.* **37**, 425

SCHUR, MAX (1966) *The Id and the Regulatory Principles of Mental Functioning*. International Universities Press Inc, New York

WAELDER, ROBERT (1960) *Basic Theory of Psychoanalysis*. International Universities Press Inc, New York

CHAPTER II

Psychic Conflict and the Dynamic Steady State

In developing the concepts of a dynamic mental apparatus, it is necessary again to remind the reader that the grouping of mental functions into id, ego and super-ego represents a useful, but none the less arbitrary set of categories. Although these groupings have a characteristic internal consistency which is specific to each individual personality (and, therefore, they may be conceived of as having a 'structure'), nevertheless, each of these 'structures' consists of a variety of different functions, not all of which are equally active at any one time.

Therefore, in the material to follow, when mention is made of 'the id drives', it should be understood that all of the drives are not necessarily active to the same degree or intensity at the same time. Likewise, when describing 'ego-processes', this may again involve a selectivity, so that at any specific time certain ego-functions may be more active than others. And the same holds true for the super-ego.

Psychic Conflict

This division of psychic processes into id, ego and super-ego permits a systematic conceptualization of the various contradictory psychological forces and functions present in the mind at the same time. Since these forces may have contradictory or mutually incompatible goals, situations of psychological conflict will arise. This may be a conflict within the mental apparatus itself (intra-psychic conflict), or there may be conflict between the individual organism and the external environment. More frequently there may be combinations of these, so that conflict may exist between the organism and the external environment which is also related to an intra-psychic conflict.

To be more specific, an id drive seeking direct gratification by the original object of the drive in accordance with the pleasure principle, may be in conflict with a super-ego prohibition against the expression of this drive or the use of this object. An id drive might also be in conflict with the ego itself, by virtue of the ego's internal perception or fantasy of danger (aside from moral punishment) involved in gratifying such a drive. Such an id drive might also come into conflict with ego perception of the demands of external reality. There is also the possibility of conflict between the ego processes and external reality in terms of the demands that reality may make upon the organism, or in terms of the ego's attempt to modify or alter the external reality situation in accordance with the organism's own needs and wishes. Intra-psychically, there may be instances where super-ego demands create a situation of conflict in terms of the ego capacity to meet them. And, there may also be situations where the effect of reality upon super-ego processes might involve a conflict situation.

Dynamic Equilibrium

The major overall function of the ego is the maintenance, in spite of these various contradictions and stresses, of a state of internal adaptation within the mental apparatus, and of adaptation between the organism and its environment. The ego, as the central, organizing, co-ordinating and integrating group of functions of the mind, operates in accordance with the reality principle and the secondary process and attempts to maintain this total system in balance. This balance is analogous to the concept of a dynamic homeostasis, as originally described in physiology by Cannon.

However, the nature and intensity of the various forces impinging on the ego from the internal drives and the external environment, as well as the processes within the ego itself, are constantly shifting and fluctuating. As a result, the equilibrium established by the ego is not a fixed and static one, but rather a constantly oscillating and shifting dynamic steady state within certain limits.

An analogy on the physiological level would be the regulation of blood sugar, which is not kept at a once-and-for-all constant level, but rather is influenced by a variety of factors. These include the state of the pancreas and its secretory functions, the effects of various other hormones, the time interval since the ingestion of food, the amount of physical exertion that has been carried out, the state of digestion and absorption, the functioning of the liver, etc. All of these factors may be operative simultaneously or in sequence to raise or lower the level of blood sugar, but as the level shifts beyond certain threshhold points, compensatory mechanisms are called into play which tend to re-establish the sugar level within the normal range. The final result is not a single fixed level, but one which fluctuates within limits from hour to hour. And it is only when the sugar level exceeds these limits in either direction and compensatory mechanisms are ineffective, that clinical evidence of a disturbance becomes manifest (hyperglycaemia or hypoglycaemia).

Long-term Change

As mentioned before, the forces involved in the psychological equilibrium are also in a state of continuing fluctuation and change, both of a short-term and long-term nature. Changes which are of a long-range nature will have a slower impact on the state of the equilibrium.

For example, there are changes in the quality and intensity of id drives relating to specific phases of psycho-sexual development throughout the childhood period. During the latency period, particularly as related to sexual drives, drive intensity is relatively diminished, thus modifying their impact upon the ego in terms of its adaptive task. With the development of puberty and physical maturation, there is again an intensification of sexual drives which throughout the phase of adolescence puts a significantly greater stress on the ego and its controls. At the other end of the biological scale, with the involution of sexuality and sexual drives, there will again be a significant and steady change in the impact of these drives on the ego's adaptive mechanisms.

The same types of long-range shift and change may occur in super-ego function where, for example, in the adolescent phase of development there tends to be a shift away from the older parental attitudes and an identification with the peer group and subsequent influence on super-ego forces. Likewise, if an individual moves from one group or society to another, there may be significant shifts in super-ego identifications which will have an impact on the super-ego forces impinging on the ego's adaptive capacity.

Within the ego itself, there are also long-term changes in the direction of increasing maturation and capacity, which will influence the nature and stability of adaptation and equilibrium as the organism matures. But during the involutional and senescent period, in response to such things as vascular changes within the brain which in turn have an effect on ego functions such as memory, judgment, motility and integration, there will be another group of changes to which adaptation will be necessary. The same is true for changes in ego functions such as perceptual acuity, and motor ability. And, the relative loss of ego functions by virtue of such changes may significantly affect the ego's capacity to maintain a stable and effective state of adaptation.

Short-term Change

Shifts in the forces impinging on the ego from within the mental apparatus and from external reality will also occur over brief time spans and influence the nature of the dynamic equilibrium. The intensity of id drives will be sharply different before and after gratification, and in the interval during the build up of drive tension towards another drive discharge there will again be shifts and changes in the strength of the drive. For example, the intensity of a sexual drive in a situation of sexual stimulation or excitation will be sharply different compared with the intensity of such a drive immediately after orgasm. There will be similar vicissitudes in terms of aggression and the aggressive drives, which may at times be specifically stimulated in response to a variety of external or internal factors.

The demands of reality on the ego and the total organism are never constant, and as the various reality stresses impinge or subside, the adaptive tasks will change.

Even the influence of super-ego forces may vary over brief times, as in the situation where an individual becomes a member of a group or a mob, or in celebrations, where there may be a temporary renunciation of internal super-ego prohibitions in favour of an identification with the group and the group morality at the moment.

The functioning of the ego itself will also vary within short time-spans, so that such factors as fatigue, illness, delirium, intoxication, sleep, trauma, prolonged conflict or stress, may all influence the integration and overall functioning of ego processes.

Adaptation

Successful adaptation, however, requires that the ego be capable of integrating, controlling and effectively dealing with all of the various constantly changing forces that impinge from the internal as well as the external environment. This entire system must be maintained as a dynamic steady state involving a minimal degree of tension and conflict, and a maximal degree of need satisfaction and effective interaction with the environment.

Theory of Anxiety

Anxiety and other affective states play a major role in the process by which this adaptation and homeostasis are accomplished, so that the theory of anxiety must now be considered.

Although Freud considered 'the birth trauma' to be the original prototype of the anxiety experience by virtue of the organism at birth being flooded with an entirely new set of stimuli, this remains a conjecture and cannot be clinically established at present.

However, the observation of infant behaviour suggests the following sequence of events. Drives (i.e. hunger) or other stimuli reaching threshold intensity (i.e. pain) awaken the child from sleep, and are experienced by him as a mounting tension, distress, discomfort and generalized un-pleasurable stimulation which cannot be controlled by the child and hence require an external object (mother) for gratification of needs and reduction of tension. In the absence of the gratifying object, the drives and tension mount and the child reacts with a generalized psychomotor response of the diffuse and non-specific crying fit and motor discharge. With the gratifica-tion (or relief) provided by the external object, there is a reduction of tension to the point that with full gratification and decrease in the un-pleasurable stimulation, the child is able to return to sleep, which then persists until such time as drives or stimuli again reach threshold intensity and the cycle is repeated.

These repetitive experiences of being flooded by excitation which the infant is unable to control, and which are increasingly painful and un-pleasurable until drive satisfaction occurs, are considered to be prototypes of subsequent anxiety experiences.

As the infant matures and there is a further differentiation of self from object with an increasing awareness of helplessness and dependence on the object for need and drive gratification, the child now begins to experience fear over separation from the object. At this time the child's relationship to reality is still a primitive and archaic one, and the relationship to the mother is perceived by the child in terms of the primary process, involving a variety of possible distortions.

The details of these very early object relationships and their subsequent development are beyond the scope of this discussion. However, in general, the mother is perceived at times as a gratifying, need-satisfying object from whom separation is experienced with fear. At other times, she is also perceived as a bad, unpleasant, painful, external object which is to be feared, particularly at times of unsatisfied drive tension. With further ego maturation and development, and interactions with the mother, these external fears become increasingly more specific, focused around such issues as separation, the withdrawal of love and punishment.

Gradually others in the child's environment also become involved in the child's concepts of punishment, pain and external threat. As the child moves into the oedipal phase of development, these threats are also influenced by the distortions of the child's primary process mode of thought, and by the projection of his own fears, fantasies and impulses on to the parental figures. These fears, threats, distortions and possibilities of punishment or loss of love are initially perceived by the child as coming from outside, and hence are perceived by him as an external fear. As further ego development occurs, there is a progressive internalization of the relationships to these objects. With continuing incorporation of the parental images internally, and identification with them in ego development, as well as the super-ego identifications and the internalization of super-ego processes, what was originally feared as an external threat is now experienced internally in the form of anxiety.

In other words, annihilation, loss of love, punishment, castration, the invasion of the body, disruption by excessive stimulation, etc., gradually come to be experienced as internal threats and expectations which are not directly related to the behaviour of the parental objects. The intensity of such internalized fears (anxiety) will be roughly proportional to the nature and intensity of the fantasied expectation of punishment or of the danger situation.

The types of primary process conflicts, fantasies, modes of thought, distortions, and danger situations, and the ubiquitousness of their occurrence is illustrated by the study of mythology and of children's fairy tales. These stories represent a common sharing and disguised working-over of some of the primary process conflicts of infancy and childhood, and common themes can be found in the mythology of widely different cultural groups.

Fear originates in response to an external threat, whereas anxiety is related to the experiencing of an internalized threat. The fears which were originally experienced as relating to external objects or events now, by virtue of being internalized, are experienced as anxiety.

Anxiety may then originate from several sources within the mental apparatus. *Instinctual anxiety* results from the anticipation of flooding of the organism by excessive tension and stimulation from its own drives, and is related to the early infantile experience of mounting drive tension with absence of gratification. *Ego anxiety* results from the internalized perception of a danger situation which was once thought to be external, and was responded to by the various fantasies and distortions of the primary thought processes in the infant and young child. *Super-ego anxiety* results from the internalized threats of punishment or loss of love on moral grounds, now experienced by the individual as a sense of guilt. In those instances where the individual fails to live up to his ego-ideal, there results a form of super-ego anxiety experienced as shame. Fear related to *realistic external danger* situations is still perceived by the ego, and will be proportionally related to the nature and severity of the external danger situation.

Signal Anxiety (including guilt and/or shame)

With continuing ego development and further maturation of the functions of intelligence, memory and reality testing, there occurs an increasingly complex use of thought as a trial action. These developing capacities for thinking permit the child increasingly to anticipate future experiences. With such an anticipation, there will be an accompanying anticipatory awareness of anxiety if the future experience involves a situation perceived as dangerous, or carrying the threat of punishment, or loss of love.

This anticipatory awareness of anxiety comes increasingly to have a signal function. It signals that a situation of potential danger or threat is developing as the result of a change in the balance of forces within the individual or his environment. Unless the dynamic steady state is re-established with avoidance of the impending danger situation, the anxiety will continue and will mount as the danger situation is approached more closely.

The ego responds to this signal of anxiety in an attempt to avoid this increasingly unpleasant affect, and eventually to avoid the danger situation so signalled. This requires that integrative or adaptive mechanisms be instituted to deal with the conflict situation which has been stimulated, and thereby to re-establish a state of dynamic equilibrium. When a stable dynamic equilibrium has been re-established, and the situation of danger or threat thus averted, the anxiety signal disappears.

Ordinarily when the ego can respond effectively and take appropriate action to modify a dangerous external reality situation in such a way that the danger is avoided or overcome, then the signal of fear disappears. On the other hand, if the individual is faced with a situation of realistic danger which cannot be mastered or avoided, there may be a persistence of the signal of fear as long as the danger situation exists (i.e. the combat situation in wartime). If there is an overwhelming external threat or massive stimulation of the ego from the reality situation, reactions of panic may occur, resulting from the ego's inability to deal with the overwhelming external danger.

Through its perceptual, integrative, self-observing and synthetic functions, the ego is consciously and unconsciously aware of id drives seeking gratification, of internalized super-ego prohibitions and of the demands of external reality. The ego is also aware of fantasies and associations related to the various internalized danger situations. There is also a scanning function of the ego, involving self-observation and an awareness of the state of ego integration and function.

A change in the function, intensity, or stress in any of these groups of forces impinging on the mental apparatus may disrupt the currently existing dynamic equilibrium, with subsequent experience of signal anxiety as a result of the disruption. If attempts to re-establish and maintain a dynamic equilibrium are quickly successful, the anxiety signal subsides. If such attempts are incompletely successful, the signal of anxiety will persist or quickly recur. If the attempts are completely unsuccessful and the individual is being irresistibly driven towards a situation he perceives as extremely dangerous, reactions of panic may occur on the basis of such an internalized danger.

Other Signals

Although the affects of anxiety, guilt, shame and fear have been the ones most extensively studied and their signal aspects most clearly understood, there are also other affect states which serve a signal function. Affects such as pride, confidence, contentment or joy will likewise be experienced by the ego in an anticipatory fashion, and may then lead to ego integrative and synthetic processes designed to establish or to maintain a state of equilibrium in which experiencing of such an affect may continue. Their signalling function would in general be the same as that played by the unpleasurable affects described above, but in an opposite direction. The pleasurable affective signals have been less carefully and extensively studied by psychoanalytic theorists and practitioners since they are less frequently involved in psychopathology than are the unpleasurable affect states.

Ego Mechanisms of Defence

Some of the important ego functions which play a central role in the establishment and maintenance of a dynamic equilibrium are the psychological mechanisms of defence, which will now be considered in detail. By virtue of the prolonged biological dependency of the infant and child, and also by virtue of the relatively long period required for the maturation and development of the various ego apparatuses, there is an inevitability of psychic conflict in the human being. The mechanisms of defence are ego functions which are developed and established in each individual as part of his psychological maturation, to deal with and resolve intrapsychic conflict, as well as conflict between the organism and the environment. The nature and intensity of the mechanisms that are used will vary significantly from one individual to another, but the analysis of normal as well as neurotic or disturbed behaviour indicates the ubiquitous existence and operation of such mechanisms. In other words, these unconscious ego mechanisms of defence occur in normal as well as in psychopathological states although, as will be developed later, the operation of these mechanisms plays a central role in psychopathology.

The final effect of the operation of all the ego defence mechanisms is to maintain the unconscious nature of the drives and drive-derivatives which must be effectively dealt with to avoid anxiety, and to help maintain the organism in a homeostatic state of dynamic equilibrium, both intrapsychically and with the environment.

These mechanisms are unconscious ego functions, and when fully successful, the individual is not only unconscious of that which was defended against, but also is not aware of the operation of the mechanism itself. In other instances, the individual may be unconscious of that which is defended against, but conscious of the final effects of the operation of such a mechanism. For example, the person may be aware of the existence of a character trait, but not be aware that this represents the functioning of a defence mechanism. Or, he may be aware that a particular incident has been forgotten, but not be aware of the active ego defence mechanisms involved in the process of forgetting.

Generally speaking, any of the various ego functions may be utilized in the service of defence against conflict, and against the experiencing of anxiety. However, a particular group of ego processes is usually conceptualized more narrowly as the mechanisms of defence. As physical and psychological maturation occurs, the capacity for defensive ego functions and the complexity of such functions will increase. It therefore is expedient to consider the defence mechanisms from the standpoint of ego development and psychological maturation, and in the sequence in which they mature and become available for use as part of the overall integrative processes.

A large variety of such mechanisms has been described but in this discussion consideration will be given only to some of the more prominent and common ones.

One of the earliest and most primitive of the ego's mechanisms is that of *denial*. This involves the attempt to ward off the perception of a sensory stimulus from either the external or the internal environment. Although stimulus intensity has reached or surpassed the usual threshold of perception, it is not recognized in conscious awareness.

A prototype of denial is the child's experience with perception when he learns to control perception voluntarily (i.e. by closing his eyes). 'Since I cannot see you, you cease to exist.'

A simple example of denial is the child who puts his head under the bed covers when afraid, or closes his eyes during the frightening parts of a movie (the 'ostrich with its head in the sand' type of behaviour), in which the attempt is to avoid the danger situation by not recognizing its existence. The denial of an internalized percept could be illustrated by the person who is unaware of experiencing a particular feeling, although others may clearly recognize outward manifestations of its existence.

With maturation of the ego and the capacity for fantasy, there develop more elaborate forms of denial in which fantasy may be used to contradict an unpleasant or anxiety-provoking perception. For example, a small child may fantasy himself to be a powerful and omnipotent giant in order not to perceive his true weakness and helplessness, or he may use fantasy to avoid recognition of a threatening reality, and try to shape it more in keeping with his own wishes, as seen for example in certain fairy tales (i.e. Jack and the Beanstalk).

Other primitive ego mechanisms are *projection* and *introjection*. The prototype of these psychological mechanisms is the physical and physiological act involved in the nutritional process. The use of the mouth as an organ for testing reality is commonly observed in the young child. The child puts anything and everything into its mouth and tests it on the basis that it is either something pleasant to be eaten or chewed upon, or is something unpleasant to be spat out.

The physiological act of eating food serves as another prototype of the psychological mechanism of introjection (taking-into-one's-self), by which various experiences, ideas and images become represented within the mind. The early anxiety-provoking situation which fosters and stimulates the use of this mechanism in the young child is separation from the object (mother) on which it is dependent. The mechanism originally involves a psychological attempt to incorporate this object within the self and thereby deal with the anxiety over separation.

Introjection involves the psychological incorporation of the whole object by the mode of the oral taking-in process. This contrasts with the mechanism of identification which develops later in more discrete patterns of imitation. Simple evidence of the existence of this mechanism is seen in such expressions as: 'I love you so much I could eat you up'; or, the expression: 'I cannot stomach that'; or the expression: 'He will swallow everything he is told.' Another example would be in the behaviour of primitive tribes in regard to cannibalism, where the individual eats a fallen enemy, partly with the goal of acquiring that person's good and valued characteristics for himself. A further example is the Sacrament of Holy Communion where the symbols of the body and blood of Christ are taken in via the oral route.

The mechanism of projection, which involves the psychological act of externalizing on to the non-self those things which are unacceptable within the self, has its prototypes in the nutritional process and spitting out, refusal to take in or pushing away. Another contribution from basic physiological processes to the psychological act of getting rid of something that originally was within the body is the act of defecation and the elimination of faeces which the child originally considers as part of its own body. This tendency to externalize unpleasurable or tension-producing internal percepts or ideas will result in the child distorting his perception of the external environment in accordance with the effects of such projection.

An example of projection in children and in primitive tribes would be the concepts of animism and attributing of human motivations or capacities to inanimate or non-human objects. Simple examples of projection would be the blaming of someone else for one's own failures, or the attributing to others of one's own ideas or impulses.

Projection is one of the basic mechanisms involved in a group of psychological tests in which non-specific stimuli are presented to the individual for study. Since the stimuli do not permit a 'right' answer, his interpretations and responses must be based on the externalization of internal mental processes.

One aspect of the developing thought processes of the young child, particularly around two to three years of age, is that of magical thinking, and with it the development of the mechanism of *undoing*. This is a mechanism in which an unacceptable impulse, drive or drive-derivative is offset and counteracted by a direct or indirect magical act, gesture or thought. The character of this mechanism is that an unacceptable or potentially dangerous and warded-off impulse reaches consciousness in the form of an act, a direct thought, an indirect and disguised thought or a negative thought, and having reached consciousness, is then offset by the act which constitutes the undoing. Another characteristic is that this mechanism is effective only for the particular impulse at the moment, and carries no lasting or permanent capacity to ward off similar impulses in the future.

For example, a girl sitting across the table from her prettier sister had the thought, 'I wish all her teeth would drop out and then she wouldn't be so pretty'. She immediately jumped up, poured a glass of milk and insisted that the sister drink it to undo her hostile wish since milk is good for teeth. Other examples would be such magical gestures as knocking on wood, crossing one's fingers, not stepping on cracks in the pavement, etc., all of which are performed after the individual becomes conscious, at least in a negative form (i.e. 'I hope nothing bad happens') of the possibility of an unacceptable impulse, fantasy or drive-derivative. This type of magical thinking is observed in the play of small children, and likewise may be seen in many of the ritualistic and sacrificial customs of primitive tribes.

Another mechanism originating in about the same period of development and related to undoing, is the mechanism of *reaction formation* (sometimes called over-compensation). By this mechanism a drive or attitude is turned into the opposite of the original, involving a relatively permanent change in ego processes, and an ongoing modification of the ego itself. This will often involve the development of character traits associated with social usefulness and acceptability, and the use of the mechanism may thus be further reinforced by rewards from the environment. Reaction-formation generally results in a more lasting and permanent defence against the original drive or impulse, rather than an intermittent one as in the mechanism of undoing.

Common examples of this mechanism include the replacement of the wish to be dirty by an attitude of cleanliness, or the wish to be dependent by an attitude of enforced and continuing independence. Hostility, aggression or cruelty may be replaced by exaggerated friendliness, gentleness and attitudes of pity or concern. The stronger the original impulse, drive or attitude, the more intense must be the reaction formation if it is to serve successfully as a defence.

Isolation is a defence mechanism in which mental processes are separated into their component parts, and the associated connections between these parts are blocked from conscious awareness. In one form of isolation, the affect and the drive quality associated with an unacceptable impulse may be split off from the ideas or thoughts related to such an impulse. As a result, the drive or drive-derivative may emerge into conscious awareness in the form of a thought, but it is not accompanied by the associated emotional feeling or sense of drive pressure. Such thoughts are often experienced as 'silly', or foreign, and the individual does not feel them as a 'true' part of himself.

A further form of isolation is the mechanism of *intellectualization*, in which the individual may consciously be aware of a coherent and integrated series of thoughts related to unacceptable or conflictual psychic processes,

4

but again without the feelings or sense of personal conviction that should accompany them.

Another form of isolation is that in which a thought or series of thoughts related to an unconscious, unacceptable impulse is separated from further associated ideas or thoughts and is experienced in consciousness as unconnected and unrelated to the rest of the person's mental life.

Another defence mechanism is that of *regression* by which there occurs a return to an earlier mode or level of psychic function. Regression may occur in the nature of the ego processes themselves with the use of less mature mechanisms of adaptation and adjustment, and the return towards primary process thinking. The most common example would be the ego processes involved in normal sleep. Here the usual waking cathexis of reality must be given up, permitting the individual to return to a more narcissistic ego state with increasing withdrawal so that sleep may occur, and there is a return towards primary process thought as illustrated by the ego activity in dreaming. Similar ego regression occurs during daydreaming and fantasy, where cathexes of reality are loosened in favour of more intrapsychic, wish-fulfilling mental activity.

The same type of process occurs when watching a magic show, or a play or movie. In these activities there is a partial and deliberate giving up of reality testing (to be enjoyed, the show is not experienced as an exhibit of sleight-of-hand, or as a group of people saying and doing things they have been told to do by the author, or as a series of lights and shadows projected on a white screen) and a temporary acceptance of the portrayed fantasy as real. Another normal example would be social behaviour at a party, where the individual who is 'in the party spirit' may enjoy games or other activities he would consider 'childish' in other settings.

A characteristic of such types of ego regression is that they are generally temporary, and are reversible when the total situation or circumstances demand it. This reversibility and oscillation between regression and progression is also seen in the normal learning behaviour of children, where attempts at mastery may be interrupted by 'giving up' behaviour and retreat to earlier patterns, to be followed again by renewed mastery attempts.

Another characteristic of ego regression is a selective quality, as a result of which there may be partial rather than total regression. In other words, the regression may involve only certain ego functions or groups of functions, while other functions remain unchanged; or there may be differing degrees and intensity of regression among and between groups of ego functions.

Regression also occurs in terms of id function, where the intensity of drive cathexis may shift in the direction of chronologically earlier forms of instinctual gratification, or where there may be a shift towards earlier types of object choice. Examples of this would include the older child who, when faced with a conflict or frustration, resorts to thumb-sucking, or reverts to soiling or enuresis, or to a diffuse temper-tantrum and destructive rage. Such id regressions are usually associated with some form of ego regression although the relationship between the two forms of regression is not necessarily fixed or constant.

Somewhat later in childhood further mechanisms of defence develop, one of which is *repression*. The drives and drive-derivatives are continually seeking conscious awareness and discharge through ego function and have a cathexis of psychic energy pushing towards such gratification. In the act of repression, the ego functions maintain a quantity of psychic energy in opposition to the drive cathexis, known as an anti-cathexis. As a result, the drives, fantasies, memories, related affects and other associated phenomena are actively excluded from conscious or preconscious awareness, and remain at unconscious levels. In order to maintain the repression, the psychic energy involved in the anti-cathexis must be continuously applied, and hence this energy remains bound in the defensive process and is not available to the ego for other functions.

Repression is an unconscious ego mechanism but is related to another mechanism known as *suppression* which occurs consciously. In suppression the individual is consciously aware of his active attempt to put something out of his conscious mind, to try to forget, to think of other things, or to hold back the expression of his thoughts or feelings. He is aware of the pressures of his own impulses, thoughts and feelings, and of attempting to maintain a barrier against them.

In repression the individual is *not* consciously aware of imposing this barrier but he may be aware of the result of such activity, namely the absence from conscious-preconscious mental activity of that which has been repressed. This may be a general and non-specific gap (i.e. the person who has no memory of his life before a particular time) or it may be a more selective and specific absence (i.e. a particular incident or memory that is lost while other memories from the same period are retained). Repression may also occur against current specific or general drives and drive-derivatives (i.e. the person who in spite of conscious effort to the contrary 'forgets' something in his current stream of mental life). In instances where repression is fully successful, however, there may not even be a conscious awareness of the absence or gap.

The mechanism of *displacement* involves the concept that a drive or drive-derivative seeking discharge and gratification through an inappropriate or unacceptable object may be permitted a partial discharge if the object cathected by the drive is changed and a more acceptable object is substituted. This mechanism thus permits a partial discharge of drive tension on to the substitute object.

The substituted object may be human, infra-human or inanimate, or it may be some other part of the individual himself, but it must have an associative link or connection with the original object of the drive if it is to be successfully utilized. There is a spectrum in the degree of consciousness in the use of this mechanism, ranging from the partially conscious awareness at the time (i.e. the individual who is aware of 'working off' pent-up feelings in substitute activity); to the individual who is aware of the occurrence after the fact (i.e. the person who later becomes aware of the irrational nature of his reaction); to the individual who is unaware of any irrationality until it is pointed out to him; and to the individual who, when the irrational reaction is pointed out, does not accept it as irrational but rather still feels his reaction to be justified.

Displacement may at times be intermittent and in response to a specific conflict situation, or it may be maintained or used repetitively. Common examples among children would include such things as the child's destruction of a toy in a temper-tantrum against the parents, or the child's positive love and attachment towards a favourite blanket or stuffed animal.

Another mechanism which is related to displacement is that of *rationalization*, a mental process by which an individual attempts to ascribe and explain some aspect of thought or behaviour by motives or reasons that are more acceptable to himself than the true ones. By seeking such a more rational and acceptable explanation, the attempt is to remain unaware of the true or complete unconscious motivating forces, and to attempt an explanation chiefly in terms of secondary process logic.

To be effective, this mechanism requires that its existence and use be unconscious (if an individual is conscious of 'lying' to himself, the mechanism fails to hide from himself the existence of other motives) but the result of its operation is to provide a conscious and acceptable explanation. The greater the contribution of reality factors to the rationalization, the more effective it will be in hiding other less acceptable motivations.

Another mechanism is that of *identification*, by which an individual effects an internal modification of himself and his mental processes in an attempt to deal with his relationship to objects within his environment. This mechanism is related to the previously described mechanism of introjection, but differs from it in that introjection involves the more primitive concept of a total incorporation of the object based on the oral mode of taking-in. Identification, on the other hand, involves a more selective or partial internalization and change through the mode of imitation of the object in more circumscribed or specific attitudes, aspects, functions or behaviour. Identification may be a deliberate and conscious process in the individual, but it also may occur unconsciously.

At times identification may derive from the wish to be like the object through the impelling force of love and positive attitudes, but at other times the identification may be based on fear, hostility and the negative aspects of the relationship. In either event, identification results in a structural change of ego and/or super-ego functions, although the permanence of such change is variable.

Whereas the major effects of identification occur in childhood, and the objects are usually the parental figures, there will be subsequent shifts and changes in the nature of identifications as development towards maturity continues, each identification leaving an imprint. This process of imitation leading to internalization and structural change is an attempt partially and vicariously to gratify a drive or drive-derivative associated with the loved or hated object, or to use the object as a means of resolving a conflict.

Common examples of identification occur in children's play where the child imitates and at times very closely mimics the behaviour of adults, through its play with toys and dolls, playing house, putting on articles of adult clothing, etc. This same mechanism also occurs in adolescence, for example, but then the object is most often the peer group, accounting for some of the adolescent fads in clothing, manners and behaviour.

Another mechanism is that of conscious or unconscious *avoidance*, by which an individual seeks to keep threatening or potentially dangerous objects or situations at a safe distance. When the threat or danger is an external one, the individual is fully conscious of the avoidance. When the threat or danger arises from unconscious associations between the external object or situation and the individual's unacceptable drives, the avoidance is partly unconscious. At times the individual may not recognize that active avoidance is occurring, and may understand the phenomenon as the result of 'a normal like or dislike'. At other times the individual may be consciously aware of anxiety and the active avoidance, but be unconscious of the reasons for these.

The most advanced and mature type of defence mechanism is that of *sublimation*, which involves a progressive change and modification in both the object and the aim of a drive. Such changes may allow a partial discharge and gratification of the unconscious drive, but in a useful and socially acceptable form.

Generally speaking, sublimations provide the most stable and effective form of defence mechanisms. They provide a form of drive-discharge and partial gratification. And the form and object of the discharge are socially acceptable, and hence are reinforced through the individual's own ego attitudes, as well as through the reactions of others in the environment.

An example would be the child whose original drive may have been to mess, and smear himself with faeces. There may be a progressive change in object, from faeces, to mud, to clay, to oil paint. And there may be a progressive change in the aim of the drive from the wish to smear and be dirty, to the wish to manipulate and mould, and eventually to a point where the original aim of smearing and being dirty is no longer part of the expressed drive.

These ego mechanisms of defence have been considered singly and in isolation from one another for purposes of description and discussion. Actually they do not operate independently, but are used in various patterns and groups, and each individual makes use of a variety of such mechanisms.

The same mechanism is not always used against the same drive, and as ego maturation and development of latent ego apparatuses continues, the patterns of defence take on increasing complexity. Mechanisms which originally developed in a particular psychosexual phase may be utilized as defences against drives from earlier or later phases of development. Several mechanisms may be used simultaneously against a particular drive. And several different drives may be simultaneously defended against by a particular mechanism. The use of a particular mechanism may provoke other unconscious conflicts for which further defences must then be instituted, thus creating a 'layering effect'.

A useful analogy in conceptualizing the richness and variability of defensive patterns is to compare the individual defence mechanisms with the individual letters of the alphabet. Variations in the sequences and combinations of the basic units permit a complex and extensive variation and individual style in the form of defence organization that develops.

In summary, the increasingly complex combinations and permutations of ego functions permit extensive and widely varied patterns of defence and integration in the attempt to establish psychological homeostasis and maintain the dynamic equilibrium.

SUGGESTED READING

FREUD, ANNA (1946) *The Ego and the Mechanisms of Defense.* International Universities Press Inc, New York

FREUD, SIGMUND (1916) *Introductory Lectures on Psychoanalysis.* Standard Edition of Complete Psychological Works, Vols. 15 and 16. The Hogarth Press, London

FREUD, SIGMUND (1926) *Inhibitions, Symptoms and Anxiety.* Standard Edition of Complete Psychological Works, Vol. 20. The Hogarth Press, London

JONES, ERNEST (1953) *The Life and Work of Sigmund Freud.* 3 Vols. Basic Books Inc, New York

RANGELL, LEO (1955) On the psychoanalytic theory of anxiety. *J. Am. Psychoanal. Ass.*, **3**, 389

RANGELL, LEO (1968) A further attempt to resolve the 'problem of anxiety'. *J. Am. Psychoanal. Ass.* **16**, 371

RAPPAPORT, DAVID (1960) *The Structure of Psychoanalytic Theory-Psychological Issues.* Monograph 6. International Universities Press Inc, New York

WAELDER, ROBERT (1967) Inhibitions, symptoms, and anxiety: forty years later. *Psychoanal. Quart.* **36**, 1.

CHAPTER III

Psychic Determinism and the Continuity of Mental Life

In the previous two chapters it has been emphasized that the structural hypothesis of the mental apparatus represents an arbitrary grouping of psychic functions in accordance with an accepted set of definitions, and that it has no separate existence of its own. Into this theoretical framework was introduced the concept of intra-psychic conflict, resulting from the co-existence of opposing sets of functions and forces within the mind. The idea was also developed that one important task in the growth and development of the organism is the establishment of ego processes as a controlling, regulating and integrating apparatus which will maintain a dynamic state of adaptation, both within the mind itself and also between the organism and its external environment.

Character

An apparent contradiction must now be introduced. Although these groups of functions have no separate existence of their own and do not correspond to any physical or physiological structure, they nevertheless have an internal consistency within each grouping which permits a conceptualization of them as 'psychic structures'.

This internal consistency within the parts of the mental apparatus exists in the following way. Within certain general limits, the qualitative nature of the id forces and drives are similar in all individuals. However, there are significant quantitative differences between individuals, in terms of innate, biologically determined energy capacities and potentials, as well as differences in drive intensity resulting from the vicissitudes of developmental experience. Once a pattern and hierarchy of predominant id drives has been established, it tends to persist within broad limits for that individual. The nature and the effects of the various repressed memories, which become functionally a part of the id, will differ sharply from person to person, but within the individual himself, these also tend to remain constant.

This same internal consistency will be manifest in terms of super-ego functions, once the concepts of reward and punishment, right and wrong and the various ideals have been established by and for the individual. Although somewhat modifiable, they tend to persist within broad limits, and the nature and intensity of these forces varies significantly from one individual to another.

In terms of the central organizing role of the ego, economy of psychic functioning requires that in order to carry out the manifold integrative functions, it is necessary that each situation should not be met as an entirely new one.

The ego's integrative and defensive functions become increasingly automatic, and to this extent there will develop patterns of integration or defence which are characteristic for the individual ego. As a result of learning and practice, the developing child begins to adopt characteristic modes of integration, behaviour and conflict solution, and when faced with the impact of the various forces within the mental apparatus, the individual will tend to react in a way characteristic to himself (ego structuralization).

This combination of a usual mode of adjustment, defence, integration and adaptation, as well as a persistent pattern and hierarchy of drives and moral values, is what is commonly called *character*, and varies significantly from one person to another. During the course of individual development a large number of forces have an increasingly specific impact on the nature and development of character.

Genic Determinants

Some of these are genic, in the sense of an inherited biological endowment, based on constitutional factors. This is manifest from the standpoint of the drives in terms of differences among individuals regarding specific drive intensity. Direct observation of newborn infants and young children indicates such variations in basic drives, which are apparently independent of experience and are constitutionally based. For example, in the feeding behaviour of newborns, some are observed to be relatively easily and quickly satisfied, whereas others appear to have a much stronger inherent oral drive towards both nutrition and suckling. The same is true in terms of their response when drive satisfaction does not occur, where some infants tend to have a persistent and intense response to frustration, and others are relatively more quiet and manifest a less sustained or massive reaction when drives are frustrated.

From the standpoint of the development of the various ego apparatuses, there will also be significant differences between individuals on the basis of inherited constitutional factors. Such things as intelligence, motor control and co-ordination, capacities for perception and discrete perceptual differentiation, and even such things as ultimate physical size and body appearance are all factors which have an effect on the individual's total adaptation and ultimate choice of adaptive mechanisms.

For example, an individual with a congenital defect in intelligence will by virtue of his constitutional endowment, be incapable of using some of the more complex psychic mechanisms that are available to the individual with normal or superior intelligence, regardless of emotional or reality experiences in the course of development. Or, an individual with highly endowed motor control and co-ordination (i.e. 'the natural athlete') will more likely make extensive use of these functions in his adaptation than will the individual with inferior physical development and motor capacity.

Experiential Determinants

Given a particular genic and constitutional endowment, the life experience which the individual organism undergoes in meeting its specific environment will also play a significant role in terms of ultimate character structure. The nature of the experiences to which a child is exposed will vary, and is never the same for two different people.

For example, even among siblings, the total impact and nature of the early feeding and need-satisfying gratifications in relationship to the mother may be sharply different, and will be influenced by such things as the mother's state of mind at the time. This, in turn, may be influenced by the many other variable factors in the mother's environment, and by the nature of the mother's specific interactions with the child, but the effects on the child may be in the direction of a more or a less gratifying overall experience. The experience of drive frustration or gratification will also vary in response to relative drive intensity. A particular mother may be quite capable of gratifying and satisfying the drives of a particular infant or child when these drives are in the lower range of intensity, but the same patterns of mothering behaviour may be inadequate in providing drive gratification and satisfaction to an infant with a relatively stronger innate drive intensity. Psychologically traumatic experiences and the vicissitudes of everyday life, which occur differently in the life of each organism, will also have an effect on the total developmental picture, and again there will be significant variations even among siblings.

Not only is the nature of the life experience important, but the age at which particular types of experiences occur will be significant in terms of the total impact of the experience on the developing organism. For example, the age and state of ego development at the time of such common experiences as separation from the mother, illness, death of a key figure, surgical operations, family moves, birth of a sibling, etc., will influence the effects of such experiences on personality development and character formation. The child will interpret and react to the experience in accordance with his own mental processes existent at that time.

The personality and character of the objects in a child's environment and the nature of their interaction with the child during the developmental years will also play a role in ultimate personality and character development. These are the objects which are psychologically internalized through the child's identifications. This will have an impact on ego development and the mechanisms of integration adopted by the child, and will also play a role in terms of super-ego formation, and the internalization of the environmental demands as represented by the parents. Although it was emphasized earlier that super-ego formation is influenced by the child's projection of his own impulses and drives on to the parental objects and that these are then reinternalized as prohibitions from the environment, nevertheless the reality of the parental attitudes is still an important factor. There will be a difference in the ultimate nature of the super-ego where the parents have been rigid, harsh or punitive, as compared with situations where the parents have been permissive, or, at the other extreme, corrupt in their concepts of morality.

Another factor in the ultimate choice and importance of the types of mechanisms adopted by the child will be the reinforcements offered by the environment for particular patterns of adaptation. The child, in seeking to adapt to or resolve a conflict, may try a number of the different mechanisms at its disposal by virtue of ego development and the apparatuses that have already matured. When these mechanisms effect a resolution of conflict and hence a reduction of unpleasurable affect, or when use of these mechanisms stimulates rewards and positive reinforcements from environmental objects, there will be a tendency towards a more characteristic and self-sustaining use of such mechanisms which again will have an impact on character formation. For example, if cleanliness is extremely important to the parental objects, then the child's utilization of a reaction-formation of cleanliness and inhibition of soiling may be strengthened through the parental approval.

Clinical observation suggests that the nuclei of character formation are laid down in the infantile and early childhood phases, and that during the latency period there is a further entrenchment and strengthening of these characteristic modes of adjustment and adaptation which ultimately lead to the development of a more fixed and stable character formation.

Character formation is thus a reflection and ultimate result of the interaction between the child's constitutional endowment, and the nature of his psychological experiences, all of which have been integrated into a generally consistent pattern of psychic functioning, reflecting the impact of id, super-ego and ego processes operating simultaneously.

Repetition Compulsion

Another factor influential in the organization and motivation of behaviour is the *repetition compulsion*. This is a descriptive rather than an explanatory concept. It is based on the frequent clinical observation that individuals tend to re-establish and repeat childhood situations and relationships that were traumatic, conflicted, or frustrating. When this tendency was initially recognized it seemed to contradict the pleasure principle. However, with the development of ego psychology these repetitions of old frustrations and traumas could be understood as the individual's attempts to achieve belated mastery of the psychic trauma, and to obtain delayed gratification in the current version of the old situation.

In this connection the observed compulsion to repeat old traumas is related to a tendency in the mind to seek an *identity of perception* in situations of pleasurable drive gratification. This in turn means that once an object has been firmly cathected with drive energy, this cathexis tends to persist. This in turn influences and often limits the possible subsequent objects available for the satisfaction of such a drive, and makes drive displacement more difficult. In psychological theory this is analogous to the biologically observed process of imprinting in lower species.

The repetition compulsion occurs unconsciously and frequently leads to life situations that are in opposition to the reality principle, thus adding another force which must be integrated by the ego in maintaining adaption.

Levels of Behaviour

The final result of all these multiple and complex interacting forces is human behaviour at various levels. This may be in the form of behaviour which is externally observable and hence readily accessible to direct observation, measurement, verification and relatively objective study.

Another large area of human behaviour, however, is purely subjective, not capable of direct observation, and requires the individual himself to describe it for an observer. These phenomena include such things as thoughts, feelings, fantasies, memories, internal associations and motivations. Although the reporting of such phenomena may involve distortions which make verification by the observer more difficult, they are none the less real for this, and any general theory of behaviour must, if complete, include an understanding of these subjective human experiences and their vicissitudes.

Continuity and Determinism

From the previous discussion it is now possible to arrive at a concept of mental life as a continuous process of adaptation and adjustment, both within the mental apparatus itself, and between the organism and its environment. These adaptations involve a constantly fluctuating and oscillating dynamic steady state, in which the various elements of subjective and objective experience and behaviour result from an interaction of *all* the active forces, past and present, that impinge on the organism.

Such a concept takes into account the significance of constitutional endowment, and other inherited factors, as well as all of the various life experiences to which the individual has been exposed.

In assessing the impact of life experiences on the individual, it is necessary to distinguish between the more or less *objective reality* of such experiences as they occurred, and the *psychic reality* for the individual. The latter is sharply influenced by the subjective experience and personal interpretation of the individual at the time and in retrospect, and hence may be quite different from the objective reality.

Of the two forms of reality, it is the psychic reality of an experience which will have the greater impact on the individual and his subsequent reactions and development. For example, in young children a surgical operation may be medically necessary and may objectively reflect parental love, and concern for the welfare of the child. However, the child's interpretation of the procedure, and hence the psychic reality for the child, may involve concepts of punishment, mutilation, lack of parental love and protection, etc., and it is *this* psychic reality which may determine the ultimate impact of the experience on the development of the child and his personality.

Mental life and behaviour may thus be viewed as the end result of a continuous interaction between all the various complex forces from outside and from within the organism as integrated through the organism's individual apparatuses. There is a long-range continuity, in that behaviour at each phase or stage of development is based on and evolves out of previous developmental stages and modes of adaptation. Hence at any point in time, subjective and objective behaviour is influenced by all that has occurred before in the individual's total life experience. This leads to the *genetic approach* which involves the concept that complete understanding of current behaviour requires an understanding of its historical antecedents, including those of the remote past and the very earliest childhood developmental experiences.

There is also a short-range continuity of mental life, leading to the *dynamic approach* to behaviour, which holds that current behaviour must also be understood as the result of the interplay of all the current forces within the mind (each of which has been genetically determined), and that these current forces will continue to exert an influence on behaviour as long as their activity persists.

The *economic approach* involves concepts of psychic energy and variations in the relative intensities of forces within the mental apparatus, even though as yet these cannot be precisely measured. It involves the concept that where opposing forces co-exist, their net effect will be a reflection of their mutual interaction and their intensity relative to each other, analogous to the vector concept of physical and mechanical forces.

The logical conclusion from the genetic, dynamic and economic approaches is the concept of *psychic determinism*. This hypothesis holds that all the phenomena of mental life and behaviour are selectively determined by the simultaneous interaction of all the active past and present forces and experiences of the individual, both conscious-preconscious, and unconscious. Nothing in mental life occurs in a random or unselected fashion, and theoretically, if given a full enough understanding of the individual's total experience and mental organization, all psychic phenomena are eventually understandable in genetic, dynamic and economic terms.

Normality and Mental Health

An attempt will now be made to conceptualize the state of normality or mental health. Since this is a relative phenomenon, and there are no absolute criteria, the first question will be whether to use a statistical norm or mean based on population surveys, or whether to use a more theoretical concept of an ideal which is approached by only a relatively few individuals. Within the context of the present discussion, the latter approach will prove more useful, particularly as a basis of comparison in the theory of psychopathology and psychotherapy.

Mental health and emotional maturity can only be considered in relative terms since it consists of more than the mere absence of specific psychological symptoms. Since conflict and stress arising both internally and externally are ubiquitous accompaniments to human life, one criterion of health is the capacity to maintain mature adaptation in the face of whatever conflicts or stress the vicissitudes of life may bring. Those things which constitute a stress will often have a specific quality and will vary greatly from individual to individual, dependent on the nature of overall integration and development, and on the nature of specific past experiences and conflicts. So that what is stressful for one individual may not be considered a stress by another.

The evaluation of the capacity for adaptation to stress involves not only the current level of conflict at any one time, but also the ability of the individual to deal effectively with even greater future anticipated or unpredicted stress without decompensation. Again it must be emphasized that this increasing stress may be internal, external, or both, but the basic concept here regarding mental health is that of psychological reserves to maintain adaptation.

This concept would be analogous to a person with rheumatic heart disease with mitral stenosis, murmurs, cardiac enlargement and EKG changes, who currently does not have any symptoms of heart failure. Although 'healthy' in the sense of having no symptoms and feeling subjectively well, such a person has a lowered reserve of function, and even though he might go through life without developing heart failure, the likelihood of his ultimately developing such symptoms is greater than in an individual who does not have such underlying pathology.

In such a concept of mental health, everyone would have a potential 'breaking point', since it is not possible to increase stresses indefinitely without reaching a point where adaptation fails. But the higher the individual's threshold to disruption of adaptation from stresses, the healthier he would be considered; and the lower the individual's threshold of tolerance, the less his reserves, and hence, at least potentially, the poorer his mental health.

During the psychosexual developmental sequence of the ideal normal personality, there will have been a progressive maturation of drives so that the aim of the individual's drives will be in the form of age-appropriate instinctual gratifications. Although there are various points of fixation in psychosexual development, both for sexual and aggressive drive energies, the main bulk of these instinctual energies will be involved at the level of genital primacy and full heterosexuality, a stage reached only after the physiological development of adolescence. There will be some continuing pre-genital attachments and drive energies, but ideally they will be relatively less important in overall drive economy, will occur chiefly in sexual fore-play rather than in end-pleasures, and will also form the basis of effective sublimations. The effect of ego and super-ego forces on the drives in this ideal state will be such that derivative drive discharge will be effective and gratifying but will occur within the framework of the reality principle.

This developmental sequence could be illustrated by the young child, in Western society, whose attempt to discharge sexual tension through masturbation at age 4–5 years would be an age-appropriate form of drive discharge, whereas genital sexual intercourse at that age would not be. However, at age 24–25 years, heterosexual genital intercourse would be age-appropriate and masturbation would not. In the very young child oral needs and gratification of total dependency are a dominating force and are age-appropriate, but in the mature adult they should be relatively less important and not be the predominant form of pleasure. In a 2–3 year-old child the expression of aggression in response to frustration in the form of physical violence or attack is age-appropriate and expectable. But in the healthy adult, aggressive discharge occurs more appropriately in verbal form, or in sublimated activities such as work, and physical violence is reserved for situations where it is realistically necessary.

Super-ego function in the ideally mature personality involves a firm and well-established *internalized* code of morality and values, in terms of ideals of aspiration, and of prohibitions and punishment. Although such functions would have originated in infancy and childhood from the psychic incorporation of authoritarian figures and the child's distortions of these objects as discussed earlier, in the ideal state there would be a significant degree of conscious awareness of the origins and development of these value systems. This would result in an increasingly conscious selection of which values to keep and which to modify, and in a group of super-ego functions which are appropriate to the reality principle, and are firmly perceived by the individual as an internal part of himself. One gradient of maturity is the degree to which these functions are internalized, since this permits a greater degree of self-regulation of behaviour, rather than regulation through continued dependence on external environmental authority.

The role of the ego in the ideal of maturity has already been alluded to in the discussion on maintenance of adaptation to stress, and the concept of reserves. This results from a variety of ego functions operating harmoniously and in an integrated fashion, and includes a maximal degree of conscious awareness of the various forces within the mental apparatus, as well as a conscious awareness of the operation of the ego mechanisms themselves.

It also involves the capacity to seek and maintain relationships with real objects for age-appropriate drive discharge and satisfaction, and the capacity effectively to modify the environment in accordance with the organism's needs but in keeping with the reality principle. However, in situations where environmental modification within the reality principle is not possible, there should be the capacity to tolerate frustration and anxiety if necessary, without fixed regression.

In the ideal state, conflict resolution occurs consciously with the use of conscious repudiation of unacceptable drives rather than unconscious defences against them. However, where there is not a full conscious awareness of conflict in the ideal ego, a wide variety of mechanisms for conflict solution would be available, with a flexibility of choice of appropriate ones for a specific conflict based on a total assessment of the situation, rather than a stereotyped and repetitive use of particular mechanisms.

The ideal state would also include a firm sense of identity and self, and the maximal degree of development of the indvidual consistent with his innate abilities and limitations.

In summary, ideal ego function involves a minimal amount of psychic energy bound in unconscious defensive functioning, and instead a capacity for modification of libidinal and aggressive energy through effective sublimations and neutralization. This permits drive energy to be available for conscious and reality-oriented ego activity and adaptation.

As mentioned earlier, this concept of ideal mental health is seldom completely fulfilled but various partial approaches to this ideal do occur. Behaviourally and descriptively, in an ideal normal personality there is adequate libidinal and aggressive drive discharge, with the achievement of genital primacy manifested in the capacity for full heterosexual love. There is also the capacity for other types of object love (such as children, friends, parents) and achievement of stability and permanence in such object relations. The normal personality is also free from neurotic suffering in the form of anxiety, morbid guilt or neurotic symptom formation, and has the capacity to work and be productive in whatever areas of conscious choice the individual has made, with the achievement of gratification through this activity.

Values and Relativity

It is apparent that these attempts to conceptualize normality involve a series of value judgments for which there may not necessarily be a universal acceptance. For example, the judgment that maturity and freedom of action are more ideal than immaturity and acceptance of external authoritarian control will be influenced by the 'cultural set' of the observer (i.e. in a Western democracy versus a Communist dictatorship versus a primitive tribal culture). The judgment that heterosexual love is more mature and ideal than homosexual love has been disputed in those cultures where homosexuality is widely practised. And even within heterosexual love, the concept that its most mature and ideal form involves the capacity to feel full sexual desire *and* tenderness for the same object is disputed in certain cultures where these forms of love are customarily directed towards different objects (i.e. the 'wife versus mistress' type of relationships).

How long and how intensively does the 'ideally normal' individual attempt to modify the environment in keeping with his own needs and ideas ? And, at what point does the healthy adherence to an idea or ideal in spite of opposition become stubbornness and obstinacy ? When does honest and direct expression of opinion or feeling become rudeness or lack of sensitivity toward the feelings of others ? At what point does personal satisfaction and need fulfilment become selfishness ?

The judgment of normality also involves an assessment of the *subjective experience* and requires the participation of the individual himself in describing these experiences to the observer. Such things as the capacity to experience love, the degree of sexual fulfilment, the investment of interest or energy in any particular activity, the various motivations behind a piece of behaviour, etc., can be only partially estimated by an outside observer. External behaviour which may appear 'normal' to an observer may have very different meanings, depending on motivation, and on the nature of the subjective feelings, thoughts or fantasies that accompany it. For example a man may work overtime at his business or profession out of a sense of ambition and wish for success. However, the same external behaviour may be a manifestation of a sense of guilt, or of a masochistic need not to have other pleasurable experiences, or of a wish not to spend time with his family, etc. Only an exploration of the subjective elements can establish the full meaning of the behaviour.

The concept of mental health thus cannot involve universal absolutes, but instead must include a variety of judgments, and a scale of relative values which will be influenced by the social, cultural, and personal environment of the individual, and by the personal, theoretical, and cultural orientation of the observer. Mental health or normality is therefore best conceptualized as a relative phenomenon.

SUGGESTED READING

ARLOW, JACOB A. (1956) *The Legacy of Sigmund Freud.* International Universities Press Inc, New York

ARLOW, JACOB A. (1961) Ego psychology and the study of mythology. *J. Am. Psychoanal. Ass.* **9**, 371

BERES, DAVID (1968) The humanness of human beings: psychoanalytic considerations. *Psychoanal. Quart.* **37**, 487

ENGEL, GEORGE L. (1962) *Psychological Development in Health and Disease.* W.B. Saunders Co

ERIKSON, ERIK H. (1950) *Childhood and Society.* W.W.Norton & Co Inc, New York

FREUD, ANNA (1965) *Normality and Pathology in Childhood.* International Universities Press Inc, New York

HARTMAN, HEINZ (1958) *Ego Psychology and the Problem of Adaptation.* International Universities Press Inc, New York

HARTMAN, HEINZ (1939) Psychoanalysis and the concept of health. *Int. J. Psycho-Anal.* **20**, 308

HARTMAN, HEINZ & KRIS, ERNST (1945) *The Genetic Approach in Psychoanalysis—Psychoanalytic Study of the Child,* Vol. 1, International Universities Press Inc, New York

OFFER, DANIEL & SABSHIN, MELVIN (1966) *Normality: Theoretical and Clinical Concepts of Mental Health.* Basic Books Inc, New York

SECTION II

Psychopathology

CHAPTER IV
Symptom Formation

Introduction

In the previous chapters the concept of mental functioning was evolved around the central issue of a dynamic steady state resulting from the interaction of all of the different forces within the mind. The central position and role of ego functions in the maintenance of such a state of equilibrium was emphasized, as well as the concept that unpleasurable affects (particularly anxiety and guilt) serve as signals when there is a disruption of this equilibrium. Pleasurable affects likewise serve as signals to the ego, in these instances to continue and maintain the current dynamic equilibrium, or to establish an equilibrium in which such pleasurable affects may be experienced. The concept of psychic determinism in mental life was also described.

Essentially the attempt was to summarize the general psychoanalytic concept of mental functioning and overall theory of human behaviour. Psychopathology and the development of psychological symptoms may be conceptualized in these same terms, and result from disturbances or distortions in the mental processes involved in this dynamic psychological equilibrium. Since a rational approach to psychotherapy must be based on a conceptual understanding of the underlying psychopathology, the theory of psychopathology will now be developed within the framework of the general psychoanalytic theory of behaviour.

Conflict

It must first be emphasized again that conflict is an ubiquitous phenomenon in human life, both in terms of intra-psychic conflict as well as in terms of conflict between the organism and its environment. The nature and the intensity of these conflicts vary from person to person and from time to time within the life-span of the individual. There may be intervals in which an individual is relatively less involved in intra-psychic conflict, or intervals in which he is relatively free of conflict with his external environment while maintaining the intra-psychic conflicts.

49

Psychopathology is related not only to the presence and intensity of conflict, but also to the way in which the individual reacts and adapts to those external and intra-psychic conflicts that he faces.

The presence of emotional reactions in themselves is pathognomonic of psychopathology or of neurotic symptom formation. For example, a soldier going into combat is very likely to experience fear, and someone who has recently lost a love-object through death will very likely experience grief and all of its accompaniments. In fact, in either of these situations the absence of an emotional reaction (the soldier going into battle without fear, or the individual not experiencing grief after the death of a loved person) would be more indicative of an underlying disturbance.

Non-neurotic adaptation and resolution of a conflict will involve at least partially conscious awareness of the existence of such a conflict, be it intrapsychic or in terms of the organism's relationship to its environment. In addition, there will be a utilization of secondary process thought and logic in the resolution, which will be undertaken within the framework of the reality principle. And, there will be minimal use of unconscious ego defence mechanisms, and minimal occurrence of fixed regression, or restriction and inhibition of other ego functions.

In other words, at a descriptive level, this will involve a reality-oriented attempt to resolve and modify the situation in such a way that the conflict is eliminated; or to use conscious repudiation and control of unacceptable internal drives or drive-derivatives; or to tolerate frustration of such drives until reality-oriented opportunities for gratification present themselves. At times a conflict may be temporarily or even permanently insoluble, in which case the normal individual will accept and learn to deal with his conflict without secondary elaboration, or regression leading to neurotic symptom formation, even though he may be unhappy with his current state.

Fixation

It is necessary now to introduce another concept for the understanding of psychopathology, namely that of *fixation*. It has already been emphasized that during the course of psychological development from infancy onwards, conflict is inevitable. In fact, in ideal amounts and at appropriate ages, conflict serves to stimulate further ego development in terms of mastery, and the capacity for adaptation, and tolerance of frustration.

Ideally, however, each successive stage of conflict for the child will be resolved, at least in large measure, as psychosexual development proceeds in a relatively orderly fashion from one phase to the next. This would mean that the infantile and childhood conflicts leave relatively little residual psychic energy involved in infantile drive and drive-derivative expression or in the defences against such infantile drives. And the main sources of psychic energy would remain available to the developing organism for use in the on-going process of growth, adaptation and interaction with age-appropriate objects in the environment.

In practice and in clinical experience, however, this is seldom completely the case, and usually there persist nuclei of unconscious infantile and childhood conflictual disturbances which have not been fully resolved. This may come about through excessive or premature frustration of drives, or through excessive stimulation and gratification of such drives beyond an optimal intensity. It may also occur in situations where excessive gratification of an earlier drive occurs in a setting of conflict over expression of a later-developing drive, and thus the former is included in the attempt at conflict solution for the latter. This results in infantile and childhood instinctual drive and drive-derivative pressures seeking a continuing expression and gratification through the repetition compulsion. Accompanying this will be the infantile and childhood super-ego forces and fantasies existing at that period in relationship to such drives. There will then also be psychic energy maintained in the defensive and integrative processes against such infantile and childhood drives and drive-derivatives, with the result that there will be a partial persistent infantile and childhood organization of drives and of defences against such drives.

Where there has been a greater-than-normal unresolved infantile or childhood conflict with persistence of the unchanged drives and defences, such a persistence is known as a point of *psychic fixation*. Fixations may occur at various levels of development, in the nature of the id drives that have persisted in a relatively unchanged state, in the super-ego prohibitions, and also in the nature of the ego processes and level of ego development for integration and adaptation to such conflicts. As will be seen, such points of fixation have significance subsequently in terms of the development of psychopathology.

Neurotic Symptoms

In the discussion to follow, the term 'neurotic symptom' will be used in its broadest sense. It will refer to any disturbance or distortion of psychological function which is based on factors and forces outside the conscious awareness of the individual, and which is not primarily related to the reality principle and the secondary process.

The sequence of events in the development of a neurotic symptom or character trait may be delineated as follows. An individual functioning at a particular level or mode of adaptation, and currently in a stable dynamic equilibrium, is now confronted by an intensified unconscious conflict which disrupts the pre-existing dynamic steady state. This may occur by virtue of an intensification of an id drive, a change in the ego's integrative and adaptive capacity, a change in super-ego forces, or by an experience in external reality which is associated with an unconscious conflict. With such a disruption of the dynamic steady state there is a threatened return of the unconscious drive or drive-derivative into consciousness, seeking discharge and gratification and motivating the organism towards the punishment threatened by the super-ego or the danger situation anticipated by the ego.

The danger situations to be avoided exist in the forms of the primitive primary process fantasies which were experienced in childhood, then repressed, and therefore unconsciously continuing to the present time. Examples of such dangers might include fantasies of bodily destruction or invasion, the loss of various parts of the body, being devoured by the object, inflicting or experiencing pain and suffering, death and dissolution of the self or of the object, etc. Super-ego fantasies from the same period might include such things as violent physical punishment for wrong-doing, the loss of love and acceptance by the needed object, helpless abandonment by the person the child depends on, images of inferiority or inadequacy, etc. The specific fantasies vary in their detailed elaboration from one individual to another, but the intensity of the signal affect is a function of the severity and proximity of the unconsciously anticipated threat.

As the previously repressed mental processes and conflict come closer to consciousness, there will be increasing signal anxiety experienced by the ego as the danger situation is approached and the dynamic steady state is further disrupted. When the danger situation involves the expression of an impulse morally prohibited by the super-ego, the signal of anxiety will be experienced as a sense of guilt. When it involves a failure to approach or fulfil the demands of the ego-ideal, the signal will be experienced as a sense of shame. In all instances there is an intensification of ego functions to re-establish a dynamic steady state of control and adaptation, in order to avoid the unpleasurable affect of mounting anxiety, guilt or shame, and to avoid the danger situation so signalled.

If the ego functions are promptly successful and effective, the previous equilibrium is restored and the anxiety signal disappears. This sequence of events may take place in a very short time-span, and the individual may be conscious only of a momentary disruption and anxiety signal.

If prompt re-establishment of equilibrium does not occur, secondary ego mechanisms of integration and defence must be called into play, and other previous defences may be strengthened and used more extensively. The attempt then is to establish a new level of equilibrium, and to solve the unconscious conflict by use of a compromise. The elements in the compromise involve a partial gratification of the unconscious drive in a derivative and disguised form, and a simultaneous partial satisfaction of ego and super-ego demands regarding the drive.

The neurotic symptom represents the manifestations of this compromise-formation in the attempt at establishing a dynamic equilibrium in the face of an unresolved unconscious conflict.

Compromise-formation

Study of the neurotic symptom itself will reveal various admixtures of the unconscious drive and drive-derivative on the one hand, and the prohibition and defences against the drive on the other. The id drive or drive-derivative may be expressed as a behavioural act, or as a fantasy or as a combination of both. The behaviour and fantasy may occur in a positive form, or as the negative of an act or fantasy, and both may be disguised to varying degrees. These acts and fantasies which represent the drive may be present at conscious, preconscious or unconscious levels of awareness.

The ego and super-ego judgments and prohibitions concerning the drive also are present in the neurotic symptom in that the impulse or drive is not directly or completely expressed, and also the individual now suffers through the disability, the inhibition and discomfort imposed by the new compromise-formation, and through experience of guilt, pain or other forms of unpleasure.

Thus in an attempt to re-establish a dynamic equilibrium and thereby avoid a threat or danger, and reduce the unpleasurable affect signal, the ego now establishes a new compromise-formation in which there is a partial gratification of drive through an act or fantasy, and at the same time a partial gratification of ego and super-ego requirements. As a result of this compromise-formation a new dynamic equilibrium is established, resulting in the reduction of the signal of anxiety *but now including the new compromise-formation which is the neurotic symptom.*

There will be significant variations in the nature and the experiencing of the new compromise-formation. In some instances, the compromise will show greater conscious elements of the drive and drive-derivatives, whereas in others it will be the defensive and prohibiting forces which appear predominant and the drive may be expressed only indirectly, or through unconscious fantasy formation. However, in the detailed analysis of any neurotic symptom, there can be discerned the impact of the different intra-psychic forces expressed in disguised, distorted or derivative form.

Regression

In attempting to resolve the current unconscious intra-psychic conflict which stimulated the disruption of the dynamic steady state, one important defence mechanism utilized by the ego is that of *regression*. This may involve an ego regression in terms of the defence mechanisms or modes of integration utilized, as well as an id regression in terms of the relative intensity of drives and drive-derivatives. These two streams of regression need not correspond to each other in depth or extent.

The degree and level to which regression occurs will be influenced by the intensity of the points of previous psychological fixation which occurred during psychosexual development. It will also be determined by the existence of significant unconscious associations between the current precipitating conflict situations, and the pre-existing unconscious conflicts at the points of fixation.

The current regression will usually be to the point of major psychic fixation, and this in turn results in a further intensification of the unresolved infantile and childhood conflict. Regression may occur to the level of the pre-existing major pathogenic conflict, in an attempt at belated mastery of the original conflict now revitalized during symptom formation. At other times, however, the level of regression may be to a point chronologically earlier than the pathogenic conflict, representing an attempt to achieve earlier (pregenital) gratification of drives and simultaneously to avoid facing the now-intensified pathogenic conflict. The net effect is that the individual is now confronted not only with his current conflict at his chronological age level, but also with a revitalization of the previously repressed unconscious infantile and childhood conflicts. These are now expressed in the form of derivatives whose content is related to the current chronological age and life experience of the individual. With the reawakening of infantile conflict, there is also a similar regression in terms of super-ego processes. The primitive, archaic unconscious super-ego concepts of punishment are likewise re-experienced in the form of derivatives whose nature and content are related to the patient's chronological age and current experience.

In essence the individual is unconsciously again driven to seek satisfaction of infantile and/or childhood wishes, and to re-establish the earlier relationships to the infantile and childhood objects. The pleasure principle demands for such drive satisfactions are accompanied by the unconscious primitive fantasies of danger and/or punishment that existed at the time these drives originally occurred. And the entire process comes into conflict with the individual's current realistic goals and expectations of himself.

Regression may continue to various levels, and if the conflict cannot be contained and an equilibrium established at a more advanced level of development, then a further and subsequently deeper regression will occur. This may continue until such time as conflict containment and the re-establishment of a dynamic equilibrium through the neurotic compromise-formation is 'successful'.

The distinction between this form of regression during symptom formation, and 'normal regression' mentioned earlier (the concept of 'regression in the service of the ego') is the degree and ease with which the regression is reversible. One characteristic of 'normal' regression is that it is easily reversible at the conscious volition and will of the individual, and ultimately its usage is in the service of the secondary process and the reality principle. In neurotic regression, there is less conscious voluntary control of the regressive process itself, and neurotic regression tends to be more fixed and less reversible.

The unconscious goal of neurotic regression is also different. Its chief function is an attempt to avoid current psychic conflict and the reality principle, in favour of the primary process, the avoidance of current discomfort, the pleasure principle, and the gratification of infantile and childhood wishes. The fact that this regression miscarries and the individual is eventually faced with a further intensification of conflict (as a result of the reawakening and re-establishment of the infantile and childhood conflict situation) may be considered 'accidental'. This is analogous to various processes in physiology where regulatory mechanisms may overcompensate and may produce new pathology in an attempt to adapt to stresses.

Clinical Examples

This conceptualization of psychopathology can best be understood by the use of clinical examples.

A married man of 40, whose work involved writing technical manuals on the latest signalling and electronic devices, became aware of some homosexual fantasies and impulses. With these he experienced acute discomfort and anxiety, which intensified as the homosexual fantasies became more discreet and frequent, and he found himself increasingly preoccupied with them. (In response to a number of factors in his current life which need not be enumerated here, there is a threatened eruption and a 'return from repression' of a previously unconscious homosexual impulse which is seeking discharge gratification. As a result of this disruption in the previous dynamic steady state, the patient now experiences the increasingly intense signal of anxiety.) The anxiety continued for about a month, during which time the patient became increasingly uncomfortable in a variety of different situations, particularly relating to other men. 'Finally I realized what was happening.' The patient began to believe that someone had perfected a new, and as yet unknown, signalling device by which thoughts could be transmitted to other individuals. He believed that for reasons unknown to himself, he had been made the object of the experiment, and that the homosexual fantasies and thoughts were being transmitted and induced into his mind through this new device by other unknown people. As he became increasingly 'aware of this explanation' and convinced of its validity, the patient's free-floating anxiety diminished sharply, and he now became increasingly preoccupied with thoughts about the nature of the signalling device and his attempts to find out who was doing this to him. (In his attempts to deal with the conflict evoked by the return of the unconscious homosexual impulse and to avoid the unpleasure of increasing anxiety, there is a steady *regression* of ego function with the increasing use of the primitive mechanism of *projection* to defend himself against the awareness of the nature and origin of the homosexual thoughts. In other words, the patient now attributes the homosexual fantasy and impulse to the external world, thereby avoiding conscious recognition of it as his own. He now perceives the homosexuality as forced upon him by an external source, and having now externalized the conflict, he attempts to seek an escape through increasing withdrawal and elaboration of his delusional thinking. A new dynamic equilibrium has been set up in which the psychotic delusion of influence represents a compromise between the unconscious homosexual drive-derivative, now expressed in the fantasy 'they are turning me into a queer', and the prohibition against such a drive expressed in the thought 'someone else is doing this to me and I am struggling to avoid it'. The specific content of the projected delusion is a function of the patient's personal life experience (the fact that he is involved in work with various new electronic and other signalling devices) but the motivation for the projection and construction of the psychotic delusion is the avoidance of anxiety and recognition of his own unconscious intra-psychic conflict.)

A 14-year-old boy with a full blown obsessional neurosis described among his many compulsions the need repetitively to check water faucets to be sure that they were turned off. His thoughts were that if the faucet were to leak, the sink might overflow, the apartment might be flooded, and his parents would drown. Being sure that the water faucet was turned off meant protection of his parents from the peril of drowning. He would experience repetitive anxiety which would mount until he had checked to make sure that the water faucet was turned off, at which point the anxiety would subside, only to recur again a short time later. (In this symptom the id drive is one of aggression directed against the parents and expressed in the disguised and derivative fantasy of the parents' death by drowning. The ego mechanisms operative include *projection* of the aggressive wish through the fantasy of the leaking faucet, so that the threat is seen as coming from outside the patient and he feels himself to be the defender of the parents against their destruction. As a result of the mechanism of *isolation*, the fantasy of drowning is perceived by the patient himself as a 'silly and ridiculous idea', since the aggressive and hostile affect accompanying the idea of the parents' death has been split off from the idea itself, thus permitting the thought to emerge into consciousness as a 'silly' idea. In spite of these efforts at defence, there is a continuing build-up of aggression against the parents, disrupting the dynamic steady state, and provoking further the signal of anxiety. The further mechanism of *undoing* is now instituted, as the result of which the patient repetitively must check to be sure that the water faucets are turned off. The compromise of drive and defence is also manifested in the act of checking the faucets where he first turns the water on, thus representing the wish to harm the parents, and then turns the water off, representing the avoidance and defence against the wish. At this point the equilibrium has momentarily been re-established and the signal of anxiety subsides. The fact that this is ineffectual in any permanent sense is indicated by the recurrence of the entire symptom complex a short time later. However, the neurotic compulsive symptom of checking the water faucets is part of the total dynamic equilibrium, and represents one of the ego's unconscious attempts at solution of the unconscious intra-psychic conflict relating to aggression directed against the parents.)

A 34-year-old married woman with several children was baking a cake for her daughter's birthday and became involved in an angry argument with her father over some of his irrational ideas and demands. She felt guilt and anxiety over her anger and tried not to express it. At the same time, it turned out that the cake was a failure, and she baked cup-cakes instead. That night she had a sudden thought, accompanied by much anxiety, that she may have put the wrong ingredients into the cup-cakes, and since she could not precisely recall every step of the baking procedure, she had an increasing concern that somehow she had put in something wrong. For the next 4 years before presenting herself for treatment, the patient experienced acute and severe anxiety whenever she had to cook for her family or give her children medicine, and had an intense need repetitively to check the ingredients of the food, and the dosage and labels of the medication. She had a constant fear that she might poison her family or give her children the wrong medication or an over-dosage. In addition, she experienced acute anxiety when driving alone in the car for fear that if she were not able to account for every moment of her trip, she might have hit and seriously injured someone without knowing it. Upon arrival at home, she would have a compulsion to get down upon her hands and knees and look under the car 'to make sure that there was not a body there'. Previously the patient had done all these things without any conscious concern or effort. In spite of her severe anxiety and discomfort, the patient was nevertheless aware that her ideas were 'silly', and that others might laugh at her for them, and hence she hid her disturbances even from her husband. In spite of recognizing the irrationality of these thoughts, she nevertheless was unable to withstand the anxiety if she did not follow the compulsion repeatedly to check the medicine and food recipes, and to look under the car. (In a setting of current, intense conflict with her father, there was the mobilization of an unacceptable aggressive impulse against the father and a threatened disruption of her pre-existing dynamic equilibrium. This mobilization of intense aggressive feeling against her father was associated with other pre-existing unconscious intra-psychic conflicts over the management of aggression, and hence presented a conflict she was unable to resolve effectively in accordance with the reality principle. There followed a *regression* with further intensification of conflicts in relationship to her own aggressive impulses, and with this regression, the need for further defensive elaboration in the attempt to deal with the conflict at unconscious levels. The id drive is manifested by her constant pre-occupation with thoughts of injuring or destroying someone else, including those whom she loves. For example, in her behaviour with the car, she has the fantasy that she has actually run over and killed someone, and has dragged the body all the way home. The ego defences instituted against awareness and expression of such drives include *isolation*, by which the idea can emerge into consciousness as a fantasy, but the affects of anger, aggression, murder or destruction do not accompany the fantasy. This use of isolation also permits her to think of these ideas as 'silly and ridiculous', but the driving quality of the wish is evidenced in her inability to put such thoughts out of her mind, and this requires further defensive elaboration to maintain a dynamic equilibrium. Another defence thus instituted is the ego mechanism of *undoing*, represented by the repetitive need to check over and over on the dosage of the medication, the ingredients of the recipe and the need to get down on her hands and knees and look under the car. With the establishment and repetitive use of the compromise-formation by means of which the drive and the prohibitions against the drive are expressed simultaneously in disguised forms, a new dynamic equilibrium has been established which now includes the neurotic symptoms, and as long as she carries out the neurotic compromise there is a temporary reduction of anxiety.)

An emotionally unstable and immature 18-year-old girl left home for the first time to go to college in another city. After 2 or 3 days she became increasingly anxious and showed a general disorganization of her behaviour. She developed a sensation of tension in her neck, and within a few days her head was turned to the left and she was unable to move it. The hysterical torticollis persisted, and a physician found no evidence of organic disease. After 2 weeks she was sent home from college. When she came for treatment, she was bright, alert, fairly cheerful and showed minimal signs of anxiety, although verbalizing her conscious wish to be cured of her symptom. During the course of her treatment, it was established that she had been unsure about leaving home, uncertain about herself, and frightened at the thought of what she might do when away from her parents, particularly her mother. At college she had been assigned a room with three other girls, where there was close proximity in dressing, undressing and sleeping together in the same room. She was stimulated towards homosexual activities using her mouth and involving such wishes as suckling and biting the other girls' breasts. As these impulses came closer to consciousness, her anxiety increased and her torticollis developed. (In the setting of a current conflict over leaving home, there was a mobilization of passive and dependent yearnings opposed to the patient's ego-ideal and her conscious wishes to grow up and be independent of her family. As part of her attempted solution of this conflict, there was further *regression* with remobilization of the previously successfully warded-off homosexual wishes and fantasies, and a threatened return of such wishes to consciousness and possible gratification in the dormitory setting. This disruption of psychic equilibrium mobilized the signal of anxiety which mounted in its intensity as the drives further escaped from repression. Through the mechanism of *displacement* and through the *symbolic act* of turning her head to the side, the patient 'turns away from' the unacceptable

6

impulse and object. The torticollis represents a compromise-formation and attempted solution of the unconscious intra-psychic conflict over her oral sexual wishes towards women. The id drive-derivative is expressed through the unconscious fantasies and wishes to use the mouth sexually, and the ego and super-ego prohibitions against these unacceptable wishes are expressed in the turning of the head to the side so that the mouth cannot be used in this way. The symptom also resulted in her being removed from the situation of conflict by being forced to return home to her parents. The concept that this has been a 'successful' neurotic compromise-formation is illustrated by the fact that when she presented herself for treatment, there was little overt anxiety and she manifested characteristic and cheerful 'la belle indifference'.)

A 55-year-old woman with a long history of intermittent depression had always been energetic and successful in business. She was married to a man who had been sexually impotent for 5 years, and was consciously aware of considerable sexual frustration, but nevertheless in other areas she was functioning effectively. Her husband died abruptly of a heart attack and the patient underwent a fairly severe grief and mourning reaction which had begun to abate after 4 months. She then became aware again of her sexual tension, but felt she had no acceptable way of gratifying her sexual wishes. On a trip to another city, she rode from the airport in a taxi with a strange man towards whom she was consciously sexually attracted, and he invited her for a drink which she declined in spite of her temptation, being aware of the likelihood that this would end in a sexual affair. After her return, she attended a business meeting at which she was the only woman and several of the men indicated a definite interest and attraction to her. As these men showed their attention and gave her compliments, she was increasingly uncomfortable and anxious. Several weeks later in a supermarket she met a married man whom she and her husband had known for a number of years. He approached her and indicated in a rather direct way his sexual attraction for her and his wish that they might be able to arrange a liaison. The patient experienced acute discomfort and anxiety, left the store hurriedly and from then on developed a fear of going out of the house alone which rapidly crystallized into the phobic symptom that 'I'm afraid to go out by myself because something terrible may happen'. From then on she refused to leave the house alone, and demanded that some member of her immediate family be with her at all times. (This patient was in a conflict between her intense sexual drives to the point of being sexually aroused by comparative strangers and tempted towards promiscuous sexual activity on the one hand, and the fact that such impulses were unacceptable to her on the other. She had been seeking to preserve her memory and loyalty to her dead husband, and the thought of herself as a sexually promiscuous person was completely foreign and guilt-provoking. This conflict was intensified by the sexual stimulation and temptation to which she was exposed when she left the house alone, and with the increased stimulation there was anxiety over possible loss of control of her own sexual desires. The phobia involved the *displacement* of conflict away from the patient's own sexual drives and on to the situation of leaving the house, and a *projection* of the danger as coming from the external environment rather than her own sexuality. In addition there was increasing *regression* with dependency on the family to control her behaviour. The phobia served the attempted solution of intra-psychic conflict, expressing the id drive-derivative in the form of the unconscious fantasy of sexual contact if she leaves the house alone, as well as the super-ego prohibitions against such gratification of drives, and the regressive ego need to have someone else responsible for controlling her behaviour.)

A 27-year-old man had a fear of going to the movies which had been present since adolescence. He could be comfortable only when sitting in the last row of the theatre and on the aisle, and if not, he found himself anxious and restless, with a repetitive need to excuse himself and go out into the lobby. He was also aware of anxiety when attending business meetings unless he could find a chair which could be pushed against the wall. Initially in treatment he had no explanation for these symptoms, but gradually became increasingly aware that his fear was of an attack from the rear by an unknown assailant. Eventually this was expressed by him as a fear of a sexual assault through an anal rape and was related to other fantasies of a passive homosexual nature. (This phobic symptom represented the unconscious fantasy of homosexual assault from the rear, which, however, was unacceptable to the total personality. Through the ego mechanism of *projection*, the defence against awareness of such an impulse was maintained by attributing it to someone outside. This was further supported by *displacing* it to the situation in which he was sitting with someone behind him. In these ways he was able to avoid conscious awareness of the underlying homosexual wish, and by phobic *avoidance* behaviour, he was able to stay away from situations in which the unconscious wish was stimulated. This phobic symptom had been a stable part of his level of psychic equilibrium for 10–12 years, and in spite of the conscious inhibition and restriction of freedom that the neurotic compromise imposed, it had served the function of unconscious containment of the homosexual conflict.)

A 37-year-old married man manifested a repetitive and uncontrolled need to visit prostitutes and to indulge in mouth-genital relations with them, in spite of the fact that he experienced significant guilt and anxiety after each such contact. During treatment he expressed the fantasy in such contacts that the prostitute had recently been engaged in sexual relations with another man, and that the other man's semen might still be present in the vagina of the prostitute. (In this piece of neurotic behaviour, the compromise-formation involved the unconscious id wish for mouth-genital relations with a man, while the super-ego prohibitions were represented by the avoidance of direct homosexual contact through what consciously appeared to be heterosexual behaviour. In this way the nature of the homosexual impulse remained unconscious through *displacement* to the prostitute, who dynamically was not the object of the drive, but rather the vehicle by which the patient unconsciously had oral contact with the semen of another male. In this behaviour, the patient was *'acting-out'* the unconscious wish. Through these mechanisms, the expression of the id drive was sufficiently disguised to keep the nature of the original drive-derivative unconscious, and through the anxiety, guilt and subsequent fear of venereal infection, there was a gratification of the super-ego demand for punishment. Although the patient had conscious wishes to stop this behaviour, it must be seen as an unconscious attempt to resolve his *more disturbing* conflict over homosexuality.)

Variation in Symptom Structure

Although the admixtures of drive and defence will vary greatly in the proportions of each that is present in the final neurotic symptom, the impact of id, ego and super-ego processes can be seen in all such compromise-formations. In some symptom formations, the derivatives of the drives appear to predominate in the form of 'driven' behaviour with relatively little inhibition, as manifested in certain types of 'acting-out' neurotic behaviour. The ultimate of such drive expression is at times seen in psychotic or psychopathic illness where the drive may be expressed in an undisguised form (i.e. a child who murders his parents; the individual involved in overtly incestuous sexual relationships, etc.).

In other instances of symptom formation, the defensive and prohibiting forces appear to predominate, and the id drive may be expressed only in the form of a derivative unconscious fantasy. The individual is then conscious only of the absence of a rational explanation for his symptoms or behaviour (i.e. a phobic woman who becomes anxious and avoids all contact with men, in whom treatment reveals an intense urge toward sexual promiscuity).

In keeping with the economic approach, the more intense the unconscious drive, the greater will have to be the defensive ego operations if the drive is to be controlled. And, in mirror fashion, where the operation of very intense and rigid ego defences is observed, the presence of equally intense unconscious drives can be inferred.

When the compromise-formation has been 'successful' in the unconscious attempt to resolve or control the intra-psychic conflict, a new stable equilibrium results which includes the neurotic symptom. As a result there will be little overt, consciously perceived anxiety, except in the symptomatic situation. Hence many individuals can remain reasonably comfortable and learn to adapt to their neurotic disabilities (i.e. a person with a circumscribed phobia of cats who can arrange his life to avoid contact with them; or an individual with anxiety in any close emotional contacts who devotes his life to a career and avoids marriage or close friendships).

In other instances, however, the utilization of ego defence mechanisms is not fully successful in re-establishing a dynamic equilibrium. For these patients continuing free-floating anxiety persists, and there may be a 'spread' of neurotic symptom formation involving larger and larger elements of ego function and overall adaptation.

Hierarchy of Conflicts

Another general characteristic of neurotic symptom formation is that of a hierarchy of unconscious drive and defensive integrations. The utilization of certain types of mechanisms may evoke further conflict against which other defensive mechanisms must be instituted, resulting in a 'layering' and an increasing complexity of psychopathological formations.

For example, in each of the clinical illustrations described above, the unconscious drive which evoked the conflict and precipitated the symptom formation (i.e. homosexuality, murderous aggression, adult heterosexuality, etc.) was itself based on an intra-psychic organization of drives and defences related to still 'deeper' unconscious conflict situations and ego attempts at their resolution or containment.

The following is another example of such layering in the hierarchy of defensive integrations. A 32-year-old single man developed the symptom of psychic sexual impotence as the result of a variety of unconscious conflicts relating to heterosexuality. These included his fantasies of an attack on himself by the woman, as well as his own sadistic fantasies of hurting and mutilating the woman during sexual relations. The impotence served as an unconscious attempt to avoid these conflicts by making sexual relations impossible. The impotence itself, however, provoked further feelings of shame and conscious sexual inadequacy, and a conscious fear of relating emotionally to women lest he find himself in a potentially sexual situation and be unable to perform. This secondary need to avoid women further increased his isolation from them, and intensified his fears of homosexuality since he was thus more comfortable with other men. The homosexual fears in turn led to increasing conflicts with men, so that when he felt emotionally close to another man he would be forced to break off the relationship because of mounting anxiety related to the unconscious fantasy of homosexual relations with such men. The final result was an extreme withdrawal both from men and women, and the symptom of emotional isolation for which the patient eventually presented himself for treatment.

Multiple Determination

Through the principle of condensation, a specific neurotic symptom or compromise-formation may simultaneously serve as the attempted solution of more than one unconscious conflict, and thus may be 'over-determined'. The larger the number of conflicts so expressed, the more important will be the specific compromise-formation in the individual's overall dynamic psychological equilibrium. For example, the young woman with torticollis described earlier also manifested a variety of voyeuristic and exhibitionistic conflicts, as well as coprophilic and coprophagic impulses, in addition to the oral homosexual wishes described before. The symptom of torticollis also expressed a compromise between the sexual wish to look, and the avoidance of this wish by turning away. It likewise expressed the wish to be looked at, since because of her neck symptom attention was focused on her, but at the same time in an unpleasurable and consciously distressing fashion, thereby satisfying super-ego demands. Simultaneously it also served as the symbolic defence against the wish to smell and eat faeces through turning the head away, while the coprophagic impulse itself was expressed initially as an unconscious fantasy, and only subsequently became conscious during the course of treatment.

Neurotic Character Traits

This same type of neurotic compromise-formation may occur in the continuous or repetitive use of ego defence mechanisms, but result in ego-syntonic character traits, rather than ego-alien neurotic symptoms. In other words, stable neurotic compromise-formations may at times result in patterns of behaviour or feeling which the individual himself experiences as 'normal' and part of his consciously desirable personality. The observer may recognize them as symptomatic of a neurotic conflict, while the patient himself may feel them to be healthy, and may wish to maintain them unchanged.

For example, a 22-year-old married woman with an obsessional character disorder manifested the typical intense need for cleanliness, neatness and orderliness, and experienced typical severe anxiety when confronted by any type of disorder, mess or dirt. The intensity of this was illustrated by a need to have two sets of bedroom slippers and two bathrobes. One set of slippers and bathrobe was restricted to use only before her nightly shower, while the other set could be worn only immediately after the shower due to her conscious concern that should she wear the clean set before the shower, it might become contaminated. Although she recognized that her needs for cleanliness were greater than those of her husband and friends, the patient herself did not perceive these disturbances as neurotic symptoms, but rather thought of her husband and friends as unpleasantly messy and dirty people while she herself merely wished to keep 'properly clean'. (The compromise formation here involved the expression of the id drive-derivative through the constant conscious preoccupation with dirt, filth, germs and disease, albeit in a negative form. The ego and super-ego prohibitions were manifested through the defence of *reaction-formation*, resulting in excessive cleanliness, and the mechanism of *undoing* as manifest in the double set of slippers and robe. The entire compromise-formation was then supported and reinforced by the further mechanism of *rationalization*, by which she attempted to avoid awareness of her behaviour as neurotic.)

A 34-year-old man had suffered repeated traumatic separations from his mother in infancy and early childhood. He developed a characteristic personality pattern of never allowing himself to feel dependent or attached to anyone, lest he be separated from them and thus experience pain and distress. Although married with children, he consciously felt and behaved in such a way that 'if my wife or kids ever died or left me it wouldn't matter much'. He insisted that this was 'the only smart way to live' since he then could never be emotionally hurt by anyone. (This man *displaced* his conflicts and disappointments from his mother to all subsequent relationships and *projected* his expectations of rejection to the new objects. He also developed a *reaction-formation* against any dependency wishes, and used *denial* to ward off any significant interest in objects. Although aware that his character was influenced by his relationship to his mother, he *isolated* the affects associated with those experiences and then *rationalized* the effects of his character pathology.)

At other times character pathology may be manifested by traits or behaviour patterns which the person himself dislikes or finds distressing but which he is unable to change. For example, a 30-year-old woman had much unhappiness and conflict in relationship to her mother as a child. She hated her mother and vowed as a child that she would behave differently when she grew up. She was depressed and frightened to realize that in a great many ways her behaviour 'is a carbon copy of my mother's', and was particularly horrified to find herself doing to her daughter the very things her mother had done to her as a child. (The chief mechanism illustrated here is one of unconscious *identification*, in spite of conscious wishes to the contrary.)

Patterns of Defence

The possibility of the co-existence of a variety of different unconscious intra-psychic conflicts of different intensities adds to the complexity of the defensive and integrative ego processes necessary to maintain the dynamic equilibrium and the unconscious nature of these conflicts. The same ego mechanisms may be used in establishing compromise solutions to various different intra-psychic conflicts. But a variety of different mechanisms may also be used in the attempted unconscious compromise solution of the same conflict when it occurs in different settings or forms.

Where such compromise-formations are 'successful' in re-establishing the disrupted dynamic equilibrium, there tends to be a relatively stable and persistent pattern of neurotic symptom or character formation with minimal free-floating anxiety. Where the neurotic compromise-formation is unsuccessful or only partially successful in re-establishing the dynamic equilibrium, there will tend to be persistent free-floating anxiety and a more fluctuating and unstable pattern of integration and symptom formation.

In each instance, however, a study of the neurotic symptom or character trait itself will reveal the simultaneous presence of the various intra-psychic forces, resulting from an attempted compromise solution to an unconscious intra-psychic conflict. This attempt to reintegrate the entire system into a new dynamic equilibrium now includes the neurotic symptom or character trait.

The major significance of this will become apparent in the section on psychotherapy since it means that both the therapist and patient are confronted by a paradoxical situation. Namely, the symptoms for which the patient comes to treatment and for which he consciously seeks help and relief, are unconsciously wanted and needed by him in his struggle to establish and maintain a more comfortable dynamic equilibrium in the face of his unconscious intra-psychic conflicts. Therefore he will have an unconsciously ambivalent attitude towards attempts to remove such symptoms, since if the symptoms are taken away too quickly or forcibly, the patient will again be confronted with the intra-psychic conflict for which the symptom was the unconscious attempt at a compromise solution.

SUGGESTED READING

ALEXANDER, FRANZ (1948) *Fundamentals of Psychoanalysis.* W.W.Norton & Co Inc, New York

ARLOW, JACOB A. (1963) Conflict, regression, and symptom formation. *Int. J. Psycho-Anal.* **44**, 12

ENGLISH, O. SPURGEON & PEARSON, GERALD H.J. (1937) *Common Neuroses of Children and Adults.* W.W.Norton & Co Inc, New York

FENICHEL, OTTO (1945) *The Psychoanalytic Theory of the Neuroses.* W.W.Norton & Co Inc, New York

FREUD, SIGMUND (1949) *An Outline of Psychoanalysis.* Standard Edition of Complete Psychological Works, Vol. 23. The Hogarth Press, London; or W.W. Norton & Co. Inc, New York

KUBIE, LAWRENCE S. (1967) The relationship of psychotic disorganization to the neurotic process. *J. Am. Psychoanal. Ass.* **15**, 626

NEMIAH, JOHN C. (1961) *Foundations of Psychopathology.* Oxford University Press

NUNBERG, HERMAN (1955) *Principles of Psychoanalysis.* International Universities Press Inc, New York

REDLICH, FREDERICK C. & FRIEDMAN, DANIEL X. (1966) *The Theory and Practice of Psychiatry.* Basic Books Inc, New York

WAELDER, ROBERT (1930) The principle of multiple function. *Psychoanal. Quart.* **5**, 19

CHAPTER V

Reality and the Choice of Neurosis

Introduction

In this discussion of psychoanalytic theory, emphasis has been placed on the role of the ego in the maintenance of adaptation, both intra-psychic and in relationship to the environment. It is now necessary to develop the concept of the role of external reality factors in the overall dynamic equilibrium, and to elaborate the various ways in which the interaction between intra-psychic forces and external reality are manifested.

When an external event or relationship does not have significant associations to unconscious intra-psychic conflicts, there will tend to be realistic and non-neurotic adaptation or conflict solution. The individual's subjective and behavioural responses will be essentially proportional to the reality of the external event or relationship, and object choice and the interactions with such objects will tend to be reality-oriented in accordance with the secondary process. Emotional responses of a pleasurable or unpleasurable nature will occur, but will be proportional and appropriate to the nature of the external event.

The psychic energy available and utilized in these realistic interactions with the external environment still comes ultimately from the unconscious id drives. However, the object and aim of these drives will have been successfully modified by the various integrative mechanisms of the ego to permit the establishment of a stable intra-psychic equilibrium, and to permit reality-oriented drive expression in non-conflict-producing forms.

Traumatic Events

A possible exception to this general statement would be the traumatic neurosis (i.e. war neurosis) in which the individual is subjected to massive threatening stimulation from the external environment, beyond the capacity of the ego to integrate it. However, the fact that other individuals exposed to the same configuration of external stresses and events did *not* develop a traumatic neurosis indicates that the reaction cannot be understood purely in terms of the external stress and event. The nature of the intra-psychic processes of the individual who faces such major external stress must also be taken into account.

The same would be true for less overwhelming reality stresses such as marriage, the birth of a child, death, accidents, illness in a loved person, loss of a job, economic disruptions, failure of an examination, situations of experimental stress or whatever other reality factors the individual may face. To each such situation a particular individual may react and respond differently from someone else, and therefore the total explanation of the individual's behaviour cannot be found purely in an understanding of the external event itself.

Impact of Reality

The mutual dynamic interaction between external reality and the intra-psychic organization is manifested in a variety of ways.

External reality provides objects for the discharge and gratification of pre-existing id drives, and choice of external objects is influenced both by the nature of the drives, and by the integrative and defensive ego functions. External objects may also stimulate or intensify unconscious id drives, leading in turn to pressure for discharge and satisfaction.

The external environment and reality events in the individual's life will also influence the overall form and nature of psychological development and ultimate intra-psychic structure, as described in earlier chapters.

External reality may also serve as the precipitating event for the development of neurotic symptom formation, or may serve to entrench and intensify an already established neurotic disturbance. A favourable and supporting external reality, however, may serve to offset or oppose neurotic adaptation or the development of symptoms, and may tend to decrease the total impact of intra-psychic conflict.

External reality may also serve in the functions of defence through providing objects and situations for displacement, projection, rationalization, acting-out and other ego defence mechanisms, whereby the nature of the basic conflict remains unconscious.

Finally, external reality may influence intra-psychic functioning by providing or by discouraging the secondary gain from neurotic symptom formation.

A. Object Selection

The selection of external objects for gratification of the various drives and drive-derivatives, and the type of interaction in which the individual engages with such external objects will be a function of the nature and intensity of the drives, and the nature of the ego mechanisms by which drive discharge is achieved. Hence the mature individual tends to make 'healthy' object choices in terms of interactions based on the secondary process and the reality principle, with minimal unconscious distortion.

On the other hand, the existence of unconscious, neurotic intra-psychic adaptations will make it necessary for the individual to seek objects in the external world which will be compatible with or support such adaptations. In such a case, object choice will be determined more by unconscious intra-psychic factors than by the reality principle and conscious ego functions.

In other words, the ego continually scans the reality situation seeking for objects on which to displace or project the drives and drive-derivatives, or for use in the defence against the drives. The stronger the unconscious drive which is seeking gratification, or the more intense the defence against such a drive, the greater will be the need to make this type of neurotic object choice in the external world. When such objects are available, the individual will tend to become repetitively involved with them in a stereotyped fashion.

For example, a patient with a strong unconscious masochistic need for suffering and punishment repetitively sought out situations and people in the external environment to gratify this need, and interacted with them in such a way that punishment and disappointment were repeatedly forthcoming.

A young woman with great conflict over sexuality, found herself acutely anxious and uncomfortable in the company of men towards whom she experienced sexual attraction. She eventually chose for her husband the man among her suitors who was least attractive and stimulating to her sexually.

A woman with a strong attachment to an alcoholic father had consciously determined that she would at all costs avoid ever marrying a man for whom alcoholism was a problem. When being courted by her husband-to-be, she was aware that he frequently took her home unusually early in the evening, and living in a small town, she heard rumours that he had been seen drinking in various local bars until late at night. She consciously discounted such rumours, did not confront her fiancé with them, and was eventually 'surprised' within a short time of their marriage, to find that he was a moderately severe alcoholic.

The point to be emphasized is that the individual chooses from the reality that presents itself, and the vicissitudes of his life experience, those external objects or situations through which there can be an expression of unconscious intra-psychic conflict. This may occur through the expression of an unconscious drive-derivative displaced on to the reality object in such a way that the drive is partially gratified, or through ways by which the object can be utilized to help in the defence against the expression of such a drive. The more that object choice in the environment is based on unconscious intra-psychic conflict, or attempts at conflict resolution, the greater will be the potentialities for disruption and disturbance in external relationships. And when two individuals use each other for complementary unconscious purposes (i.e. a dependent person with someone whose needs are to have others depend on him; a masochistic character whose mate has a sadistic personality; etc.) long-term but characteristically neurotic relationships and interactions may occur. The more that such choice of external objects is on the basis of the reality principle, the more likely is it that the adaptation and relationships will be relatively healthy and stable.

B. Impact on Development

In Chapters II and III, some of the forces were described by which the reality objects and events in the individual's life influence the development and structure of the personality.

A large variety of other reality factors beyond the immediate family unit will also mould and influence the development of the individual, and the forms by which conflicts related to the human condition are integrated.

Psychoanalytic interpretations of anthropological studies and data demonstrate the important impact of cultural factors on the modes of adaptation to human conflict. For example, many of the infantile and childhood drives which are unconscious in Western adults may be recognized in the customs, rituals and taboos of primitive societies. And attitudes vary greatly among cultural groups regarding such things as childhood sexual play, nakedness, infant feeding practices, defaecation and faeces, menstruation, childbirth, family structure, etc.

Such cultural differences will be significant determinants of whether or not a particular drive becomes the source of a psychic conflict. And the culture will tend to provide both opportunities and limitations for methods by which psychic conflict may be expressed, contained, ritualized or integrated. To some extent too great deviation from cultural norms is one signal of the existence of a neurotic adaptation.

Social factors within a given culture will also play a significant role in the methods and modes by which conflicts of an intra-psychic nature are expressed or integrated. The relatively recent development and interest in community psychiatry has led to an increasing emphasis on the relationship between social, educational, or economic forces and the development of mental disability or illness.

Factors such as economic deprivation, changing patterns of family structure, absent or negligent parents, limitations of social opportunity, etc., make it more difficult to provide optimal satisfaction of basic human needs in the developing child. Educational deficiency or lack of optimal stimulation and experience, if occurring at crucial phases of development, may result in ego arrest or in failure to develop effective specific ego functions. Educationally, culturally, socially, or economically deprived parents are models for identification in the developing child. These adults also serve as super-ego introjects and specific value systems or anti-social parental attitudes are thus transmitted to the next generation.

Successful adaptation in Western society frequently involves postponement of immediate gratifications of drives in favour of increased frustration tolerance and sustained effort toward reaching long-range goals. If the social situation itself blocks the possibility of achieving such long-range goals, impulsive behaviour with low frustration tolerance becomes more characteristically acceptable. Social forces which mobilize intense aggression, or which encourage and emphasize direct drive discharge place an additional adaptive and controlling burden on already stunted ego functions. Integrative or adaptive demands which are beyond the capacity of the ego to achieve or to maintain tend to evoke an affect of helplessness or hopelessness, and may then provoke regressive behaviour patterns.

Social factors and forces which mitigate against the achievement of such affect states as pride, confidence, security, and hopefulness likewise tend to disrupt long-range adaptive patterns and to make the breakthrough of regressive drive expression more likely. At that point the search for pleasurable affect states and relief of psychic tension makes such regressive behaviours as the use of alcohol, narcotics, sexual promiscuity, physical violence, direct pre-phallic drive discharge, etc., more likely. And if the social mores of the group condone or encourage such behaviours, and the search for objects of identification is among the social group, such character patterns are further enhanced and established.

However, it must be remembered that all of these various behaviours and character patterns may also occur in individuals exposed to very different types of social forces. The essential issue is the impact that such social forces exert on the individual relating to drive satisfaction or frustration, and to the development of ego and super-ego structures for control, integration, and adaptation. These social, economic, cultural and political factors and forces should be understood as contributing primarily to the elaboration and form in which intra-psychic conflict is expressed, rather than in and of themselves being the primary source of such conflicts.

C. Precipitating Events

When a reality stress or event serves as the precipitating factor for the development of neurotic symptom formation or decompensation, it acts as a triggering mechanism by virtue of a series of associations between the reality event itself and a pre-existing unconscious conflict or an unacceptable drive stimulated by the external event. In such a situation, the neurotic decompensation may appear consciously to be in response to the particular external stress. However, the fact that the same external stress may have a different significance for another individual, indicates again that the neurotic disturbance is the result of the specific associative connections between the external stress and the pre-existing unconscious intra-psychic conflict.

This concept can account for the fact that some neurotic disturbances are precipitated by what appear to other observers as relatively minor or insignificant stressful situations. Such precipitating situations have a specifically enhanced unconscious meaning for the particular individual. This has been analogously described as a 'key-lock mechanism', where the lock represents the configuration of the dynamic intra-psychic equilibrium already existent, and the key is the specific precipitating event which has particular meaning through an associative link to the intra-psychic state.

Not infrequently the individual is unaware of the unconscious associations between the external event and the intra-psychic conflict, so that the reaction to the precipitating event escapes conscious recognition by the patient. This concept also permits understanding in an established neurotic disturbance of the acute or intermittent exacerbations of symptoms which the patient may experience as unexplainable.

A 26-year-old woman complained of a recurrence of her depressive feelings, without apparent cause. 'It came on as I was getting ready for bed after watching TV'. Inquiry about the TV programmes indicated that one had dealt with the theme of violence and a person being beaten, while the other dealt with a fatal attempt at suicide. At the time of watching these programmes, she was unaware that both had relevance to her own feelings and reactions in relationship to her own father who had committed suicide when she was a girl. The recurrence of her depressive feelings was related to her unresolved reaction to the father's death, triggered by the external reality of the content of the TV programmes.

In other situations, an external reality event may serve as the precipitating factor in a neurotic decompensation by blocking or interfering with the use of ego mechanisms which previously had been important in the maintenance of a dynamic equilibrium but which now, by virtue of the event, can no longer be utilized.

For example, a 50-year-old man, who previously had made use of extreme activity and independence as a reaction-formation against his passive-dependent wishes, developed a myocardial infarction and as a result had to stay in bed and be passively taken care of. He was therefore unable to make use of the previous ego defence of reaction-formation through excessive independence. This disrupted his intra-psychic equilibrium, with subsequent experience of anxiety and development of further neurotic symptoms.

It follows, therefore, that depending on the nature of the unconscious drives and drive-derivatives, and the nature of the defensive and integrative mechanisms utilized by the individual, the vicissitudes of reality and the relationships of the individual to his external environment may at times precipitate or further entrench patterns of neurotic disturbance.

D. *Reality in the Defensive Process*

A favourable reality situation may have the opposite effect of a buffer against neurotic disturbance, and may help to maintain a relatively comfortable psychic equilibrium as long as the favourable external situation persists. For example, a 39-year-old scientist with a severe work inhibition was nevertheless capable of modest scientific achievement by virtue of his relationship to the department chairman. The chairman was willing to take the patient's poorly organized, inarticulate notes and manuscripts, and essentially write the final scientific paper, something the patient felt incapable of doing for himself. This arrangement permitted the patient greater comfort and stability in his neurotic adaptation, and a reduction in the impact of his neurotic conflicts. The same was true in his financial arrangements, where the favourable reality of his father being wealthy and willing to support him with large gifts of money permitted a form of comfortable passive-dependent adaptation which would not have been possible if the father had happened to be poor.

External reality may also provide the vehicle whereby, through the use of various ego mechanisms, an unconscious internal conflict or disturbance may be externalized and then dealt with as if the external disturbance were the chief source of difficulty. At times this may result in an apparent reduction of intra-psychic disturbances and neurotic symptom formation. However, responses to the continuing intra-psychic conflict will tend to recur when or if the external event or stress is resolved. For example, a 40-year-old man had for many years complained about his wife's frigidity and therefore his lack of sexual outlet. The wife finally underwent psychotherapy, was cured of her frigidity, and she began to make healthy sexual demands upon him. At this point the man developed severe sexual impotence. (As long as he could project, displace, and rationalize the sexual difficulty to his wife, he could avoid awareness of his own sexual conflict and anxiety. When the external situation changed and he could no longer use these defences, his own sexual problems became manifest.) This formulation also helps in the understanding of instances where an individual may withstand a major or intolerable external reality situation without neurotic symptom formation or decompensation (i.e. the prisoner of war or concentration camp), and then develop such disturbances when rescued and the external reality situation involves less stress or greater gratification.

E. Day Residue

This scanning of external reality by the ego, and its impact on the psychic equilibrium, is illustrated by the occurrence of a 'day-residue' in the formation of a dream through the dream work. Of all the many thousands of perceptions and experiences that each individual undergoes in the course of a day, a particular one is chosen by the ego for use in dream formation.

Such a choice is based on the unconscious association between the external event or percept and the intra-psychic conflict expressed in the dream. The external event becomes an object for the displacement either of the drive-derivatives or the defences, and as such may be utilized by the mental apparatus in the adaptation to intra-psychic conflict. On the day of the dream, if this particular percept or event had not occurred, there would have been a further scanning of the various other percepts or events, and the selection of some other one which could serve the same dynamic function to be the 'day-residue'.

F. Secondary Gain

Another area in which neurosis and reality interact is the issue of the *secondary gain* of the illness. The primary gain of illness has already been elaborated in terms of attempts at intra-psychic conflict solution through the unconscious compromise-formation and re-establishment of a dynamic equilibrium.

Establishment of such a primary compromise-formation may subsequently result in influencing or modifying the patient's environment or the attitudes towards the patient in the objects with whom he interacts, in a way that provides further gains or benefits to the patient. Examples would include the individual who, by virtue of being neurotically ill, now receives a different or more gratifying type of attention, or is now excused from the performance of unpleasant or difficult tasks which would otherwise be expected of him. The most extreme form of this is the malingerer who consciously simulates various symptoms in order deliberately to influence the environment in a way more favourable to himself.

In the neurotic individual, the symptoms are developed unconsciously as described before, and the possibility of secondary gain is not a significant factor in symptom formation, but rather something of an 'added bonus'. However, secondary gain may tend to perpetuate and entrench the neurotic symptom formation established as a result of other unconscious forces, and hence may make it more difficult for the individual to give up his neurotic adaptation in favour of a more mature one.

Factors in the Choice of Neurosis

Throughout the development of these theoretical formulations the concept has been emphasized that normal and pathological psychic functioning exist on a continuum, and that many of the unconscious conflicts involved in the psychopathological disturbances also exist in a milder form among normals. Likewise, many of the integrative and adaptive mechanisms, the use of which contribute to the development of psychopathology, may also be seen in normal mental functioning, although used in a somewhat different fashion.

Since the qualitative nature of the intra-psychic conflicts and the mechanisms of adaptation are non-specific in terms of the spectrum of normal to pathological, and likewise are not specifically restricted to various nosological entities, the question arises as to the nature of the factors that determine the final choice of neurosis.

This choice of neurosis will be the end result of the interaction of a variety of genetic and dynamic forces. Although some generalizations are possible, the full and complete understanding of the development and content of a neurosis in any particular instance must still rest on the establishment of the relative importance of the various factors relevant to that particular case.

A. *Constitutional Factors*

Constitutional factors play a significant role, although the details of the mechanisms by which such constitutional forces exert their influence are as yet largely unknown. In the first place, constitutional factors play a role in terms of differences in relative drive intensity. Among newborns there are significant differences in the apparent intensity of drives, as well as in the intensity and nature of the response to frustration of these drives. The observation of some infants being more readily satisfied than others, and of some infants manifesting a massive and sustained frustration response, whereas others appear more readily to accept frustration and show less response, is probably a reflection of innate constitutional differences. In addition there may be constitutionally greater or lesser intensity of specific drive activity manifest in terms of general biological energy and functioning, or in terms of specific differences in intensity among the various drives. For example, there appear to be differences in the innate intensity among individuals of oral, anal and phallic strivings, over and above the effects of experiential factors.

Constitutional factors are also significant in terms of the nature of the various autonomous ego functions and the ego apparatuses as they unfold during development. Such factors as memory, intelligence, motor-skill, heightened or disturbed perceptual capacities, etc., are all influenced by constitutional endowment, and will ultimately influence the nature of the mechanisms that the individual is likely to use, and thus the nature of the ultimate adaptation he is able to make. Even such things as size, physical attractiveness, body configuration and the nature of secondary sexual characteristics may influence the nature and form of the conflicts that an individual faces, and the adaptive mechanisms he uses in dealing with such conflicts.

Somatic constitutional variations or predisposition towards specific physiological or anatomical deviations in various organ systems may likewise influence the nature of the ultimate psychological and psychosomatic adaptation.

Similarly, among the various psychiatric nosological entities there may be constitutional predispositions towards disruption or disturbance of a specific nature (i.e. constitutional factors in schizophrenia, or manic-depressive psychosis). In dynamic terms, such constitutional factors would ultimately operate through distortions or disturbances of integrative ego functions or of drive intensity, as these influence overall adaptation.

Finally, the nature of the individual's own biological functioning, and his relative susceptibility or immunity to certain types of disease and of biological degenerative processes will influence the nature of his total adaptation and choice of neurotic symptoms. This may occur indirectly through the effects that such disease or degenerative processes have on the modes and methods of adaptation that are available.

There may be more direct effects in instances where the physiological or anatomical disturbances affect the central nervous system directly (i.e. epilepsy, encephalitis, cerebrovascular arteriosclerosis, senile dementia, etc.). In these latter instances some of the manifestations of disturbance will be specifically determined by the nature of the underlying process, but some will also be a function of all of the experiential factors to be elaborated.

B. Experiential Factors

The other major group of factors involved in the final choice of neurosis is the total experience and life situation of the individual during the course of development. These experiences include such things as the specific nature of drive frustrations and gratifications, and the way in which the infant and young child adapts to and resolves the inevitable conflicts. The nature and intensity of psychosexual fixation and the degree to which such fixation influences subsequent psychological development will be of major importance in determining the level to which regression may occur later in life during neurotic symptom formation.

Object Relationships

Another major determining factor in the life experience of the individual is the nature of object relationships, where the earliest infantile and childhood experiences serve as prototypes for subsequent relationships to objects in the external environment.

As elaborated earlier, these objects serve as the means by which gratification or frustration of drives may occur, and the child's relationship to such objects will tend to be repeated in subsequent life situations and experiences with other individuals. The earliest object relationships also are crucial in providing the developing child with objects for identification, and hence for the development of the child's own ego and sense of identity. These identifications will have a significant effect on the nature of the integrative mechanisms the child comes to utilize in the attempts at conflict solution and adaptation.

The early objects are also important in that they may permit or encourage certain types of instinctual drive expression while prohibiting others, and they may also encourage or reward certain types of defensive ego functions while punishing or preventing the use of others. In this way the parental objects also exert a significant effect and influence on the nature of the integrative mechanisms through which the child seeks and achieves adaptation and homeostasis. As illustrated earlier, the type of psychic mechanisms and the intensity with which they are utilized is significant subsequently in relation to the development of neurotic symptoms or character traits.

The presence or absence of such objects, particularly early in life, will be crucial in terms of ultimate ego development, and significant separations or loss of such objects will influence the final level of ego maturation and modes of integration. The individual will also be influenced in the same ways through life by interaction with subsequent objects in later phases of psychological development. Although such later interactions and identifications will influence the final mode of adaptation and adjustment, the effects will not be as intense as those occurring in the earliest object relationships.

These same patterns of identification and of reinforcement through environmental responses will play a significant role in super-ego formation. As one of the developing psychic structures, this will have a major impact on the nature of the conflicts that occur, and the nature of the adaptation and mechanisms that become necessary for their containment or resolution.

Trauma and the Vicissitudes of Life

Another important factor in the ultimate choice of neurosis is the nature and intensity of the various inevitable traumatic experiences and situations to which the individual is exposed, and which may evoke various types of adaptations or responses.

What must be emphasized here is not only the external reality of a traumatic event or experience, but also the internal psychic reality of such an experience. This psychic reality will be partly a function of the age of the person at the time when the traumatic event occurred, and partly a function of the way in which the environment and environmental objects help him to integrate or deal with the traumatic event.

For example, surgical procedures in childhood may have varying psychological effects and thus cannot be compared directly in their psychic significance without taking account of the other factors involved. In a normal 2-year-old child, their impact is likely to be around the anxiety over separation from the parental figure, and fantasies of abandonment or object loss, etc., since these are among the primary intra-psychic experiences and fears undergone by a child at that age. In a normal 5-year-old child who is involved in the oedipal phase of development with conflicts over sexuality, a surgical procedure will more likely be responded to in terms of fantasies of castration and possible punishment for sexual impulses. A normal 10-year-old child at the latency phase of development will be more likely to respond to the event primarily in terms of its external realistic impact and such things as pain, discomfort and the fear of the surgical procedure itself.

Traumatic events may leave significant effects in terms of persistent unresolved conflict situations, and points of drive or ego fixation, which in turn may have a subsequent impact on the ultimate choice of neurotic symptoms.

Another group of factors and forces are the accidental vicissitudes of life and the impact that these may have on the individual's total experience. Some experiences will tend to reinforce stability and will tend towards decreasing intra-psychic distortion and disturbances, and may hence be supportive of more healthy or more mature adaptations and integrations. Other experiences may have the opposite effect of increasing the stress to which the individual is exposed, or specifically stimulating and fostering further intra-psychic disturbance and overall instability and disruption of the dynamic equilibrium.

Verification

A full and comprehensive formulation of the origin and meaning of neurotic symptoms requires an integrated understanding of all the factors mentioned above. This is theoretically possible only after extensive study and investigation (usually at the conclusion of the treatment) and even then large gaps in specific understanding often still remain.

In clinical practice, however, it is necessary to make a number of early generalizations and inferences regarding the choice and meaning of various neurotic symptom or character formations, since the pressures of the clinical and therapeutic situation require prompt decisions or interventions in the interests of the patient's treatment. The use of such inferences and generalizations as a working hypothesis regarding the choice of neurosis is valid in the clinical setting, as long as it is recognized that they remain inferences until such time as the data from the specific patient confirm or negate them.

SUGGESTED READING

ALEXANDER, FRANZ & ROSS, HELEN, ed. (1952) *Dynamic Psychiatry*. University of Chicago Press

ARLOW, JACOB A. (1969a) Unconscious fantasy and disturbances of conscious experience. *Psychoanal. Quart.* **38**, 1

ARLOW, JACOB A. (1969b) Fantasy, memory and reality testing. *Psychoanal. Quart.* **38**, 28

HENDRICK, IVES (1958) *Facts and Theories of Psychoanalysis*. 3rd Edition. Alfred A.Knopf, New York

NOVEY, SAMUEL (1966) The sense of reality and values of the analyst as a necessary factor in psychoanalysis. *Int. J. Psycho-Anal.* **47**, 492

ROHEIM, GEZA (1950–1968) *Psychoanalysis and Anthropology*. International Universities Press Inc, New York

TARACHOW, SIDNEY (1962) Interpretation and reality in psychotherapy. *Int. J. Psycho-Anal.* **43**, 377

CHAPTER VI

Classification

Introduction

The problems of nosology of psychopathology and the classification of psychiatric disturbance are areas in which there is still disagreement, and as yet no single completely satisfactory system has been evolved. The currently used system of classification as exemplified in the Standard Nomenclature of Disease, published by the AMA, represents an advance over previous attempts in such classification but still contains a number of limitations for the dynamic approach to psychopathology.

Such a system implies a static, once-and-for-all concept of psychopathological entities, and makes it difficult to account for the clinically observed fluctuations and shifts in intensity and in the nature of the presenting psychopathology. Another implication of such a static concept is that all individuals who are classified as belonging to a particular nosological group will be essentially comparable to each other. This implication is contradicted by clinical experience which demonstrates that marked differences may occur among individuals who, on the basis of their major presenting symptoms, are placed in the same nosological category.

Such a static classification also is based on the major conscious presenting symptomatology, and does not take account of the underlying psychic conflicts and mechanisms which have resulted in the formation of symptoms. This results in an implied limitation in the use of such a system for comparison of the various similarities that exist in the psychic organization of individuals who may otherwise fall into different nosological categories. Clinical experience indicates that many of the same psychological mechanisms and conflicts which are present in one psychopathological entity may likewise occur in other entities although with different emphasis, duration or intensity. For example, some of the same mechanisms used by the normal individual during the process of dream formation may be seen in the psychotic individual during the formation of some of his psychotic symptoms. Any system of classification which does not permit an understanding of such similarities as well as differences is therefore incomplete from a dynamic point of view.

82

These concepts of flexibility, change and difficulty in establishing fixed or static classification of psychopathological states are particularly striking in the various attempts to establish diagnostic entities in the disturbances of childhood and adolescence, where there is even less consistency and structuring of pathology than in the adult patient.

A Psychodynamic Approach

Psychoanalytic theory and dynamic psychiatry are not at present capable of presenting a complete system of nosological classification. The material in the following discussion is intended as a supplement to the usual systems of nosological classification, and although not replacing them, there will be a heuristic value in using it conceptually as an addition to the theory of psychopathology, and in the approach to psychotherapy that will be described later.

Spectrum of Regression

Within the theoretical framework of psychic functioning and adaptation which has been developed, it is possible to conceptualize psychopathology as occurring on a spectrum of disturbance ranging from normality at one end, to psychosis at the other. The axis along which such a spectrum exists is that of the level and intensity of psychological fixation or regression, and the ease or degree to which such fixation or regression is modifiable. The fixation or regression may involve ego processes, id drives and super-ego functions, although as described earlier, the various forms and manifestations of fixation and regression need not all occur simultaneously or to the same degree.

The concept of such a spectrum is not related directly to the aetiology of the psychopathology, but would encompass a variety of different aetiological forces and factors. It is intended primarily as a dynamically descriptive formulation for understanding the level of psychological integration, the nature of the psychic mechanisms, and the content and latent meaning of the symptoms through which the underlying psychopathology is expressed.

This concept of a fixation-regression spectrum of psychopathology is also not directly related to the prognosis of any particular patient in response to therapeutic intervention, which again is in accord with the clinical observations and data. Individuals are frequently observed whose presenting psychopathology is not severe or extreme in the form of distortions or symptom formation, but whose prognosis for change is poor by virtue of the irreversibility of the fixation or regression, and the rigidity of the ego's defensive integration. Patients are also encountered whose presenting symptoms may be extreme and disruptive, but whose capacity to recover from the more severely regressive level of integration is greater, thus giving a better therapeutic prognosis.

In considering the various points or groups in this spectrum, it must be emphasized that as in any such concept, there will be relatively well-defined groups and phenomena at the central points of each zone, but that where one zone merges into another there will be a less clear and less discreet differentiation.

A. Normality

Maturity and normal behaviour are not absolute concepts and instead reflect a range of psychic activity and behaviour within which there will be a significant variation, as discussed in Chapter III. The variations may be in terms of overall integration and function, or in terms of any of the specific psychic functions or behavioural manifestations.

The concept has been emphasized that many of the psychic conflicts and mechanisms occurring in the various psychopathological entities are also to be found in the mental life of normals, although their intensity and their integration into the overall mode of psychic functioning is different. Normal mental functioning has been described earlier but may be dynamically summarized as involving a stable equilibrium at a relatively mature level of psychosexual development, with the use of effective sublimations and maintenance of a state of adaptation within the reality principle.

B. Personality Disorders

Dynamically closest to the concept of normality is that group of disturbances known as the Personality Disorders, of which there is a large variety of types. These disorders may involve varying intensities of disturbance from mild to severe. They may at times be generalized and involve the total personality and all of the different aspects of psychic integration, or in other instances they may involve only circumscribed aspects of personality structure and behaviour, with other psychic functions maintained at relatively mature levels.

The general characteristic of this group lies in the concept that in each instance a particular mode of integration, and a particular group of psychic mechanisms have been used repetitively in attempts at adaptation to conflict throughout the individual's life. As a result, adaptation tends to be stereotyped and based on the unconscious repetition compulsion with fixation at varying points of conflict in psychosexual development.

The manifestations of personality disorders result from the intensified use of various ego mechanisms in the attempted solution of unconscious conflicts, and these produce a modification of the ego itself which then tends to persist throughout the individual's life. These may be some of the same mechanisms which contribute to the development and function of the normal personality, but their use is more exaggerated in the character disorders. Likewise, in personality disorders the intensity of unconscious conflicts is greater, but qualitatively many of the same unconscious conflicts exist in the normal personality in an attenuated, or better integrated form.

For example, when does the normal and ego-adaptive need for neatness, orderliness and a well-organized approach to life become the demanding and intensely involved need for cleanliness, a rigid schedule, and the inflexibility of the obsessional character? At what point does the normal wish to be attractive, outgoing and vivacious become the exaggerated, dramatic, seductive and provocative type of exhibitionism associated with an hysterical character structure? At what point does the normal ability for effective action to modify an unsatisfying external reality situation and make it more gratifying, become the 'acting out' of the neurotic character disorder? When does the normal capacity to tolerate frustration and postpone gratification, become the unconscious need for punishment by remaining in an unhappy situation as manifested in the masochistic personality?

These questions illustrate the difficulty in clearly delineating any dividing line between normality and personality disorder. The difference results from the intensity of conflict, the level of fixation and the pattern and stereotyped way in which defence mechanisms are used.

Within the group of personality disorders, the neurotic manifestations may be either 'ego-alien' or 'ego-syntonic', depending on their intensity and on the nature of the total integration. Some individuals will see their character traits as unpleasant and consciously unwanted, but be unable to modify them and essentially adopt the attitude 'I can't help it, and I don't like it, but this is the way I have always been'. Other individuals, however, will see their character traits as more syntonic with their overall personality integration, and will not think of themselves as neurotically ill, even though the outside observer may discern repetitive neurotic patterns or sharp deviations of function due to the type of adaptation to unconscious conflicts.

Patients with various personality disorders may show significant degrees of psychic fixation or regression, but the level of integration and nature of the mechanisms used are essentially constant and consistent throughout the individual's development and later life experience. Even though the specific behavioural manifestations will vary in relationship to the patient's physical and psychological development and current life situation, the dynamic motivations behind the behaviour will be essentially the same throughout.

For example, the adult sociopathic character disturbance will often present the pattern of delinquent behaviour in adolescence, and of low tolerance to frustration and outbursts of aggressive or destructive behaviour in latency, and intense temper-tantrums when subjected to frustration in earlier childhood. At each successive level of physical and chronological maturation, the psychic mechanisms utilized in dealing with conflict are essentially the same, although their effects may be different and more dramatic as physical and social development proceeds.

Similarly, the obsessional character will frequently have been observed to be extremely neat and careful of himself and his toys as a child, rather inhibited and meticulous in his work in school, frequently emotionally distant or remote from his friends and peers during latency and adolescence, and usually emotionally inhibited while choosing a particularly rigid or controlled mode of life as an adult.

Or a patient with a passive dependent type of personality disorder may show a variety of submissive and dependent reactions to authority figures at all chronological periods of development, or a dependent reliance on substances such as food or alcohol, or withdrawal from competition and self-assertion in a variety of different circumstances.

The point to be emphasized is that the manifest behaviour may show considerable variation in its impact, depending on such things as the patient's age, physical development, life situation and reactions of those in his environment, etc. But the unconscious dynamic meaning behind the manifest behaviour will be relatively similar and will be a reflection of the level of fixation and the continuing use of the same ego-integrative mechanisms.

C. Neurosis

The next group in the spectrum is that of Classical Neuroses. Clinical experience indicates that in cases of classical neurosis there is always a pre-existing characterological disturbance, even though the individual himself may not recognize this, or may be aware of it only in retrospect after the onset of his neurosis.

The onset of the neurosis itself involves a further degree of regression from the previously established level of function of a personality disorder. This occurs in response to the precipitating events or conflicts which disrupt the equilibrium, as described earlier in Chapters IV and V. There follows a further decompensation and neurotic breakdown, and establishment of a new dynamic equilibrium for the individual at a more regressed level of psychic functioning than previously.

In the case of classical neurosis, the basis of the disturbance in the form of an unconscious intra-psychic conflict pre-exists the onset of the neurotic symptom complex, and hence has been latently present in the form of some disturbance in overall personality function. Facing the unresolved intra-psychic conflict which precipitates the neurosis, the individual then undergoes a further regression with a reawakening of the previously latent conflict, as described earlier. In other words, in classical neurosis there is observed a significant degree of regression from the pre-morbid level of function and integration, even though the previous level was itself a deviation from so-called normal personality.

Again an apparent exception to this is the case of a traumatic neurosis primarily in response to massive and overwhelming external stimulation, in which the contribution of an underlying personality disorder is relatively less significant. Even here, however, it must be inferred that the individual was, by virtue of previous character structure and integration, susceptible to the development of a neurotic regression in the face of this external conflict, since others exposed to the same external situation do not necessarily develop the same degree of symptomatic neurotic disturbance. Parenthetically, the greater the contribution to the regression in a traumatic neurosis from the external stress, and the less the contribution from the internal personality organization, the more quickly will the regressive response be resolved when the external precipitating stress or situation is modified.

A 27-year-old man with the acute onset of a phobic neurosis in a situation of current conflict described himself as previously having been 'perfectly normal and healthy, without any complaints or disturbances'. During the course of his treatment, however, it was established that from latency onwards he had experienced a generalized feeling of inhibition; tension and discomfort with people; a sense of shyness, fear and avoidance in relationship to girls; a conscious fear of being the best in any group, and instead a determination to be near but never at the top in any achievement he undertook; and a compulsive need always to be 'on the go' and away from home, particularly when his parents were there, as he was comfortable only if alone in the house. He himself did not consider these reactions as symptoms, or as manifestations of any disturbance. To an observer, however, they represent the evidence of a significant personality disturbance which existed prior to the onset of the acute neurosis.

A 39-year-old married woman complained of a very intense preoccupation with cleanliness, contamination, washing rituals and other compulsive symptoms which had been present for 5 years, reaching the point where she had 'driven my family crazy' with the severity of her symptoms. She indicated that this was of sudden onset following a summer vacation, and that she had been well prior to the development of her neurosis. Relatively superficial questioning, however, established the fact that throughout her life she had been excessively preoccupied with cleaning and cleanliness. She took the curtains down and cleaned them each week, cleaned and straightened every drawer and wardrobe in her house at least once a week, and was preoccupied with straightening pictures and keeping boxes straight in her bureau drawers. As a girl she had been unable to enjoy her dolls and toys, and instead had great involvement in their cleanliness, orderliness and in keeping them well cared for in bureau drawers and cabinets, rather than risk messing them up or damaging them during ordinary play.

These clinical examples illustrate the concept of classical neurosis as occurring in an individual with a pre-existing personality disorder, even though the latter may not be of major disruptive proportions. In response to a precipitating conflict there is a disruption of the dynamic equilibrium manifested in the personality disturbance, with further regression and the utilization of new or more active defence mechanisms, thus establishing a new dynamic equilibrium at a more regressed level of psychological function in which the new neurotic symptoms now play an essential part.

One of the major dynamic differences between the personality disorder and the classical neurosis is that in the personality disorders the nature and level of psychological integration is relatively fixed, and persistent throughout the course of the individual's disturbances. In a classical neurosis there is evidence of a specific decompensation and intensification of regression at the time of onset of the neurotic symptom complex. In instances of spontaneous recovery from a classical neurosis, there is usually a reversal of this regression and return to the previous level of neurotic character distortion.

Some individuals with character disturbances may manifest psychological fixation at more primitive and less mature levels than individuals with a classical neurosis, but such fixation is essentially constant in the character disorder, and the pattern of acute decompensation and regression is generally not present.

D. Psychosis

At the lower end of the spectrum of regression are the Psychoses. In these states, the nature of the psychological disturbances and the elaboration of the symptoms is a function of the extreme degree of regression, in which there is a return to the use of primitive psychic mechanisms and overall level of ego integration and function.

With this there is a greater return to conscious primary process thinking, with partial giving up of the secondary process and increasing disturbances in reality testing, with subsequent disruption in the adaptation to reality. In addition to the disruption and fragmentation of ego structure in the regression, there is also a drive regression with return towards a more narcissistic organization, which causes a further elaboration of the regressive psychotic symptomatology.

E. Borderline States

Lying between neurosis and psychosis on the scale of regression are the so-called 'borderline states', in which the level of adaptation fluctuates, with oscillation between positions of dynamic equilibrium involving a greater or a lesser degree of regression. With these shifts in the level of regression there are corresponding changes in the nature of the conflicts and of the mechanisms utilized to maintain equilibrium, and in the ratio of primary to secondary process thinking, and in reality testing.

In other words, these are individuals who at times give way to more severe degrees of regression to overt psychotic levels, but who likewise are capable of more quickly reverting from the regressive level of organization than are patients with a fixed or classical psychosis. These are people whose capacity to maintain adaptation at neurotic levels of regression is limited, and in response to relatively less intense stress or conflict they undergo greater degrees of regression and transient psychotic symptom-formation.

Other patients considered within the borderline category may never manifest the specific clinical stigmata of psychosis. But they are so severely disabled by their intense symptoms, disturbances in object relationships, distortions in perception of self, and general maladaptation that their level of function is closer to the psychotic than to the neurotic.

F. Organic Disturbances

Any organic process which interferes with the function of the brain (i.e. tumour, infection, trauma, intoxication, vascular disturbance, etc.) may produce psychological symptoms or disturbances. The clinical patterns of such disturbances show a wide variation which may include intensification of previous symptoms or character traits, or the development of specific new neurotic symptoms, borderline states, or a variety of psychotic phenomena.

The organic interference with cerebral function (regardless of the specific cause) tends to impair such processes as perception, memory, judgment, intellectual capacity, etc., all of which are component functions of the psychological structure of the ego. As a result, in the psychic organization ego functions are secondarily impaired and the previous level of psychological integration cannot be as easily maintained. With this disruption of the ego, drives and drive derivatives previously controlled may now come closer to consciousness or even be released. The same sequence of psychological events occurs as in symptom formation (described in Chapter IV), with the disabled ego seeking to establish a new psychic equilibrium.

The final clinical picture in the organic syndromes is thus a result of the degree and rate of development of the ego disturbance caused by the organic process, and the nature, intensity, and organization of the pre-morbid drives, conflicts, and state of adaptation.

Aetiology

Current evidence would suggest that in many of the psychopathological states, the primary aetiology is a psychogenic one. In some conditions, however, constitutional and/or organic factors are more prominently implicated in the aetiology, although the precise nature of such factors is still obscure.

For example, a large body of data has been accumulated to suggest that constitutional, biochemical and/or neurophysiological factors may play a significant role in the aetiology of such conditions as schizophrenia and manic-depressive psychosis. And in such disturbances as cerebro-vascular disease, the various intoxications and infections, brain tumours, psychomotor epilepsy, endocrine disorders, etc., the presence of an organic aetiological factor is well established.

However, the full understanding of the origin, meaning and variations in the specific psychological symptoms and disturbances in such conditions cannot be achieved through a study of the organic factors alone. For example, the same intoxicating amount of alcohol taken by the different people at a party will result in variable patterns of behaviour among them, both qualitatively and quantitatively.

Even in those conditions where an organic factor can be demonstrated, a full understanding makes it necessary to consider the individual's genetic psychological development and current dynamic level of psychic integration. Whatever the nature of any organic aetiological factors may ultimately prove to be, their influence on psychopathology and behaviour will have to occur through their effects on the final common pathway of the mental apparatus, and the level of psychological adaptation.

The concept of various regressive levels of psychological adaptation within the theory of mental function and psychopathology which has been evolved, makes it possible to ascribe psychological meaning to the specific manifestations of the psychopathology, regardless of aetiology.

Rate of Regression

The rate at which regression occurs will likewise influence the manifest clinical picture. In some instances, there is a very rapid process of regression in which the individual appears very quickly to have developed an acute and overt psychotic episode. In other instances, the rate of regression is considerably slower, with steady decompensation from more advanced levels of integration. Often in such cases there are repeated attempts at establishment of a dynamic equilibrium at various successively more regressive levels, by virtue of the fact that the equilibrium cannot be maintained at the more advanced level. These are the individuals in whom the psychosis is frequently ushered in by apparently neurotic or 'pseudoneurotic' symptom formations, but when these mechanisms fail, the conflicts persist, and there is further and deeper regression. Clinical observation indicates that in situations where regression occurs slowly, the individual has more opportunity to test and develop other compensatory mechanisms, whereas in situations of acute and rapid psychological decompensation this is less frequently true.

8

Fluctuation of Regression

The concept of relative levels of regression also permits an understanding of the clinical phenomenon in which a patient may be examined at various times and diagnosed as falling into different categories of psychopathology. The examiner at any one period in time is observing a 'cross-section' of psychic function at the particular level of regression existent at that moment. This level of regression may fluctuate in either direction, so that at a different point in time the examiner may see a significantly different clinical picture. These shifts in the level of regression will be reflected in the nature of the ego functions and defence mechanisms utilized in establishing the dynamic equilibrium, and this in turn produces the changing manifest clinical picture.

However, in the individual case there are usually points of major psychosexual fixation to which the individual tends to regress during symptom formation, subject to the various fluctuations in level described above. For example, if an individual has once manifested the propensity for regression to psychotic levels, the likelihood of a subsequent regression to this same level in the face of conflict or stress is greater than in an individual who has been capable of establishing a stable dynamic equilibrium at the level of a neurotic regression. Conversely, there are individuals whose ego defences are so rigid and fixed (i.e. the obsessional character) that any regressive movement is met by sharply intensified efforts at maintenance of the rigid defensive structure. The significance of this will be elaborated in the section on psychotherapy.

Neurosis as Way of Life

These conceptualizations on the nature and origin of neurotic symptoms and character disturbances permit the following further formulation. Given a particular individual's genetic development, and given his current dynamic cross-sectional interplay of intra-psychic and environmental forces, his neurotic symptoms and character traits (used here in the broadest sense) represents a method of adaptation and 'way of life'. Regardless of the conscious degree of restriction, lack of fulfilment, symptomatic disturbance and suffering, this adaptation represents the best and most effective level of integration and function that the individual has been capable of achieving *on his own*. As such, it is needed by him to prevent what *he* perceives as a greater danger situation, or a more disruptive and maladaptive level of integration and function. In other words, in spite of conscious distress, the psychopathological state serves a positive unconscious function for the individual.

Furthermore, within units larger than the individual himself, such as family, work or social groups, there will be a variety of group integrations and adaptations based on the dynamic interaction between the individuals who make up the group.

As described earlier, each individual scans his environment and seeks relationships with available objects either for the gratification of intrapsychic drives or for reinforcement of the defences against such drives. Therefore, states of adaptation between individuals and within groups may be based on unconscious neurotic factors and forces, and the entire group may seek to maintain the adaptation resulting from the interaction of the forces represented by the individuals that make up the group. The recognition of this dynamic interplay of forces between members of a family, and of the impact on family structure that may be produced by a major change in one of its members, has led to the development of family therapy. Here the family as a whole, rather than one or more of its individual members, becomes the unit for treatment and the interactions within the family are the chief focus of attention. However, it must be remembered that these interactions are also a function of the various psychic forces within each of the members.

Where such interactions are interlocking and mutually complementary, group structure will be enhanced, group adaption maintained, and in spite of major neurotic symptoms or behaviour patterns the life of the group persists. Conversely, if members of a group have the same neurotic needs and each is looking for the same unconscious satisfactions which are not being met, or if personality patterns are not complementary, the group has a tendency to disintegrate with individual members seeking such gratifications elsewhere.

The following clinical examples illustrate these issues. A passive, dependent, submissive and depressive woman was married for 40 years to a violent man with needs to dominate and control her. She complained bitterly about his behaviour and her own unhappiness, but after his death felt helpless, unable to make decisions, and needing someone to depend on. Within a year she had married another dominating and controlling man and was again complaining about his behaviour.

An alcoholic man with an intense conflict about emotional commitment and closeness was married to an hysterical and violently aggressive, competitive woman who repeatedly attacked and depreciated him. The man complained about his wife, saying she made it impossible for him to feel or show love. However, at times when the wife was warm, supportive, or loving, he would deliberately provoke a fight and then complain again about her hostility. The wife attacked him for drinking and failure to hold a job, but during his periods of sobriety and work, she became increasingly anxious, angry, and provocative, and eventually she would help to precipitate another bout of alcoholism. For the period of his acute drunkenness, she would be warm, concerned, and supportive, but then would revert to the hostile depreciation and the cycle would be repeated.

A masochistic woman with one son was married to a man who drank, beat her, brought his mistresses into their home, never took her out, etc. She resolved to stay for her son's sake, but to get a divorce when he was old enough. After the son married she divorced the husband, but while waiting for the final decree she developed increasing depression, anxiety, multiple conversion symptoms, and had many suicidal impulses. Ten days after the divorce was final she remarried the same man, and her subjective symptoms promptly subsided.

An obsessive-compulsive woman had such intense anxiety about dirt and contamination that she insisted that her family immediately change all clothing when coming into the house from outside, the house was divided into 'clean' and 'dirty' zones, and no one was allowed to go from one zone to another within the house without washing. As a result no guests or playmates could ever enter the home. Her husband and children were so concerned and guilty about her suffering that they accepted this style of life for many years until the youngest son's *bar mitzvah*. For this event the husband insisted that his relatives be invited to the home after the ceremony. This so intensified the wife's symptoms that she finally sought psychiatric help.

In contrast to these examples, a reasonably mature, responsive and effective young woman married an apparently healthy man she had known for two years. After six months the man became increasingly disinterested in sexual relations, and emotionally withdrawn from her. Eventually he was spending more and more time away from home, refusing to participate in mutual activities, and indicating directly his wish not to have married. The wife tried for two subsequent years to discuss the problems, and suggested marriage counselling or therapy but the husband refused. She was unwilling to accept this type of unfulfilling marriage and the husband's defences were challenged by his wife's expectations. She then decided to divorce him and the relationship was terminated.

In interpersonal relationships or in family groups, a change in one of the members may have an impact on the others in a variety of ways, either positively or negatively. This will influence the stability and equilibrium of the group structure, analogous to the shift of intra-psychic equilibrium within the individual as a response to change in any of the component forces.

The importance of this will be illustrated in the section on psychotherapy, since a change in one individual in response to psychiatric treatment may significantly alter the dynamic equilibrium of the group to which he belongs, and thus may either be supported or opposed by the other members of the group, depending on the nature of the pre-existing group equilibrium.

SUGGESTED READING

ARIETI, SILVANO (1967) *The Intra-Psychic Self: Feeling, Cognition, and Creativity in Health and Mental Illness*. Basic Books Inc, New York

EIDELBERG, LUDWIG (1954) *A Comparative Pathology of the Neuroses*. International Universities Press Inc, New York

GRINKER, ROY R. *et al.* (1968) *The Borderline Syndrome*. Basic Books Inc, New York

MENNINGER, KARL A. (1959) *Towards a Unitary Concept of Mental Illness—A Psychiatrist's World*. The Viking Press, New York

MENNINGER, KARL A. (1962) *A Manual for Psychiatric Case Study*. Menninger Clinic Monograph Series No. 8. Grune & Stratton, New York

RANGELL, LEO (1965) Some comments on psychoanalytic nosology with recommendations for improvement. In: *Drives, Affects, and Behavior*, ed. Schur, Max. International Universities Press Inc, New York

SECTION III

Psychotherapy

CHAPTER VII

The Strategy of the Therapeutic Process

Introduction

Both the theory and the technique of psychotherapy evolve logically from the psychoanalytic theory of mental function and of psychopathology. In earlier chapters these concepts were developed in detail, and at present they may be merely summarized. Neurotic symptoms and character disturbances are compromise-formations, resulting from an attempted solution of an unconscious intra-psychic conflict, in each of which may be recognized the impact of id, super-ego and ego forces. They represent an attempt to restore the disrupted dynamic equilibrium and to bind anxiety and other unpleasurable affects. By definition, the unconscious conflicts can never be observed directly, but their existence can be inferred from their manifold derivatives. In these derivatives there may be greater or lesser elements of the drives or of the prohibiting and defensive forces, but at all times there are simultaneous contributions from all parts of the mental apparatus.

Even in a psychotic patient where at times there occurs a more direct break-through of the previously unconscious drives, there is still some attempted disguise, so that in spite of relatively weakened ego function, the patient is still seeking to keep from consciousness the real nature and full extent of his impulses. This unconscious attempt at maintenance of repression is more evident and more effective the further the patient moves along the regressive spectrum of psychopathology in the direction of neurosis and personality disorders.

Therapeutic Alliance

All types of psychotherapy involve some sort of therapeutic alliance where the healthy aspects of the patient's ego form a partnership with the therapist in which they, as a pair, pit themselves against the neurotic or the sick elements in the patient's mental life, in an attempt to influence or change the latter. These healthy ego processes include such things as capacities for communication, self-awareness, intelligence, motivation, object relationships and overall capacity for integration and synthesis.

However, there are also aspects of ego function which oppose the process of therapy, so that although the patient wishes relief from his neurotic suffering and disability, he does not want to give up the neurosis itself since it represents his attempt to solve a psychological conflict, and as such represents the best level of adaptation he has been able to achieve on his own. The wish for relief is largely conscious and supplies much of the motivation towards therapy and the willingness to work in treatment, and to make the necessary sacrifices and effort to achieve its success. The wish to maintain the neurosis is largely unconscious, and results in the erection and maintenance of a variety of resistances to changing, and to resolving the underlying unconscious conflicts.

Resistance

This resistance comes basically from three different sources. The deveopment of neurotic compromise-formations was described earlier as the result of the patient's wish to avoid full awareness of the nature of his unconscious drives and conflicts, to avoid what he unconsciously fantasies to be a situation of danger, and thus to re-establish psychic equilibrium and reduce signal anxiety. In the therapeutic situation, the patient will try to maintain repression of the basic conflicts through the unconscious ego defence mechanisms. As the patient in therapy becomes more consciously aware of these conflicts, he at first will experience increasing anxiety, and it was partly to avoid this unpleasurable affect of anxiety that the neurosis was originally established. The patient in treatment continues in the wish to maintain the conflicts at unconscious levels and thereby avoid the 'dangerous' fantasies, and the unpleasant affects that accompany them, and hence he will resist therapeutic efforts to make them conscious.

Another determinant of resistance results from the fact that the neurosis partly represents a continuing unconsious search for gratification of infantile and childhood strivings. Although the infantile drives and objects are in conflict with the patient's conscious attitudes towards himself at his current age, and although they are accompanied by anxiety or guilt over the various infantile fantasies, these drives still press for direct satisfaction. The process of maturation and the giving up of the neurosis means that the patient must accept the frustration of his infantile wishes, and must give up the infantile pleasure principle in favour of the reality principle. Unconsciously, the patient clings to the hope of gratification of these drives, and hence he is further resistant to efforts at helping him to find substitute but more reality-oriented satisfactions.

The third source of resistance is the fear of change. To try new patterns of adaptation and new modes of reaction is often accompanied by fear. The old patterns, though unsatisfactory, are at least familiar and hence the tendency will be to maintain them and thus avoid the anxiety that new and unfamiliar behaviour patterns bring. In addition, when a patient attempts new modes of adaptation, these may be initially unsuccessful, and hence the patient will be again more prone to resort to the old and familiar ones.

All patients, therefore, have a mixed motivation in regard to psychotherapy. They have a conscious wish to be relieved of their neurotic suffering or disability, but also an unconscious wish to hold on to the neurosis itself.

Spectrum of Therapy

It is convenient to conceptualize a spectrum of psychotherapy running from supportive treatment at one end, to intensive, insight-directed uncovering psychotherapy at the other. The deepest and most penetrating form of insight-directed psychotherapy is formal psychoanalysis which involves a specialized and specific training and technique that are beyond the scope of this discussion. However, some of the principles of psychoanalytic technique are applicable in modified form to less intensive and more superficial types of insight-directed psychotherapy. It is these latter forms of insight-directed psychotherapy that will make up the other end of the spectrum in this present discussion.

The ends of this spectrum can be clearly distinguished from each other in regard to the theory of psychotherapy, and to the technique which evolves logically from this theory. In the centre of the spectrum these differences are less discreet and less clearly demarcated, so that this discussion will focus on the opposite ends of the spectrum and on the similarities and differences between supportive and insight-directed therapy.

Appropriate treatment of either variety rests on dynamic concepts of basic psychopathology and an appraisal of the patient using the insights offered by psychoanalytic theory. The actual technique of treatment can be conceptualized in terms of strategy and tactics. Strategy represents the overall plan and approach in general terms, while tactics are the immediate and specific therapeutic interactions. Strategy derives from basic theory, and tactics are derived from strategy.

THE STRATEGY OF PSYCHOTHERAPY

Setting of Goals

As will be seen in Chapter VIII on the Indications for Treatment, those patients who are to be treated supportively are often potentially capable of only limited participation or change in therapy, and hence treatment is aimed chiefly at relief or amelioration of symptoms without expectation of change in the underlying character structure, or resolution of basic conflicts. Treatment may also be aimed at producing external behavioural change within the existing neurotic adaptation. At other times the prospect of chronic psychological illness must be accepted, with the recognition that many patients must learn to live with their illness and symptoms. This would be analogous to a patient with chronic heart disease, or residual paralysis after poliomyelitis, where cure is impossible and part of treatment involves helping the individual adjust himself and his life to his disability.

Where the prospect of basic change is unlikely (for whatever reason) the therapist must recognize that the patient's level of adaptation may require his neurotic symptoms, and must be cautious about attempting to remove them too forcibly or rapidly lest he thereby precipitate a further disruption and even more disturbing level of adaptation or of symptom formation.

At times a patient may have unrealistically high therapeutic ambitions and part of the treatment may be to help him accept more limited goals for himself. At other times the goal may be merely to prevent further disability and to maintain the patient's current level of adjustment. For example, in some chronically psychotic patients, the goal may be only to keep them functioning outside of a hospital.

In some instances the goal is merely to tide the patient over an acute crisis in his life, or exacerbation in his illness, and not attempt to modify the underlying chronic psychological disturbance.

In any event, supportive therapy is generally aimed at symptom relief and overt behavioural change, without emphasis on modification of personality or resolution of unconscious conflict.

The goals of insight-directed psychotherapy are more ambitious in terms of the ultimate level of psychic function than in the case of supportive treatment. The extent and depth of change will vary, but insight therapy involves some attempt at helping the patient to achieve greater self-awareness and some degree of underlying personality change. It involves his becoming conscious to some extent of previously unconscious aspects of his own mental life, and attempting consciously to resolve and better integrate such conflicts. The immediate relief of symptoms becomes of secondary importance, on the assumption that when and if a symptom-producing unconscious conflict becomes conscious and is elaborated and worked through, the symptoms will no longer be psychologically necessary and will disappear or subside. This is analogous to the relief of fever and cough by treatment of the underlying infection in a case of pneumonia.

Other goals include some degree of overall psychological development towards maturity, with increased independence and tolerance of stress. This includes the dominance of the reality principle over the pleasure principle, and the achievement of more effective and age-appropriate drive satisfactions and gratifications.

Levels of Consciousness

In supportive therapy, the strategy is to permit the patient to maintain repression and to deal in treatment only with those elements of mental life which are currently conscious or preconscious. The therapist does not attempt to bring unconscious conflicts into consciousness, since to do so in the absence of the ego-capacity to integrate or resolve such conflicts will result in increased anxiety and further symptom formation.

On the other hand, the opportunity to ventilate, share and discuss consciously disturbing problems or conflicts can be helpful, and once these have been expressed by the patient, the opportunity for reassurance, suggestion or other intervention by the therapist is presented. The therapist may recognize that what is consciously disturbing the patient is a derivative of an unconscious conflict, but the goal is to help the patient more effectively maintain his resistances and defences against the emergence of this conflict into consciousness, and the hope is that by so doing he can be helped to a more comfortable and stable dynamic equilibrium. Relief from consciously disturbing problems or conflicts lightens the burden on the patient's ego processes, and makes the ego that much more effective in the maintenance of its various other defensive and integrative functions.

One paradox here is that in certain types of patients where repression and other defensive ego functions are failing (i.e. the schizophrenic, the borderline, or the obsessional patient) the patient may be consciously aware of psychic conflict or primary process material generally considered 'deep' and usually repressed in other types of patients. According to the concept of dealing with current conscious and preconscious material, the therapist would give such a patient an opportunity to express these 'deep' ideas, since if not permitted to do so the patient is blocked from talking about what is currently in his mind, and left to struggle with this material alone. However, the therapist would not encourage the patient to dwell on such material or explore it more deeply. In fact, once these thoughts or feelings have been expressed, the therapist may focus attention away from them, but it will have been therapeutic in the sense that the patient can then feel accepted by the therapist in spite of his bizarre, disturbing or guilt-laden thoughts or feelings.

Reassurance to the patient is most effective *after* he has revealed what is consciously troubling him. If reassurance is offered before the patient reports what is consciously on his mind, he cannot accept it since he keeps the reservation 'but the therapist wouldn't feel this way if he *really* knew what I'm thinking'. As the patient improves and defences against this 'deep' material become more effective, the therapist encourages these and does not bring up this material for further discussion.

In insight-directed therapy, technique is designed to increase the scope of the patient's awareness of his own mental processes, and to help him become conscious of previously preconscious or unconscious psychic conflicts. The extent of this bringing of unconscious and preconscious material to consciousness will vary with the intensity and depth of the therapeutic undertaking. And the elements to be made conscious include not only the drives and drive-derivatives, but also the unconscious and preconscious ego and super-ego functions.

The bringing of this material to consciousness will occur against the patient's resistance as mentioned above, but the goal of increased self-awareness requires that in spite of the resistance, the patient become gradually conscious of previously repressed psychic processes and conflicts, and of how these influence and affect his current life adjustment. After becoming conscious, these old conflicts must be resolved by making new and more appropriate conscious choices and by the development of more effective conscious mechanisms of integration.

Dynamic Use of the Therapeutic Relationship

In Chapter XII on Transference, the theoretical, strategic and tactical aspects of the therapeutic relationship will be explored. It is this relationship and the dynamic use of it by the therapist that forms the cornerstone of treatment, both supportive and insight-directed. The more that goals are insight-directed, the more necessary it is to maintain a relatively consistent, neutral, participant-observer role; the more supportive the goals, the more the therapist makes use of himself as an instrument in specific types of active interventions, designed to further the supportive goal.

A. Resistance and Defence

The failure of the patient's previous defences and threatened return of the repressed conflicts has led to a disruption of the dynamic steady state and the formation of symptoms. The strategy supportively is to help the patient re-establish more effective psychological defences, thus strengthening the repression of conflict, permitting a more stable dynamic equilibrium and reduction in level of anxiety, and thereby diminishing the impetus towards symptom formation.

One of the therapist's tasks in supportive treatment is to survey the various defences available to the patient and determine which of these can most effectively be introduced, strengthened, encouraged or reinforced. He generally permits the patient to maintain those defences already in use, unless they result in symptoms or behaviour seriously jeopardizing the patient's existence, and does not attempt too rapid alteration of important defences. He tries to help the patient more effectively use pre-existing defences which for him are familiar, rather than introduce new ones the patient is not able to use himself. But when new defences are to be introduced by the therapist, they are chosen to be compatible with the patient's overall ego structure and already existent major defences.

The following are a few examples of such an approach. With patients using isolation and intellectualization as major defences, the therapist's interventions would include intellectual explanations rather than an emphasis on emotional reactions. With obsessive-compulsive patients the interventions might include ritualistic and semi-magical instructions. Where patients have the defensive need to defy authority and maintain active control, interventions would be more casual, and would minimize the role of the therapist. If the patient already uses displacement, as in the phobic individual, the therapist might suggest new and more appropriate objects or activities for the displacement.

These examples will be elaborated in later chapters on tactics, but the strategy is based on a dynamic assessment of the patient's pre-morbid defensive patterns, and interventions are designed to best make use of these patterns in furthering the patient's ego controls and re-establishing a more comfortable and stable level of equilibrium.

In insight therapy, where one goal is to make unconscious and preconscious conflicts and mental processes conscious, the therapist gradually helps the patient reduce or give up his resistances and defences in order that conflicts can emerge more clearly into consciousness. This means interpreting resistances and defences at appropriate times and in such a way that the patient is willing and is helped to relinquish them and become conscious of that which was defended against. Initially, as a defence is reduced and the conflict comes closer to consciousness, there will be an increase of anxiety until the material is fully conscious. Once the material is subject to the ego's conscious integrative and controlling processes, there will again be a reduction in the level of anxiety.

This means that whereas in supportive therapy the attempt is to allay and reduce anxiety by strengthening defences, in insight-directed therapy it is necessary, through lowering of defences, temporarily to mobilize and increase anxiety in amounts that can be tolerated by the patient as part of the process of making unconscious material conscious.

Another difference in insight therapy is that defences against the recall of repressed memories are gradually reduced so that the patient may remember some of the earlier pathogenic experiences, attitudes and re-actions. Such recollection is one step in the ultimate resolution of the impact of such experiences on the patient's current modes of adjustment. In supportive treatment, on the other hand, no special effort at recall of repressed memories is made, and the patient is permitted to maintain his amnesias.

B. Conflict

In supportive treatment, strategy calls for an attempted reduction or removal of conscious and preconscious conflict and the therapist uses a variety of means to help accomplish this. At times it may become necessary for the therapist actively to assume certain ego functions that ordinarily the patient would carry out himself. In this sense, the therapist temporarily takes over a surrogate-ego role, in that he may actively make decisions for the patient, intervene in the patient's life, arrange for various things to be done to and for the patient, etc. The ultimate of this is seen in the situation of hospitalization, where the therapist directs and controls even the physical activities of the patient, and if required, provides the necessary impulse controls (i.e. seclusion, sedation, restraint, etc.).

Such interactions in part repeat early child-parent relationships, and as in the latter, one of the therapeutic tasks is to promote a positive relation-ship in which identification with the therapist may increase. The therapist may then gradually permit or encourage the patient to use his own ego processes, relinquishing the surrogate-ego role, but being ready to resume these functions should the adaptive task prove too much for the patient. In supportive treatment there are instances where such anaclitic relationships are maintained for long periods of time, and for some patients this type of therapeutic contact may have to be maintained indefinitely.

In the role of surrogate-ego, however, it is again necessary that the therapist's interventions be undertaken in keeping with the overall dynamic assessment of the patient's personality and the interplay of psychological forces.

In insight-directed therapy, the relationship and the therapeutic interventions are used to bring previously unconscious conflicts to the patient's conscious awareness in an emotionally meaningful way. In other words, the strategy is to re-establish and recreate the earlier conflicts which have resulted in the formation of neurotic symptoms or character traits.

Consciously confronted with such a conflict as a result of the therapeutic efforts, the patient will now be in a better position to attempt to resolve it or at least to find more effective modes of dealing with it than previously. One difference is that this is now being undertaken with the patient at a more mature and advanced stage of development than at the time of origin of the conflict. In general, his ego will have a greater tolerance of anxiety and frustration, as well as greater potentiality and available mechanisms for resolution of conflicts than were present at the developmental level where fixation of conflict occurred. In other words, the patient is older, has had more experience, has a greater potential for independent functioning, and has a greater opportunity to find new modes of adjustment and new ways of dealing with his conflicts.

Another difference between the original pathogenic conflict situation and the current therapeutic situation is that in the original setting, the patient was attempting to deal with these problems alone. Therefore, he had a greater need for prompt resolution, and there was greater likelihood of an attempt at repression and exclusion of the conflicts from consciousness as quickly as possible. In the therapeutic situation, however, he has the aid and alliance of the therapist, and thus a greater capacity to tolerate the anxiety and frustration that will be mobilized in the attempt to deal with the previously unconscious conflicts. The support and encouragement that are tacitly experienced in the therapeutic relationship also aid in the current efforts at conflict resolution. And the therapist's efforts to confront the patient with his conflicts make it less possible for the patient to go on hiding his basic disturbances from himself.

9

Because the goal of treatment is the patient's further personality development and increased independence, as well as greater tolerance of stress, the therapist does not actively intervene or advise him regarding solutions for his various problems. Instead he maintains the neutral role of participant-observer and encourages the patient to seek his own active solutions based on increasing insight and selfawareness.

C. Identification

In supportive therapy, strategy involves encouraging and promoting identification with the therapist. This is done through the establishment of rapport, the maintenance primarily of a positive relationship, and an active participation in the patient's attempts to deal with his problems. The therapist may indicate different ways of approaching them, suggest new mechanisms for the patient to use, indicate his own ways of looking at or resolving problems, reveal certain aspects of his own personality or problems, offer suggestions, etc., and in general encourage the patient to think as if he were the therapist.

This process, in part, repeats the earlier development of identification with parents and others in childhood, but presumably the therapist is offering a more stable, consistent and effective model for such identification.

The goal here is improved ego function for the re-establishment of a more stable dynamic steady state, and the role of identification in the original process of ego development has been well documented.

In insight therapy, the goal is the greatest possible degree of independent development and self-fulfilment. Therefore, the therapist would not actively encourage identification, and instead encourages the patient's efforts at self-development. In spite of this, a certain amount of identification with the therapist does occur, and it is often necessary to deal with this as a manifestation of resistance and defence against the development of a more independent sense of identity.

D. Reinforcement

In the supportive development and establishment of new or more effective ego defences or patterns of integration and adaptation, it is generally necessary to reinforce any movement by the patient in the direction of more healthy adjustment and adaptation. This means some type of interaction by the therapist which is dynamically designed to provide a meaningful 'reward' in terms of the patient's specific needs and patterns. The choice of an appropriate reward must be in keeping with the patient's specific unconscious drives and defences.

The hope in such reinforcement techniques is that as the patient successfully attempts new ego methods of adaptation, originally motivated by the reward, the gratifications achieved by using these new modes will themselves provide further reinforcement, and hence the new responses may become self-sustaining. In this way, behaviour may at times be modified without the patient becoming conscious of his underlying conflicts or motivations.

The concept of 'reinforcement by rewards' involves reliance on an external authority for motivation, control and judgment, and as such is opposed to one of the basic goals of insight-directed therapy, namely the development of independent judgment and motivation. Therefore, in insight-directed therapy the therapist does not attempt to reinforce or actively reward specific types of behaviour or change. This is designed ultimately to help the patient to establish his own more mature attitudes and motivations, based on his own judgment, experience, and increasing self-awareness.

E. Drives and Drive-derivatives

The patient initially will tend to react to the therapist in ways similar to his reactions to other people, but influenced by the realities of the therapeutic situation and the impact of the roles of patient and therapist.

The details of the subsequent development of the therapist-patient relationship and the dynamics of the transference will be discussed in Chapter XII. At this point, suffice it to say that as a result of a number of factors in the treatment situation, the therapist may become the object of the patient's unconscious drives and their derivatives, as well as the object of the patient's defences against such drives.

How this relationship is managed by the therapist will in large measure determine whether the reality elements in the relationship predominate, with the transference aspects maintained at unconscious levels, or whether there is an increasing investment and distortion of the relationship by the patient in accordance with his unconscious drives and defences, and the development of an intense transference relationship.

In supportive therapy, the strategy is to maintain a positive relationship based on conscious rapport, in which the conscious elements of the relationship are emphasized, and distortions are minimized. This may at times require gratification of the derivatives of the unconscious drives, done in the setting of therapeutically realistic interventions and emphasizing the current realistic therapeutic intent, but minimizing or leaving repressed the deeper unconscious meanings of such gratifications.

For example, in giving medication, the conscious emphasis to the patient would be on the current needs for symptom relief. The unconscious needs for tangible evidence of love, the symbolism of the medication itself, the passive receptive demands, the magic expectations of the patient, etc., would not be expressed or focused upon, but would be unconsciously gratified by the therapist.

Such derivative gratifications tend temporarily to reduce the intensity of the drives, and to promote identification with the need-fulfilling therapist, and thus relatively to increase ego capacity for defence, control of impulses, and adaptation.

Throughout supportive therapy, emphasis by the therapist is on the current conscious reality of the relationship. Transference distortion, intensification, elaboration through fantasy, etc., are minimized and controlled by techniques to be described later.

In insight therapy, the strategy is to help the patient become more consciously aware of the nature, intensity and origin of his drives and drive-derivatives, as well as the ego defences and super-ego demands against them. To this end, as the therapist becomes the transference object of the patient's drives and defences, he maintains the neutral role, and the therapy continues in a state of relative abstinence of gratification of drive-derivatives by the therapist.

This results in drive frustration for the patient, which in turn increases the intensity of the drives and their derivatives. The aim is to promote a direct and emotionally meaningful awareness in the patient of the existence and nature of his drives and of their pressures for gratification. And eventually as the patient's defences against conscious awareness are further reduced, there is an increasing degree of consciousness both of the drives and of the defences.

Frustration of drive-derivatives in the treatment situation also acts to promote the patient's seeking for more reality-oriented objects and satisfactions outside of the treatment situation.

Thus strategy in insight-directed therapy calls for relative frustration of drive-derivatives in the treatment situation. This will tend to enhance the development of a transference relationship in which the conflicts may become increasingly conscious as the first step towards definitive resolution.

F. Super-ego and Conscience

In earlier chapters the role of identification and projection in the development of the super-ego was discussed. In the supportive therapy situation, the therapist actively uses himself as a new model for such identification, depending on the nature of the super-ego processes in the patient.

This may involve active interventions and attempts at ameliorating an overly rigid and harsh super-ego in the patient. In patients with defective or incomplete super-ego formation, it may involve active, though mild, judgment and criticism. In both instances the therapist attempts to provide a relatively consistent but benign external super ego.

In either case, the hope is that identification with the therapist will also occur in terms of super-ego function, and with it an incorporation of a more realistic and reasonable set of super-ego attitudes. However, in supportive therapy, this process is dependent on continued unconscious acceptance of moral standards and ideals determined for the patient in part by an outside authority.

In insight treatment, the goal is a greater participation of conscious ego processes into what were originally unconscious super-ego attitudes. The aim is for the patient to establish his own moral code and ideals, based on conscious judgment and rational thought, rather than on unconscious, automatic responses to a past or current authority figure.

Therefore, the therapist does not provide moral judgments, punishments or rewards, and deals with the patient's attempts to elicit these as resistances to movement towards maturity and independence in super-ego function.

Summary

In summary, the strategy of supportive psychotherapy involves limited goals, and the direct relief of symptoms, by focusing chiefly on current conscious conflicts, and supporting and strengthening defensive and adaptive ego functions in an attempt to re-establish a dynamic steady state. External behaviour may be modified within the limitations of the existing neurotic state, but the nature of the underlying unconscious conflicts and personality distortions is not exposed, and organized efforts to modify them are minimized.

Insight therapy involves the attempt, in whatever degree is possible, to expose, elaborate, and then resolve unconscious conflicts and to promote more effective personality organization and development towards maturity.

Immediate symptom relief becomes secondary, in the sense that after the resolution of underlying conflict, there will be a shift in intrapsychic forces which then makes the symptoms superfluous and permits the patient to give them up.

CHAPTER VIII

Indications for Psychotherapy and Evaluation of the Patient

Introduction

The main conclusions to be drawn from the discussion on the Strategy of the Therapeutic Process relate to the significant differences in the therapeutic task for both patient and therapist in insight-directed as compared with supportive psychotherapy. As elaborated there, the goal of insight-directed psychotherapy is conflict resolution, the development of new modes of adaptation, and personality reintegration and maturation to whatever degree is possible in the particular patient. It includes the increased ability to develop latent talents, the capacity for more effective interaction with the environment, a greater freedom of choice regarding behaviour patterns, and a more satisfying sense of personal fulfilment.

Insight-directed psychotherapy therefore will usually involve a significant investment of time, effort, sacrifice and emotional significance if it is to be successful, and it frequently represents a long-term venture both for the patient and the therapist.

When insight therapy has been successfully completed, it may offer major and lasting benefit, and improvement beyond the mere alleviation of presenting symptoms, including a generalized capacity for more healthy and effective overall integration and adaptation. In instances where such changes occur, both the patient and the therapist will generally feel that the investments were worthwhile.

However, the majority of people with psychiatric and emotional disturbances are incapable for various reasons of making effective use of an insight-directed therapeutic opportunity. Many patients are unwilling or unable to make the necessary investments even to begin such treatment. In other cases, in spite of prolonged efforts, the therapeutic change may at times be minimal. In some cases such treatment may end in a stalemate with a sense of disappointment and dissatisfaction for both patient and therapist, or the patient may break off his therapy prior to its conclusion, with minimal resulting benefit. In still other instances, an ill-considered attempt at insight-directed therapy with an unsuitable patient may result in an intensification of symptomatic disturbances and precipitation of a more severely regressive or disturbing level of function. The patient may then be worse off than if he had never entered treatment in the first place.

These considerations make it essential that the type of psychotherapy which is advised and undertaken be appropriate to the particular patient's needs and capabilities, and that the implied goals are capable of being reached by this individual.

Two extreme positions are often expressed in regard to the type of psychotherapy which is indicated. One group of therapists believes that anything short of intensive and insight-directed psychotherapy is unworthy of the name, and that given enough time, effort, energy and determination, any and all patients can be benefited by insight-directed treatment. On the other hand, the opposite extreme is expressed by those who feel that insight-directed psychotherapy has nothing specific to offer and does not produce significant change, and that all patients should be treated by supportive methods without resorting to the prolonged therapeutic undertaking of an insight-directed treatment.

Neither of these extreme positions is in keeping with general clinical experience which suggests that in certain well-selected cases, insight-directed treatment is the therapy of choice. But as mentioned above, for a variety of reasons the majority of people with psychiatric illness, social deviancy, marital disturbances, character problems, acute or chronic psychosis, somatic conversion symptoms, etc., are not suitable candidates for a formal attempt at insight-directed psychotherapy. Instead they are more suitably and expeditiously treated by a dynamically oriented supportive approach.

The problem in the evaluation of patients for therapy thus rests on the ability of the examiner correctly to identify those patients for whom an insight-directed approach is likely to achieve the goals set, and thus is the treatment of choice. These patients must be distinguished from the larger group for whom supportive treatment is the therapy of choice.

Indications

Patients who are candidates for insight-directed therapy will often also respond effectively at symptomatic levels to supportive treatment. Insight-directed treatment is generally an elective procedure, and thus the problem of the indications for insight-directed treatment essentially represents formulating the factors related to therapeutic prognosis. And, in applying these to any particular case, the examiner is assessing the likelihood that if this patient were to undertake a course of insight-directed treatment, the gains which would be achieved if therapy is successful and the likelihood that such a successful conclusion will occur, are great enough to warrant the investments.

The decision in favour of supportive psychotherapy may be made on a positive or a negative basis. A positive decision rests on the evaluation that for this particular patient at this time supportive treatment is the ideal approach. A negative decision rests on the evaluation that for various reasons this patient will not be sufficiently benefited by an insight-directed approach to warrant the necessary investments, and that more limited therapeutic goals must be accepted.

Clinical Diagnosis

Part of this evaluation is the clinical diagnosis, and the nosological category in which the patient may be placed. This involves the standard diagnostic and clinical entities mentioned in Chapter VI on the Classification of Psychopathology. But as elaborated there, such a category and classification is too static to provide for full evaluation of the therapeutic potential of any one patient.

Prognosis in therapy, and thus the choice of the appropriate form of treatment, will vary considerably even among patients who bear the same clinical diagnostic label.

Dynamic Diagnosis

An effective evaluation of a patient for treatment must include a dynamic assessment of the overall level of integration, and particularly an assessment of the various structural components of the personality and the nature of the total adaptation. It is the evaluation of these factors as they relate to the overall strategy of treatment, and to the therapeutic task for the patient, which determines the therapeutic prognosis.

As described in Chapter VII, the process of therapy occurs through a therapeutic alliance between portions of the patient's ego and the therapist, working together to modify the unconscious neurotic elements in the patient's life and mental processes. One important indication for treatment will thus be the nature and effectiveness of the patient's half of this alliance. This is sometimes known as 'ego strength'. The assessment of ego strength involves both a global, overall evaluation of the nature and level of ego functioning, and also a more specific evaluation of those particular ego functions which are of primary importance in a therapeutic undertaking.

Ego Strength: General

The strategy of insight-directed psychotherapy is the attempt to remobilize unconscious and preconscious psychic conflict in the therapeutic setting, with the anticipation that through the patient's synthetic and integrative ego mechanisms, he will make use of such new awareness in establishing more effective patterns of psychological function and adaptation. Insight by itself is not necessarily effective in producing therapeutic change, and in some instances it may even be the cause of further psychological decompensation.

In other words, within an insight-therapy situation, the patient is subjected to increments of psychic stress within limits of his tolerance, and then must deal with and resolve this stress. The better the individual's overall level of adaptation and function prior to the onset of his disturbance, the better will be the prognosis. The more the patient is capable of maintaining his various activities, work and other relationships in spite of his neurotic disturbances, and the more he has been capable of meeting and dealing with the vicissitudes of his life, the more likely is it that he will be capable of tolerating and successfully dealing with the stresses of insight-therapy. The more an individual has had a general pattern of persistent effort in a goal-directed fashion, and of success in the various ventures that he has undertaken, the more likely will he be to sustain his effort during the course of the treatment, and ultimately to achieve some measure of success.

At the opposite end of the spectrum of overall ego function are those individuals whose life pattern had been one of repeated failures, ineffectual adaptation, or of major disturbance, disruption or defect in ego functions. Ego patterns will tend to be repeated in the therapeutic situation, and even though the patient may develop some awareness and insight, he may be incapable of using this insight effectively to modify his previous patterns of disturbance by virtue of his inadequate overall ego capacity. Hence, such patients are usually more effectively treated with supportive techniques.

The same is true of patients in whom psychic conflict has in the past led to repeated psychotic episodes or where hospitalization has been necessary. If the individual has required removal from his conflictual environment or relationships as the means of coping with his illness in the past, the fact that he was unable to function without the various forms of support offered by hospitalization would be an indication of an overall ego failure at maintenance of adaptation. This suggests that when again confronted with the same conflict in an insight-directed treatment approach, there may be a similar severe regression and disruption. Hence supportive therapy, aimed at improving or strengthening ego function, is usually more in keeping with such an individual's capacity.

The same would be true in a patient who is currently undergoing severe ego regression and decompensation due to the failure of defences and the poorly-controlled return of previously unconscious material into consciousness. At such a time of active decompensation, the individual needs to maintain those defences which he has, and therefore an insight-directed approach aimed at further reduction of defences is likely to intensify and increase his psychic disturbances and manifestations of psychopathology. At such times these individuals are more suited for a supportive therapeutic approach aimed at preventing further regression.

Ego Strength: Specific

A variety of specific ego functions that have a particularly important impact on the therapeutic prognosis must also be considered individually.

A. Object Relationships

As described earlier, insight-directed therapy occurs in a therapeutic alliance based on the patient's conscious rapport and willingness to trust and work with the therapist in striving towards the therapeutic goal. In this alliance the patient increasingly must confide his innermost personal thoughts and feelings. In addition, insight-directed therapy will usually involve an increasing investment of the therapist as a significant object in the patient's life, and this investment will then be influenced by a variety of transference distortions, the nature of which will be described in Chapter XII.

The important element here is that successful insight-directed psychotherapy must involve an emotional relationship between the patient and therapist which will exist throughout the course of the treatment, although varying in its form and intensity. The patient's previous capacity to establish and maintain emotionally significant ties to other people will influence his ability to enter into a meaningful and useful therapeutic relationship.

In general, the patient will bring to the treatment relationship the same general patterns of response, interaction and defence in regard to the therapist as he has manifested in his earlier life with other people. Where such past experiences and reactions have been favourable and gratifying, the same will be anticipated in the treatment situation. The more that the patient is capable of close emotional ties to other people, the more likely is he to invest emotionally in the therapist and therapeutic situation, and therefore the better will be his prognosis.

Similarly, since psychotherapy of an insight-directed nature is usually a long-term process, the greater the capacity of the patient for sustained object relationships, the more effective will he be in making use of the therapeutic situation. Even if a patient indicates that he has had a long-term but intensely hostile relationship with another individual, this is still preferable in the evaluation for treatment when compared with the person who has never consciously experienced any emotionally intense relationships.

A supportive treatment approach is generally more feasible in instances where the patient shows patterns of remoteness and failure to establish meaningful object relationships, or in instances where the patient is suspicious and requires a long period of testing of objects before investing trust in them. In such situations, it is often necessary for the therapist to use a variety of supportive techniques to establish a therapeutically useful and meaningful relationship with the patient, since these often are individuals who cannot develop this in the therapeutically neutral atmosphere of an insight-directed approach.

Likewise, in some cases when a patient has become involved in a meaningful or close emotional tie to another human being, he has been forced by his neurotic disturbances either to break this off or to destroy the relationship in some way. It would be anticipated that this will occur again in the treatment setting, and hence the prognosis for an insight-directed approach would be guarded. Such patients will often be better dealt with at the level of supportive treatment, where the therapist can respond more actively in keeping with the patient's various unconscious patterns of drives and defences, and where the therapist can become more of a 'real' object in the patient's life.

B. Motivation

Another major ego function that has direct relevance to the type of treatment to be instituted is that of conscious motivation. The strategy of insight-directed therapy calls for the mobilization of conflict, intensifying anxiety, maintaining a state of abstinence from gratification in the transference, and the recall of painful and previously repressed earlier memories.

Therefore, the patient will often try to avoid the treatment process when confronted with the inevitable difficulties, pain and frustration involved in an insight-directed approach.

The more that such unconscious resistances are offset by a conscious motivation and determination to seek the basic nature of the underlying conflicts and to elaborate and resolve them, the better will be the prognosis.

The patient's motivation need not be a ready-made concept of the impact of psychotherapy, or an intellectual understanding of the process, for it to be successful. It need be only a conscious wish to get to the bottom of his problems in a definitive way, and the individual must be willing to try to change himself.

At times such motivation may be uncertain initially, but it may be developed more solidly as the individual progresses and becomes more aware of the nature of his disturbances. In other instances the patient's initial positive motivation may weaken after exposure to the treatment situation, in which case the prognosis for insight-directed treatment is poorer.

Patients are best treated supportively if they do not wish to accept the existence of a psychological illness; or if they come for treatment primarily under pressure by their families or by other authorities; or if they are interested only in immediate, symptomatic relief and have no interest or desire to explore the underlying factors behind their illness. The same is true in patients whose main hope from treatment is to change the behaviour of other people in their environment.

Such individuals lack the necessary positive conscious motivation to offset their conscious and unconscious resistances in an insight-directed approach, and more modest, superficial and supportive goals should be set, more in keeping with the patient's expressed and felt motivations.

The assessment of motivation will be a function not only of what the patient consciously verbalizes, but also of his unconscious attitudes, expectations and implied motivation. For example, a patient may say that he wants to get to the bottom of his problems, but at the same time express an attitude of dissatisfaction if he does not get immediate advice, or relief of symptoms, or if he is expected to talk about himself and his thoughts. In such situations it is this latter, unconscious or non-verbalized motivation which will be more significant.

Initially, the patient may present himself with poor conscious motivation, but it may be possible over the course of time to help him improve or change this so that he becomes increasingly interested in obtaining more definitive treatment for himself, in which case the prognosis for an insight-directed approach will be improved.

C. *Psychological Mindedness*

Another significant ego function for evaluating therapeutic prognosis is the patient's psychological mindedness. The strategy of insight-directed therapy requires that the individual become increasingly aware of his inner emotional reactions, responses, thoughts, fantasies and ideas, and that he reflect on how these psychic processes are integrated, and related to his past experience. Thus the more a patient is initially capable of introspection and awareness of his own inner emotional life, and of the emotional life and reactions of others, the more likely is it that he will be able to carry out the therapeutic work and enlarge his awareness in the treatment situation.

Some individuals, however, by virtue of rigid defensive psychological organizations, are unaware of their own inner emotional impulses, conflicts, reactions and responses, and they tend instead to focus almost exclusively on external current realistic events. Such patients will generally have a difficult time in insight-directed therapy, and are often more suitably treated by supportive techniques, unless such psychological mindedness can be developed.

However, prospects for insight treatment are also poor in instances of extreme introspection to the point of excessive and continuous rumination, or internal awareness to the point of exclusion of reality and external life situations.

The therapeutic strategy calls for the patient ultimately to make adjustments and changes in his interactions with the external environment on the basis of the understanding and insight gained through the treatment process. Patients who continuously look inward and introspect, ruminate or fantasy, and are incapable of effective external action and interaction, may be unable to put the insights learned in the treatment situation to effective use.

In regard to this ego function, the better suited patients for insight-directed therapy are those who show a capacity for introspection, and also an ability to take effective external action based on self-knowledge and understanding.

Another aspect of psychological-mindedness which is important for the prognosis in psychotherapy is the capacity for effective verbal communication. Insight-directed treatment requires that the patient communicate his various inner psychic experiences to the therapist, and the more that the patient is able to make himself understood in words, the more effective will this process of communication be.

The more an individual is capable of expressing himself descriptively and colourfully, using various forms of imagery and non-stereotyped language, the more likely is it that he will be able to communicate his thoughts and feelings in the therapeutic setting. Contrariwise, the patient who is hesitant, blocked, has difficulty in talking clearly or coherently, and who uses only limited verbal stereotypes will have greater difficulty in effectively communicating the specific inner feelings, thoughts and ideas that are necessary for a successful insight-directed treatment.

Unless such an individual can learn to express himself more clearly in the therapeutic process, or can resolve the primary inhibition in communication, he usually does not derive as much benefit from treatment as a person who talks more fluently. However, this ability to communicate must be distinguished from glibness, which may be a negative therapeutic factor.

D. Defences

The strategy of insight-directed psychotherapy calls for the gradual reduction in the intensity of ego defences, thus permitting the emergence of previously unconscious or preconscious conflict in such a way that the individual is not flooded with major anxiety, or with the sudden intense eruption of primary process thinking. Hence another indication for insight-directed psychotherapy is the pattern and effectiveness of those ego defences already in existence at the time the patient comes for treatment.

The larger the number of psychological defence mechanisms available for use by the patient, the less dependent will he be on any one specific mechanism to maintain adaptation, and therefore, the more easily will he be able to reduce the intensity of any one particular defence. The greater the flexibility of his defensive pattern and the larger the number of mechanisms available for use, the more likely will the patient be to find more effective modes of integration as his understanding of himself increases. Contrariwise, in instances where there are only a few rigid and extensively used ego defence mechanisms, the possibility exists that by reducing the intensity of these defences in the therapeutic process, the individual's capacity to adapt may be seriously disrupted, with overwhelming anxiety.

The more the individual is capable of utilizing a variety of different mechanisms in different situations, the better will be his prognosis for insight-directed therapy. The more he relies on simple, stereotyped defensive patterns which are indiscriminately applied to all different situations, the poorer will be his prognosis and the more suitable will be the use of supportive treatment.

Some specific defence mechanisms, if used extensively, may suggest a poor prognosis in insight-directed treatment. For example, intense reliance on projection, massive denial, or major withdrawal may be suggestive of an underlying psychotic core and hence may make insight-directed treatment inadvisable. Major reliance on acting-out in dealing with psychic conflict, particularly when combined with projection, likewise may make an insight-directed, introspective, self-changing therapeutic approach extremely difficult and at times impossible, so that a supportive technique is usually more applicable in such instances.

Patients in whom currently there is an active, on-going, regressive process, and patients who without previous treatment are consciously aware of thoughts, fantasies or impulses which are ordinarily unconscious, are usually in a position of relative failure of ego defences. Hence they are candidates *at that moment* only for supportive attempts at treatment and stabilization to prevent further regression in overall psychic functioning.

In such instances of acutely failing defences, the approach of insight-directed treatment in which further reduction of defences is attempted will only lead to more extreme psychological disruption and general disturbance. Such patients may at times appear to be suitable for intensive uncovering treatment since they seem to have so much 'insight', but frequently they lack the other ego capacities to integrate and deal with such insight, and the 'insight' proves to be a function of the failing defences.

Once the process of regression has been arrested and there has been a stabilization of ego defences, further evaluation may indicate that the patient can now be more appropriately considered for insight-directed treatment.

E. Intelligence

Intelligence is another ego function which has some specific relationship to the choice of therapeutic approach. Considering the strategy of insight-directed psychotherapy and the nature of processes of introspection, psychological perceptiveness and communication which are required for successful treatment, it becomes apparent that such a therapeutic approach would be extremely difficult, if not impossible, in an individual with primary defective intelligence. Insight therapy generally requires average or better-than-average intelligence, although parenthetically, sometimes an individual with superior intelligence may use this ego function in the service of resistance.

In assessing intelligence, the attempt must be made to distinguish between primary intellectual or mental retardations or defects, and intellectual deficiencies secondary to anxiety or specific psychological conflict. The prognosis for treatment is better in the latter instance, since if the anxiety or conflict is resolved, intellectual function will improve.

F. Tolerance of Anxiety and Frustration

As described earlier, the strategy of insight therapy involves the gradual mobilization of anxiety, and the treatment is carried out in a state of relative abstinence of drive satisfaction in the treatment situation. Therefore, the individual's ego capacity to tolerate anxiety and frustration while working towards a long-term goal are important factors in the indications for treatment.

The individual who is capable of continuing to function in spite of anxiety or frustration, and who is willing to postpone immediate gratification in hopes of achievement of his long-range goals, makes a better therapeutic prospect for insight-directed treatment.

The individual who, by virtue of his behaviour or past history, indicates that he is incapable of tolerating such anxiety and frustration will usually make a poor therapeutic prospect for insight-directed treatment, since when anxiety and frustration occur in the therapeutic situation he will tend to avoid or break off further treatment. The patient whose tolerance of anxiety and frustration is low tends to do better in a supportive approach aimed at the immediate reduction of anxiety and the attempt to gratify unconscious drive-derivatives in such a way as to reduce frustration to a minimum.

However, the other extreme of the individual who has an exaggerated need to keep himself in unpleasurable, frustrating, and anxiety-provoking situations as part of his neurotic symptom complex may also be a poor therapeutic prospect, by virtue of the dynamic patterns implicit in the masochistic personality organization.

G. Alloplastic versus Autoplastic Ratio

The strategy of insight-directed psychotherapy requires that an individual become increasingly aware of his inner emotional life, and then be capable of making use of this new insight for effective modification within himself

10

and in his own interactions with the environment. For some types of patients the characteristic mode of adaptation has been primarily *alloplastic* in which efforts are chiefly directed towards influencing, moulding or changing the external environment rather than himself. Such individuals are able to consider and attempt to change themselves only after long periods of therapeutic work, and often they will break off the treatment before this occurs. Hence the prognosis is relatively poorer and by and large they are better treated supportively.

At the other end of the spectrum, however, is the completely *autoplastic* individual who attempts to maintain adaptation solely through internal change, and is incapable of attempting to modify his environment to meet his own needs more maturely. Such patients may have difficulty in putting to effective use the new understanding gained from insight-directed treatment.

Id Functions

From the standpoint of the id, it is helpful to know something about the nature of the specific unconscious drives and conscious drive-derivatives, both those involved in conflict and those related to the conflict-free sphere of function. It is also helpful to know something of the level of psychosexual adjustment and drive organization which the patient has been able to achieve in the course of his own development. In other words, we try to assess the relative intensities of the later phallic-oedipal drive organization as compared with the oral and anal pre-phallic drive organization. Although components of both phallic and pre-phallic organizations are present in all individuals, the relative intensity of each can be significant in terms of therapeutic prognosis and the appropriateness of any particular form of treatment. The more that the major level of conflict is focused at the phallic and oedipal level of development, even if there are regressions from this to pre-phallic stages, the better will be the overall therapeutic prognosis. The more that there is intense fixation at the level of pre-phallic development with a relatively weak or ineffectual oedipal and phallic stage, the more immature will be the nature of the patient's conflicts and disturbances and, hence, the more difficult the therapeutic outlook and prognosis.

Another important criterion is the overall level of drive energies available to the individual. The more limited his total energy and drive intensity, either through constitutional factors, or as the result of developmental experience, the more difficult will be the therapeutic task in modifying basic personality.

Super-ego Functions

From the standpoint of the super-ego functions, a number of issues tend to make insight-directed treatment increasingly difficult and uncertain. This includes such things as strong self-destructive impulses or behaviour, including a significant risk of suicide. It also includes such things as an extremely rigid, unyielding, or inflexible set of moral values and attitudes. At the other end of the spectrum would be the individual who has never internalized a set of useable moral values and for whom super-ego functions essentially remain externalized and not involved in intra-psychic conflict. These latter individuals frequently manifest considerable anti-social behaviour without demonstrable internal guilt or control, and hence these individuals tend to make poor therapeutic prospects for insight-directed treatment. They tend instead to act-out their conflicts in various ways, rather than to experience them as subjective states of conflict accompanied by significant subjective discomfort.

Previous Treatment

The type of response to any previous therapeutic efforts should be carefully assessed within the framework of the goals of that treatment venture. It must be remembered that the patient may distort his report, and that the previous therapist may have been a significant factor in the outcome. Therefore a detailed description of the previous therapeutic arrangements, relationship, and progress is important in assessing the patient's response. But generally speaking, prognosis is better when there has been some gain, even if limited, and it is more guarded if the previous therapy failed.

Age

Age is another factor to be taken into account in determining the appropriate method of treatment. Other things being equal, the young adult is best suited for insight-directed therapy. Patterns of response and reaction in the young adult tend to be more flexible, and less stereotyped or rigid than in the older person, and the young adult will usually find it easier to learn new modes of reaction and adaptation than will the elderly person whose capacity to experiment and try new things will often be impaired.

Insight-directed psychotherapy is frequently a long-term procedure so that the younger person who has successfully completed such a therapeutic undertaking will have a longer time to make use of the changes that have resulted within himself, and the total effect of the treatment is likely to be greater since benefits accrued in his treatment may be passed on to his children in terms of reduction of emotional disturbances in the family.

The young individual will generally have greater opportunity to make whatever changes he deems necessary in his life based on the insight and the personality changes resulting from his treatment. The chance and ability to seek and find new objects, to change or modify work or other professional activities, and to reorganize his total life situation will usually be greater than in the elderly person, whose opportunities may be sharply limited and for whom such changes may be virtually impossible.

Furthermore, the elderly person, by virtue of the insight gained through his therapy, may come to recognize important neurotic forces in such things as his patterns or choice of work, of a marital partner, or of other relationships and activities in life, and then become significantly depressed since it may now be too late in life to change them. In other words, in such instances, development of insight may result in the patient experiencing a sense of depression, hopelessness or the feeling that his life has been wasted and that he no longer has the opportunity to start over again. However, for some older people whose children are grown, and whose financial, occupational and family responsibilities are reduced, the opportunity for change may still exist and these issues must be evaluated individually.

At the other end of the age spectrum are the adolescents, where there are sharp differences of opinion as to whether or not insight-directed therapy is suitable for patients in this age group. In general, insight-directed treatment requires a degree of stability and the capacity to reflect, to stand off and take emotional distance, and to modify reactions and conflicts over a period of time. Many people feel that even normal psychological development during adolescence is too stormy and tumultuous a time in the individual's life for this type of therapy since the adolescent may be unable to take the proper reflective distance, and the total configuration of drives and defences fluctuates so rapidly and sharply. Also, the adolescent often needs to maintain and use whatever defences are available to him in dealing with unconscious conflicts, and to reduce or eliminate such defences in the course of insight-directed treatment may evoke significant further regression and decompensation.

The line of argument is that adolescents are best treated supportively until safely through the upheaval of adolescence itself and more established in a stable form and level of personality integration and adaptation.

However, others argue that conflicts are relatively closer to consciousness during adolescence and are not as heavily defended against, so that it is easier to help the patient towards an understanding and conscious awareness of the nature of his disturbances. The thought is that such treatment may improve the likelihood of relatively healthy adjustment and adaptation after the adolescent period.

There is general agreement, however, that the technique in either form of therapy during adolescence has to be significantly modified from that used in adult patients.

Nature of Illness

As described earlier, insight-directed psychotherapy usually involves a major investment by the patient and therapist, and so another factor in assessing whether or not such treatment is warranted is the nature of the illness and the degree of disturbance that it creates. In other words, is the degree of disability and severity of symptoms sufficient to warrant the investment of the necessary time, effort and money?

Patients who are currently undergoing significant regressive decompensation are usually not good candidates for an insight-directed approach since the final level of equilibrium has not yet been established, and it is possible the patient is incipiently psychotic and moving in the direction of further regression. Insight-directed psychotherapy is usually indicated only after the illness or disturbance has been stabilized to some extent.

However, it must be remembered that in an initial evaluation the patient frequently minimizes the extent of his illness, and often does not mention his more embarrassing or disturbing symptoms. It must also be kept in mind that *subjective* disability is often more intense than an objective evaluation would suggest, and the therapist must try to avoid 'playing God' with these decisions.

Neurotic symptom formations which appear as part of a reaction to a significant external stress or change in the individual's life situation are often indications more for a supportive than an insight-directed therapeutic approach. Often when the response to the external stress has been dealt with at supportive levels, the neurotic regression and symptom formation proves to be transitory and reversible, and further treatment may be unnecessary.

When the patient's response appears to be proportional to the intensity and significance of the external stress, the therapeutic attempt would be to help him reconstitute and adapt at his previous level of equilibrium. At the time of a major external precipitating stress, the individual is frequently incapable of reflecting introspectively on the nature of his reactions, as is required in an insight-directed approach, and when the immediate response to this external stress subsides, the patient's motivation will frequently change. Whereas previously he may have been interested in 'getting to the bottom of his problems', he now may be satisfied with things as they are and be reluctant to undertake any further long-term treatment measures. This might occur, for example in situations such as the death of a loved person, marriage, the birth of a child, loss of a job, financial or other failure, etc.

However, if the reaction is out of proportion to the external stress or change in life situation, or if after a reasonable period of time, the reactions to the stress have not subsided and the neurotic disturbances continue or further intensify, it then becomes more clear that the major source of difficulty is an intra-psychic one. Therefore, the patient will need to be re-evaluated as to whether or not insight-directed treatment is now indicated.

In other words, in any situation of major change in his life, an individual may have transient neurotic symptom formation, but it may not be necessary to explore the deeper unconscious conflicts in a long-term therapeutic venture. It may instead be sufficient to deal with the situation at the level of immediate support and symptom relief, with subsequent assessment of the severity of the disturbance after the change in the individual's life is not so acute or recent.

At the other extreme are those patients whose symptoms have been in existence at an essentially constant level or degree for many years, or for large parts of the person's life. The more that the neurotic adaptation and symptom formation have been firmly entrenched and 'calcified' and the more that the patient and family have adjusted to the disability, the more difficult will it be for the patient to change, and hence the poorer the prognosis for insight-directed treatment.

In assessing such a chronic illness, the prognosis is better where there is a pattern of waxing and waning intensity of symptoms, as compared with illness in which there is a rigidly persistent, entrenched and constant level of disturbance which shows no variation. The situation of waxing and waning symptomatology indicates that there is an ongoing and active response and variation in the forces impinging on the individual, and that although neurotic compromises are present, they are not so deeply entrenched as to become a fixed part of the individual's way of life.

One group of neurotic disturbances which are particularly difficult to treat are those conditions in which the major presenting symptoms in themselves provide a source of pleasure or gratification. In such conditions as overt sexual perversion, food or drug addiction or impulse-ridden character disorders, the immediate pleasure achieved through the symptoms will make it difficult for the patient to tolerate the frustration of an insight-directed treatment situation. The patient will often be reluctant to give up a known current neurotic pleasure in exchange for an unknown, and only potential, future more mature gratification. In these instances, unless the other criteria strongly favour an insight-directed approach, such patients are better treated supportively.

The same is true in the situation where the major presenting complaints largely represent ego-syntonic character traits, and hence are more acceptable to the patient, as compared with symptoms perceived by the patient himself as ego-alien.

Another problem in the strategy of psychotherapy is the situation in which there is a large secondary gain to the illness, which may interfere seriously with the patient's willingness or ability to give up his disturbances through an insight-directed approach. In such situations, supportive treatment will usually be more feasible, at least until the problem of the secondary gain has been resolved, thus clearing the way for insight-directed treatment if still indicated.

Reality Factors

Another series of factors that must be evaluated as one of the indications for treatment are the reality aspects of the patient's situation. One group of reality factors relates specifically to the possibilities of making arrangements for the patient to obtain the necessary treatment.

The strategy of an insight-directed approach requires that the patient plan for a long-term treatment contact with regular therapeutic sessions and as much continuity as possible, so that there will be minimal interruptions of the therapeutic work and relationship. The patient must be willing and able to arrange regular time for appointments, at a sufficient rate of frequency and over a long enough period to achieve the goals that are set. If there is a significant limitation to the total length of time available, it may interfere with the optimal development of the therapeutic relationship since from the outset the patient will anticipate termination. If the patient is unwilling or unable by virtue of his reality situation to make such an investment of time, the prognosis for successful insight-directed treatment is impaired. In general, supportive treatment approaches are more readily adaptable to an infrequent or irregular time schedule.

Another factor is money, and the patient's ability to pay for the necessary therapeutic time to achieve the goals of an insight-directed approach. If the costs of the treatment unduly burden and disrupt the patient's total life, it may place so great an added pressure on the therapeutic undertaking as to make it virtually impossible, and hence it may be wiser not to begin such a treatment approach. The total financial outlay in supportive therapy is generally less than in insight-directed treatment.

Another group of reality factors to be considered is the patient's total life situation and other relationships, and to what degree they are supporting of the therapeutic venture. It can be anticipated that with the mobilization of conflict and anxiety implicit in an insight-directed approach, there may be times during the course of treatment when the patient will require added encouragment, support or help from his environment, and from the objects in his outside life. If the environmental objects are unsympathetic towards such a therapeutic approach, or if they actively attempt to disrupt or sabotage it, successful therapy will be more difficult or at times even impossible.

And when a patient is involved in a disruptive, chaotic, unstable or repetitively disturbing and frustrating external environmental situation, insight-directed therapy may be more difficult or virtually impossible. The strategy for such a therapeutic approach requires that the patient stand off and take distance from himself and his problems, and observe his own inner emotional reactions, feelings, thoughts, memories, relationships, etc. If there is a continuing and major emotional involvement and pre-occupation with repeated crises, or with the external problems of his daily life existence, it may be impossible for the patient to be sufficiently introspective and reflective to permit such a therapeutic undertaking. His energies may be so taken up with such external matters that he will have very little energy or willingness left to undertake the real therapeutic task of insight-directed therapy, which involves thinking back over his life, reducing his resistances and defences, and allowing pre-existing conflicts to return to consciousness so he can successfully resolve them.

In such instances, it may be necessary to have the patient first rearrange and settle his current reality problems, at least to the point of reasonable stability. This may introduce something of a paradox, since for such a patient the chaotic and disruptive external environmental situation may result from pre-existing unconscious intra-psychic conflicts, and hence he will be unable definitely to settle these problems without having to some extent first resolved the inner conflicts. However, insight-therapy undertaken under such conditions will of necessity be more difficult and the outcome will be more uncertain.

These types of reality situations frequently require various forms of active intervention and participation by the therapist, who may at times be required to function as an alter-ego for the patient if he is to be therapeutically helpful. Since such interventions are well within the strategy of supportive therapy, this treatment approach is more often indicated.

Factors in the Therapist

Ideally, the decision as to which form of treatment is appropriate should be made on the basis of the patient's needs, capacities and therapeutic prognosis. In practice, however, another significant group of factors which frequently become part of this evaluation and decision are forces within the therapist himself. Some of these are conscious, and may be a reflection of such things as the therapist's training, or therapeutic ability. Even factors such as the therapist's current schedule and the availability of time, or his need for income, may influence this decision.

In addition, the therapist may have a variety of conscious personal reactions to the patient or to the nature of the illness. These in turn may influence him to advise intensive or more ambitious treatment for those patients whom he likes, or to advise treatment which will involve minimal contact and be of brief duration for those patients whom he dislikes.

Other less-conscious factors in the therapist may involve such things as his ability to work more effectively with certain types of patients or illnesses than others, and this will influence his choice of patients on whom to expend his time and energies.

There may be other significant and specific unconscious countertransference reactions which will influence the evaluation of a particular patient, and the recommendation of the type of treatment to be instituted. The issue of counter-transference will be dealt with in Chapter XV, but suffice it to say here that the stronger the unconscious factors in the therapist which enter into the decision regarding appropriate treatment, the more likely will it be that such a decision may not be fully in the best interests of the patient. Therefore, the likelihood of complications or failures in the therapeutic undertaking will be greater.

The more that such factors are conscious to the therapist, the greater will be the possibility of his being able to recognize the influence of such forces within himself upon his judgment. These may then be consciously offset, and a more objective decision can then be based on the reality of the patient's therapeutic capacity.

The Relativity of Indications

It must be emphasized that all of the above factors which are considered as indications for insight-directed versus supportive treatment are relative in their significance, and no single one is in itself an absolute indication or contraindication. The final decision regarding therapy must be based on a total assessment of all of these factors in the particular individual, taking account of their relative importance as they influence the ultimate therapeutic prognosis.

Usually there are admixtures of positive and negative factors in each patient which will then require assessment by the therapist as to their relative strength and significance. For example, in terms of age, reality situation and overall ego strength, a patient may be a suitable candidate for insight-directed therapy, but if he is unwilling to undertake such a treatment approach, it may be precluded. Another individual may be highly motivated towards a deep, insight-directed therapeutic approach, but if by virtue of significant ego disruption it would appear likely that insight-directed therapy might precipitate a psychotic reaction, the total evaluation would have to be in the direction of a supportive approach in spite of the patient's consciously expressed motivation.

In other words, the decision regarding appropriate treatment ultimately rests on a dynamic assessment of the various pertinent positive and negative factors, and the weighing of all of these in the light of the overall therapeutic strategy and task.

There may be instances in which the prognosis after full evaluation is that the treatment is likely to be long and difficult, with a relatively poor likelihood of success. However, an attempt at insight-directed therapy may still be warranted in spite of the poor prognosis, on the basis that if the individual is to have any chance of success or stability in his life, he must modify or change underlying conflicts and disturbances.

For example, it may be reasonable to undertake insight-therapy in spite of an adverse reality situation if the patient is to recognize his unconscious needs to get into such situations, and only then may he be able effectively to prevent recurrence of a disturbing reality. The same might be true in the individual whose capacity to be introspective and to express himself freely is impaired largely as a function of his neurotic inhibitions or disturbances. If insight treatment were to be undertaken, it would require the necessity of added time and effort in helping the patient to prepare himself for such a treatment approach. The same might be true in the individual who initially has poor conscious motivation but in whom it is anticipated that with time and effort such motivation might be developed. The expectation would again be for a longer and slower therapeutic course. On the other hand, when there is recognition that a long preparatory period will be necessary, or a long therapeutic course will be required, then such factors as a reality limitation in time or money become even more important.

Another decision which should be made by the therapist involves a quantitative estimate of the goals to be set, whether in supportive or in insight-directed treatment. The depth or degree of insight and change which can reasonably be achieved by the patient will vary significantly in accordance with the factors outlined above. For some patients only a relatively superficial understanding of current responses may be possible; other patients may be capable of a deeper genetic understanding of the conflicts.

In supportive therapy, the goal for some patients may be a full symptomatic remission, while in other patients a reasonable goal may involve only partial relief.

In other words, in setting appropriate goals for treatment, the overall assessment must reflect the therapist's conclusion as to what would be realistically possible of achievement, given his general knowledge of the strategy and problems involved in psychotherapy, and knowledge of the specific positive and negative factors pertinent in the present case.

Changing Goals

Once a therapeutic goal has been established and set, it may still require modification when and if new factors that were previously unrecognized become apparent. Not uncommonly, after the original assessment has been made and therapy has begun, a patient's motivation may change, the reality situation may be altered, or there may be factors previously hidden from the therapist which now come to light and indicate that the previously set goal is no longer the one of choice. It may be that the previous goal was too ambitious, or that the previous assessment of the patient proved to be overly pessimistic and that a more ambitious goal may now be possible.

In either case, the therapist must reassess and re-evaluate the total situation in keeping with the new information, and if necessary modify the goal and treatment approach. The main point to be emphasized is that at all times there should be a conceptualization and understanding by the therapist of his goals in treatment, based on a conscious, explicit and rational appraisal. This helps to avoid the all-too-frequent vagueness and aimlessness of therapy that may occur if goals and strategy are not clearly understood.

Therapeutic Evaluation of the Patient

In a general way, therapy begins with the initial contact between patient and therapist, and yet it is necessary that there be a careful evaluation of the patient and his therapeutic potential before a plan of treatment is explicitly outlined and agreed upon. The manner in which this early evaluation is accomplished may be significant in terms of how the therapy ultimately works out.

During these first interviews, it is important that the therapist have sufficient flexibility of approach to permit an adequate evaluation and still keep the greatest possible degree of freedom of action for therapeutic intervention.

Depending on the nature of the patient and the way in which he comes for treatment, the therapist's own activity should be minimal but sufficient to achieve the immediate goal. When patients are quickly able to express themselves, and can present their difficulties and past history in a fairly spontaneous and free fashion, an open-ended interview is optimal with questioning along general lines which follow the patient's lead. In such a setting, the immediate focusing of the patient's material through the use of extensive specific and direct questioning may set up a slanted therapeutic atmosphere and a question-and-answer type of interaction which may be difficult to reverse later on.

On the other hand, if the patient is acutely uncomfortable, anxious, or frightened at the prospect of psychotherapy, or is acutely blocked in presenting his difficulties, it becomes necessary for the therapist to structure the situation more in keeping with the patient's immediate needs at the moment, and to take a more active role in helping the patient give the necessary historical and other information. In some instances it may even be necessary immediately to focus on the patient's feelings and thoughts about such a referral for psychotherapy, and to postpone the collection of factual data and history until the patient is more comfortable in the interview situation.

The general rule would be to start with minimal activity, but increasingly to be as active as necessary to accomplish the goals of the evaluation.

By virtue of the pressure of his anxiety, symptoms and his underlying illness, the patient will frequently be understandably eager for a prompt and immediate decision as to the nature of the treatment that is indicated and the various other factors that he will have to consider. It is important that the therapist does not make premature statements or promises in this regard, and that he instead help the patient to a realization that this is a decision to be reached by both therapist and patient after the necessary evaluation and understanding of the problems. In other words, evaluation must be tentative at the beginning, since the patient may not have given enough information on which to base an appropriate recommendation.

On the other hand, the other extreme of a lengthy series of evaluation interviews without a recommendation being made may likewise be difficult, since it may keep the patient dangling in a state of uncertainty and confusion.

Clinical History

One source of data for the evaluation is the patient's own clinical history as he describes it, and a search for, and elaboration of, the material in the patient's past life which bears on those items mentioned under the indications for treatment. This is most frequently made in the context of the usual psychiatric history, and examination.

Behaviour in the Interview

In addition to the factual historical information, another important aspect of the evaluation is the way in which the patient responds and reacts to the interviewer during the diagnostic sessions. For example, the patient may verbally express the wish to understand himself better and get to the bottom of his problems, but his behaviour and attitude may indicate a demand for immediate advice, reassurance, medication or an inability to wait for the answers to his questions, all of which would be more revealing than his expressed verbalizations regarding motivation for psychotherapy.

In the assessment of psychological-mindedness, for example, the therapist is interested in what types of explanation the patient has attempted to work out for himself regarding the understanding of his symptoms. He is not so much interested in whether or not the patient has arrived at a correct formulation, but rather in the types of thoughts and ideas the patient has had spontaneously. Has he considered inner psychological or emotional thoughts, feelings or conflicts, or has he sought only to explain his behaviour on the basis of external events? Does he project his disturbances and blame others? Does he still cling to a physical explanation of his illness and disturbance? When asked about feelings or thoughts in connection with a particular incident or episode that he has recounted in the history, does the patient respond by elaboration of his inner experience, or is he incapable of exploring himself and his reactions further? In these diagnostic interviews the emphasis is not on the correctness or therapeutic usefulness of the ideas that the patient develops, but more on the ego-capacity to begin a search for such factors.

In these early diagnostic interviews, it is helpful to look for a piece of behaviour or an emotional reaction which will lend itself to a superficial interpretation, or to the establishment of a superficial connection with some other piece of behaviour, and for the therapist then to point this out to the patient. Again the emphasis is not on the therapeutic movement from such an interpretation or confrontation, but rather on an assessment of how the patient reacts to the therapist's intervention. Is he capable of recognizing the connection and elaborating it, or is he incapable of seeing any relationship and does he avoid the offered bit of insight? Does he have a need to disregard the therapist's intervention, or on the contrary, does he immediately accept it as gospel in an uncritical fashion, and make no contribution of his own to furthering the understanding?

In terms of assessing the patient's capacity for object-relatedness, how does he make use of the interview, and how capable is he of relating in an appropriate and effective way to the therapist as an object? Even such things as whether or not the patient looks directly at the therapist, or whether he shows movement in a direction of increasing confidence as the interview proceeds, will at times be more useful evaluations of the patient's capacity for an object-relationship than his reports of past behaviour.

It is frequently helpful to see the patient more than once in making a therapeutic evaluation. This allows opportunity to observe any changes in the patient's way of relating from the first session. It is also a test of his response to the first interview, and of his further spontaneous thoughts, associations, or recollections. The therapist can then assess how actively the patient works on his own, or how dependent he is on the presence of the interviewer.

The question will arise whether or not to do a formal mental status examination and examination of the sensorium. It must be recognized that such an examination, with the implications and possible interpretations that it may have in the mind of the patient, is not without hazard in terms of its impact on the ultimate development of the therapeutic relationship. The experienced interviewer learns to be alert for subtle manifestations of a thought disorder, a psychotic state, or an organic deficit as they would appear in the spontaneous communications of the patient. Where there is doubt based on disturbances in thinking, sensory misperceptions, suggestive ideas of reference, other forms of delusional thinking, confusion in communication, or where there is inaccuracy or confusion of memory or dates, a formal mental status examination becomes essential. However, where there is no evidence of these types of disturbances, the formal examination of the mental status and sensorium may tend to alienate the patient or make him feel that he has to defend himself against the therapist's questioning and, hence, interfere with the establishment of an optimal therapeutic relationship.

Contact with Others

During the evaluation, another source of information which may have bearing on the planning for the appropriate treatment is contact with the patient's relatives or others in his life. However, this approach has both positive and negative elements, and the decision whether or not to see the relatives is one which must be met flexibly in the total context of the evaluation and the patient's problems.

Arguments in favour of seeing the relatives include the fact that the relatives may be in a position to give information which the patient is reluctant to reveal, or to which, at times, the patient does not have access. Also, seeing the relatives may at times give the therapist a more objective appraisal of them as individuals, free from the distortions that will emerge as the patient attempts to describe his relationship to them.

Furthermore, the relatives are usually genuinely interested in the patient's welfare, and in assessing the therapist as the appropriate person to treat the patient, and they may be hurt, angry or unable to understand the situation if the therapist does not see them. With such feelings of being left out, they may consciously or unconsciously attempt to sabotage or disrupt the treatment, either at the beginning or later on. The relatives often are actively interested in advice as to what they can do to help the patient, and how to react to the patient during the treatment, and also in a statement as to the prognosis and other reality factors. Their commonsense feeling is that the therapist will be the best person to give them such answers, and they may be unwilling to go to someone else to get this information. Seeing relatives is a commonly accepted practice in medicine generally, and both the patient and relatives may have difficulty in recognizing that in psychotherapy this is at times unwise.

On the other hand, there may be a number of disadvantages in seeing the relatives, in terms of the effect it will have on the development of a useful therapeutic relationship. The first problem will be whether to see the relative in the patient's presence or alone. If the relative is seen with the patient present, the relative may feel inhibited or unable to express freely what is on his mind, because of the anticipated effect this would have on the patient, so that the data may not be of major significance in such a setting. When seeing the relative and the patient together, if a conflict or tension ensues between them, each may call upon the therapist to 'take sides', which may be difficult to avoid in such a setting, and at the same time, be untherapeutic if it is done.

If the relative is seen alone, the patient may have doubts and concern as to whether the therapist may not have taken the relative's side, and therefore be reluctant to trust the therapist. There may also be concern as to whether the therapist has revealed some of the confidential material to the relative and, therefore, the patient may be reluctant to trust the therapist with other and more personal confidential material. Furthermore, by seeing the relatives, the therapist implies that he is willing to get information from others than the patient and to by-pass the patient, which may again be a source of difficulty in the future. The therapist will also have indicated his interest in the relatives, whereas the patient's usual wish will be that the therapist be primarily interested in him, and this may have a retarding effect on the development of a workable and useful treatment relationship.

Furthermore, by seeing the relatives the therapist tacitly agrees that the patient is incapable of effective interaction with them, and that he requires the therapist's interventions or explanations. This attitude may foster the patient's already-present regressive feeling of himself as helpless, and may not be in his long-term therapeutic interest.

In general, the more that treatment is to be aimed at insight-directed goals with emphasis on the transference component of the patient-therapist relationship, the less advisable it is to see relatives. Instead, it is generally wiser to set the therapeutic stage with the major focus of interest on the patient alone, and with the anticipation that the patient himself should deal with his reactions and interactions to the external environment.

The more that therapy is to be supportive in nature, with the focus on the current, conscious, reality-oriented relationship between the therapist and patient, the more reason there is to see the relative if the patient or relative wishes.

If the patient is acutely disturbed, psychotic or potentially suicidal, the immediate reality of the situation and the necessity to deal with it at the level of the emergency management may make it necessary for the therapist to contact the relatives even if the patient expressly indicates his wish that this not be done.

In instances where the therapist is still in doubt as to the ultimate treatment approach, it may be wiser to postpone making the decision about seeing the relatives until the period of evaluation is over, and then actively to include the patient in the ultimate decision whether or not to carry this through.

Psychological Testing

The use of psychological tests may at times be helpful during the time of clinical evaluation, partly since such tests may be revealing of the under-lying psychodynamic conflicts and structural patterns, and also in estab-lishing a baseline of function against which the results of therapy may be compared at a later time. Some therapists use psychological testing as a routine, while others prefer to use it only at times of uncertainty or doubt after purely clinical evaluation. However, it must again be recognized that psychological tests may have an impact on the developing therapeutic situation and relationship, since they tend to by-pass the patient's conscious participation and suggest that the therapist may have semi-magical means or methods of understanding the patient. In any event, if psychological tests are to be used, they are best introduced and obtained early in the evaluation sessions where they can be logically supported as a part of the evaluation procedure. If psychological testing is introduced after treatment has been well established and after a transference relationship has been developed, it will inevitably influence the relationship in the transference and the patient will have significant doubts about the therapist's confidence in himself and in the choice of treatment being undertaken, or it will indicate to the patient that the therapist has significant doubts about the patient's capacities and progress.

Other Diagnostic Tests

At times, as part of the overall evaluation, there is need and indication for the use of EEG, or other laboratory procedure, and possibly a general medical examination. By and large, all such procedures should be done early in the course of the evaluation, since they can be easily and logically introduced as part of the initial complete work-up at that time. If they are delayed and are introduced later during the course of the actual therapeutic relationship, and particularly in the case of an insight-directed treatment

11

approach, they may often be involved in major transference distortions and lead to later therapeutic complications.

Therapeutic Trial

In an insight-directed treatment approach, the initial evaluation of the patient's therapeutic prognosis is at best a rough estimate of the treatment potential. The final evaluation of whether or not such a therapeutic attempt is indicated and feasible will rest on the patient's ultimate performance during the course of the treatment process itself.

The argument is thus raised by some therapists that the only evaluation of significance is the therapeutic trial, and the further suggestion is made that it be explicitly understood by the patient that the first interval of treatment is in the nature of a therapeutic trial to determine whether or not this is the treatment approach of choice.

In a general sense, it is probably correct that the best therapeutic prognosis can be given after a trial of actual treatment, and the therapist must be aware of the possibility that the patient's performance and reactions early in the course of the treatment experience may indicate his initial evaluation to have been incorrect. Nevertheless, there are several reasons why it is probably better that this not be an explicitly stated therapeutic trial as far as the patient is concerned. For some patients a therapeutic trial may represent the necessity that they 'pass the test' to be accepted for treatment. Contrariwise, other patients may attempt to work harder and more effectively with the immediate goal of 'passing the test', and then when told that they are accepted for treatment, they may let down and no longer feel the need to work so hard in the treatment process.

Since it is a therapeutic trial and there is no commitment by the therapist, the patient may be reluctant to work actively in this therapeutic situation, and reluctant to enter into the treatment relationship, anticipating that it may be a temporary one and, therefore, 'why should I get involved if I am not sure that it is going to continue?' If the patient is reluctant and withholds himself from the treatment relationship because of the possibility of interruption, then the early therapeutic reaction and behaviour is still not a significant trial, since the assessment of whether or not the patient can enter into a meaningful and workable treatment relationship cannot be an accurate one.

On the other hand, although it may not be explicitly stated to the patient, for the therapist the beginning of every treatment is a trial period during which he is assessing how the patient responds to the treatment that has been undertaken. If it develops that factors previously unrecognized or unexpressed now appear which make insight-directed therapy less appropriate as a treatment modality, it becomes incumbent on the therapist to change his goals, and either explicitly, or quietly through a shift in therapeutic technique, adopt a more supportive treatment approach and accept a more modest goal.

On the other hand, there are times when the therapist has begun with a supportive approach and limited goals, and then finds as a result of the therapeutic contact that the patient's motivation changes or that he shows a greater capacity than previously for an insight-directed approach. In the latter instance, this should usually involve an explicit discussion of the change with the patient and a restructuring of the therapeutic situation, since the patient should have the opportunity of deciding for himself whether or not he wants to work towards the more ambitious goal, recognizing the necessary commitment and sacrifices.

Summary

As can be seen from the above discussion, the evaluation of a patient for psychotherapy and the choice of appropriate treatment involves the dynamic appraisal of a variety of factors within the patient, both in terms of past historical behaviour and information, as well as current behaviour in the treatment situation. It also involves the awareness of a variety of factors within the therapist himself. These must all be weighed within the framework of the overall strategy of the therapeutic process.

The importance of this overall evaluation and the selection of the appropriate treatment modality cannot be overemphasized, since the ultimate outcome and benefit to the patient will in a large measure be a function of how accurate and correct this initial evaluation has been.

SUGGESTED READING

BIRD, BRIAN (1955) *Talking with Patients*. Lippincott Co
DEUTSCH, FELIX & MURPHY, W.F. (1955) *The Clinical Interview*. International Universities Press Inc, New York
FREUD, ANNA (1965) Diagnostic skills and their growth in psychoanalysis. *Int. J. Psycho-Anal.* **46**, 31
GEDO, JOHN E. (1964) Concepts for a classification of the psychotherapies. *Int. J. Psycho-Anal.* **45**, 530
HOLT, WILLIAM E. (1967) The concept of motivation for treatment. *Am. J. Psychiat.* **123**, 1388

LINN, LOUIS (1955) *Handbook of Hospital Psychiatry*. International Universities Press Inc, New York

POWDERMAKER, FLORENCE (1948) The techniques of the initial interview and methods of teaching them. *Am. J. Psychiat.* **104**, 624

SAUL, LEON J. (1957) The psychoanalytic diagnostic interview. *Psychoanal. Quart.* **26**, 76

WALDHORN, HERBERT F. (1960) Assessment of analyzability: technical and theoretical observations. *Psychoanal. Quart.* **29**, 478

CHAPTER IX

The Beginning of Therapy: the Therapeutic Contract

Initial Contact

In Chapter VIII on Evaluation of the Patient, the point was made that in a general way treatment begins with the first contact between therapist and patient, and that the way in which these initial interviews are conducted may facilitate or hamper the ultimate therapeutic response.

This may even extend to the scheduling of the first diagnostic appointment. The therapist has no way of knowing in advance how great or urgent is the patient's need and distress, and it is unwise to conduct extensive diagnostic questioning by telephone to settle such a matter without having first met the patient. But if a patient in acute and urgent distress is told that he must wait for what he considers to be a very long time before any help is offered, it may well colour his expectations of the possibility of ever receiving help from treatment, and thus interfere with establishing an optimal treatment relationship.

If a diagnostic appointment time is available promptly, this problem is to some extent obviated. However, if no appointment is available in the therapist's schedule in the near future, it is often wise to inquire of the patient whether or not he feels his difficulties are urgent. Then if the patient feels that the matter is urgent, the therapist can decide whether to make special efforts to see him promptly, or whether to indicate directly that he is currently not in a position to do so through lack of available time, but is willing to help the patient find a therapist who could see him sooner.

This approach demonstrates a sensitivity on the part of the therapist to the acuteness and severity of the patient's discomfort. Even if the patient indicates that the matter is not an urgent one, the fact that the therapist inquired about this will be helpful in establishing a trusting relationship when contact is finally made.

These same considerations hold true in a clinic setting, where at times the lengthy and complex intake process and the long waiting lists likewise may have an adverse effect when the patient and his assigned therapist finally begin their work. Patients in acute psychic distress or facing an unexpected personal crisis have difficulty tolerating the long delays in obtaining help that frequently accompany clinic intake procedures. Such patients often make immediate positive transferences and establish quick rapport to the person who responds promptly and effectively to their distress.

The significance of the manner in which the initial diagnostic interviews are conducted was also emphasized, as was the considerable variation regarding the ease and degree of organization with which patients are able to present their history and symptomatology.

From the standpoint of ultimate therapeutic response, it is important to recognize that for many patients referral to a psychotherapist may be a disturbing or anxiety-provoking prospect. At times this is based on intellectual ignorance and the patient may experience the referral as a declaration that he is 'crazy'. At other times it may be a function of poorly timed or poorly carried-out referral in which the reason for the referral has not been fully explained, or fully understood by the patient. Some physicians refer patients with statements such as 'there is nothing more I can do for you, so you had better see a psychiatrist', and the patient may come to the psychiatrist feeling that this is his last resort.

In other instances, however, referral to a psychiatrist may provoke anxiety by threatening too abruptly the various defences the patient has used against awareness of his underlying disturbance and conflict. It forces him into a situation in which he will now be called upon to face conflicts and disturbances which part of his mind is attempting to avoid. This is particularly the case in patients with somatic conversion symptoms, where many still cling to an organic explanation. The declaration of absence of organic factors and the referral to a psychiatrist challenges one of the major unconscious defence mechanisms, thereby provoking greater anxiety.

Dealing with such anxiety over referral can be therapeutic and helpful for the patient, and unless it is dealt with when present, the diagnostic evaluation will be hampered. At this point in the contact, 'dealing with it' primarily involves the therapist's getting across to the patient his recognition of the uncertainty and anxiety which the patient is feeling, and encouraging the patient to explore and express his feelings about the referral itself. This includes helping the patient to verbalize some of his misconceptions about psychiatry and psychotherapy.

Explanation to the Patient

The process of evaluation and the establishment of tentative hypotheses regarding the appropriate type of treatment have been discussed. Having made the decision regarding therapeutic goals for this particular patient, it now becomes necessary for the therapist to make sufficient explanations to the patient so that a clearly understood therapeutic agreement can be arranged between them.

Patients vary considerably in terms of their sophistication and intellectual understanding of psychotherapy, and before making such explanations it is often helpful to inquire of the patient regarding his own understanding of psychiatry and psychotherapy. In this way the level of the explanations which are made can be appropriate to the particular case.

The patient is entitled to a statement from the therapist regarding the general nature of his difficulties and the various therapeutic approaches that are available. If the therapist feels that insight-directed treatment would be the therapy of choice, it is still helpful to point out to the patient the various alternative approaches, emphasizing their positive aspects as well as limitations. Even though the therapist may recommend one approach over the others, the patient and his own motivations should be a party to the decision, and for this the patient must have some information about the alternatives. Some sophisticated patients come with an already-formed idea of the type of treatment they want, and extensive explanations may be unnecessary. However, the inexperienced or unsophisticated patient usually requires such general explanations.

The patient is also entitled to a frank explanation of what the commitment will be in time, money and effort for the various treatment approaches, in order that he may make a rational judgment, taking these various factors into account. Many patients do not understand what psychotherapy represents, and have no knowledge about the duration of treatment, the frequency of interviews or the role to be taken by the patient.

Although in his explanations the therapist may include a specific recommendation, it is important that he does not attempt to cajole, seduce or persuade the patient to accept a course of long-term insight-directed treatment, since the patient's own motivation is so important in regard to its ultimate success. Rather than start such therapy with a patient who is inadequately motivated, it is wiser to help the patient develop more effective motivation before beginning such a therapeutic course.

The more that therapy of a supportive nature is considered to be the treatment of choice, the more definite can the therapist be in specifying the approach to be used, and in departing from the more neutral position required if insight-directed treatment is to be undertaken. It is often necessary for the therapist actively to encourage or even insist that the patient enter some form of treatment. Occasionally such patients will have overly ambitious goals and will openly and directly ask for an intensive insight-directed approach. Then it may be necessary for the therapist specifically to discourage this and to emphasize the patient's more immediate needs, and postpone any insight-directed approach to some indefinite future time.

Diagnosis

Some patients ask for a medical diagnosis. When possible, this is best presented in the form of a summary taken from the patient's own description of his symptoms and disturbances, without necessarily giving a specific diagnostic label. Some patients may ask whether or not they are mentally ill, or whether they are psychotic, and it is often wise first to inquire what such terms and concepts mean to the patient, rather than to answer them as straightforward factual questions.

However, there are instances where these responses do not suffice, and the patient insists on a definite diagnosis. In such a case it is often wiser to offer a definite diagnosis rather than to be evasive, since vagueness or evasiveness may reinforce pre-existing feelings of mistrust in the patient, and may interfere with the development of a useful therapeutic relationship.

Some patients may be insistent and demanding of further explanations and will push intensively for answers beyond what the therapist feels to be appropriate or in the patient's best interests. In such a situation, it is helpful to deal with this as a manifestation of the patient's overall anxiety regarding therapy, and to focus the issue more directly into the patient's conscious awareness of his uncertainty and his fears of what will transpire. Since this type of reaction is generally a displacement from the more basic issues, it can be more effectively dealt with at the general level of its implications for the therapeutic relationship.

Process of Therapy

Unless a patient is relatively sophisticated and has a clear understanding of the process of psychotherapy, it is usually necessary to give some general explanation regarding the therapeutic process. When the treatment is to be insight-directed, it is often helpful to use material directly from the patient's past history and experience to illustrate the necessity for a better understanding so that more effective adjustments or conflict solutions can be found. This might then be followed with simple explanations that the patient's responsibility is to talk freely and not edit, even though material may be embarrassing or painful, and that the therapist will listen, try to understand and make contributions or comments as he feels they are indicated to help the treatment. In other words, in insight-directed therapy the therapist attempts to make a general statement concerning the role of the patient and himself, but it is best to keep such explanations simple, and to avoid technical or theoretical expositions.

The more that therapy is to be supportive, the more likely would the therapist be to depart from such a neutral position, and make the appropriate explanations in accordance with the overall nature and integration of the patient's conflicts. For example, if the patient has a high degree of intelligence and uses intellectualization as a prominent defence, explanations of the process of treatment might be made in technical or theoretical terms. If the patient has a passive-dependent character structure and a need to rely on a strong and omnipotent parent-figure, explanations might be made in this vein, stressing the authoritarian position of the therapist and emphasizing his powerful ability to intervene successfully. But if the patient manifests a reaction-formation against such dependency, explanations should de-emphasize the role of the therapist, and emphasize instead the patient's abilities to modify his situation with minimal outside help.

Prognosis

The patient is also entitled to an explanation regarding the prognosis for treatment in the modality of therapy that has been chosen. In considering this question a number of factors must be kept in mind. Among these are the basic concepts of psychopathology and the difference between the conscious and unconscious meanings of the patient's symptoms and wish to be well.

Since the symptom represents an unconscious attempt at resolution of an intra-psychic conflict through the construction of a compromise-formation, any promise or assurance that the symptom will be removed unconsciously represents a challenge to the patient's defences. Therefore, such a promise may mobilize anxiety as the patient anticipates facing the unconscious danger situation.

For example, to tell a patient with psychic impotence that he will be capable of erection and sexual intercourse means that treatment will cause him to put himself into the unconscious danger situation against which his symptom was created in the first place. To promise a phobic patient that he will be able to go into the phobic situation may mean to the patient that treatment will put him in the very situation of unconscious danger which he is attempting to avoid through his symptom. In this way, unconsciously, the promise of removal of symptoms may actually mobilize further anxiety.

Other factors include the realistic uncertainty at the beginning of any treatment as to the degree of success that can be achieved. There are multiple variables in the psychotherapy situation and not all of them can be foreseen. Also some aspects of the formulation of the case may have to be changed as further experience with this patient proceeds. And some conflicts or symptoms may permit only relative rather than absolute relief. Furthermore, much of the ultimate prognosis rests with the patient's continuing efforts actively to help himself. Therefore the promise of a cure may foster an attitude of magical expectation in the patient and may de-emphasize the concept that prognosis is largely dependent on the effectiveness with which he applies himself to the therapeutic task.

On the other hand, the patient's conscious suffering and desire for cure require that he be given some reasonable hope and expectation that the therapeutic efforts can be successful, since without this there would be little reason for him to enter into the therapeutic procedure. Therefore, in insight-directed psychotherapy the least threatening approach to this question is a relatively neutral one which indicates to the patient that conditions such as his have been successfully treated, but that the prognosis in any particular instance is always uncertain and is a function of many factors which will only become clear as the treatment proceeds. This gives the patient some hope, but at the same time does not threaten immediately to take away symptoms which represent his defence against an unconscious conflict.

In supportive psychotherapy there is greater rationale for departure from this neutral position, since the idea of uncovering the unconscious sources of conflict has not been stressed, and hence there is less challenge to the patient's defences. When the authoritarian role of the therapist is to be stressed, or in situations where magical expectations are to be gratified, or reliance on positive suggestion is to be used, a more authoritative and positive statement regarding prognosis may be strategically appropriate.

Even in such situations, however, it is wise to permit the patient some degree of latitude by emphasizing the idea that while definite help is available, the exact degree to which particular symptoms can be relieved is not completely certain.

Qualifications of the Therapist

Before agreeing to a particular form of therapy and a therapeutic contract, the patient has the right to know something of the qualifications of the therapist as an individual. Such questions fall into the two major categories of professional qualifications and personal or biographical attributes. Professional qualifications include such things as the nature and duration of the therapist's training, his degrees or certifications, his professional affiliations and professional status, etc. The patient may also have a variety of questions regarding the personal life and attributes of the therapist, including such things as his marital status, whether or not he has children, his religious affiliation, his interests and activities outside of the professional sphere, his attitudes towards certain social or personal issues, etc. In other words, there may be questions and curiosity about a number of things which do not relate directly to the therapist's professional competence.

A. Professional Information

In all instances the patient has a right to frank, simple and direct answers to his questions regarding the therapist's professional training, experience and status. These are important issues for the patient in making the decision whether or not he wishes to accept the therapist's recommendation, and whether or not he wishes to enter treatment with this particular therapist. If the therapist is evasive about answering such questions, or refuses to answer them, the patient may have doubts or suspicions as to why this is the case. It would not be realistic for the therapist to expect the patient to accept and trust him without recourse to such material. Furthermore, the patient may often have access to such answers through sources such as professional directories or by word of mouth from others. Therefore, in the interest of establishing a frank and trusting therapeutic relationship, it is wiser that these answers come directly from the therapist.

It should be emphasized, however, that if the patient raises these issues regarding professional qualifications once the therapeutic contract has been agreed upon and treatment is under way, the dynamics of the situation have been altered. Before answering such questions, the therapist should consider their transference implications. These questions may still appropriately require a direct answer, but usually it is wiser first to inquire as to what the question represents, and why it has not come up before, and to help the patient recognize that there may be other preconscious or unconscious meanings behind the question.

B. Personal Information

The tactical issues in managing questions and curiosity regarding the personal attributes of the therapist will be a function of the nature and strategy of the treatment goal. In insight-directed psychotherapy, one of the strategic goals is the establishment of a transference relationship in which the patient responds to the therapist increasingly on the basis of internal drives and defences, and the projection of these on to the therapist in the treatment situation. Therefore, the more reality information that the patient has about the therapist's personal life, experience and attitudes, the less can transference distortion occur, and the more will the patient be circumscribed and influenced by his realistic knowledge about the therapist. The less that the patient knows in reality about the therapist, the more will his reactions be based on a projection of his own drives or defences.

Therefore, in an insight-directed treatment approach such personal questions are usually not answered, but instead are used as a means of illustrating to the patient the way in which questions are dealt with in psychotherapy. In other words, the therapist might ask for the patient's associations as to why they are being asked, or for his associations to either answer ('What would be your feelings if I were married, and what would be your feelings if I were not?'), thereby elaborating further the patient's fantasies. This may be accompanied by an explanation that in the ultimate interests of the treament, there are times when the therapist may not answer direct questions.

In supportive psychotherapy, the strategy in the management of the therapeutic relationship is to emphasize the current reality of the relationship, to establish a positive rapport, to maintain secondary process thought, and to avoid regressive transference distortions. At times the therapist may actively use the relationship in promoting identification and in strengthening or reinforcing specific defences or defence systems.

For these reasons, answers to personal questions might be given in keeping with the therapist's understanding of the impact of such questions and answers on the total psychic economy of the patient. It becomes necessary to anticipate and predict what the patient's response is likely to be to a specific bit of information before giving such an answer, since in some instances an answer may be reassuring and strengthening of defences, whereas in other instances the same answer might have the effect of mobilizing further conflict and anxiety.

For example, in a latently homosexual individual the knowledge that the therapist is married may reduce anxiety over unconscious homosexual seduction in the treatment situation. A patient with a marital conflict may be unable to relate effectively if he knows the therapist is unmarried, since there is less possibility of identification and the patient may feel, 'What can he know, since he isn't married?' The same may be true of religious affiliation where the therapist of the same religious faith may be seen as an object of identification and support, whereas the therapist of a different faith may be seen as a potential source for the disruption of the patient's religious belief.

In general, in a supportive treatment situation there is less hesitation in answering personal questions in a definitive way, provided that such answers are in keeping with the overall understanding of the dynamic conflicts between drives and defences. Such answers may minimize frustration in the treatment setting, and will provide a framework of reality within which the patient can establish a more comfortable relationship based on rapport and on conscious secondary process thought.

Therapeutic Agreement

After these various explanations have been given and discussed, the patient must make a decision regarding therapy and the therapist. While such a treatment contract need not be strictly formal, some type of therapeutic agreement should be verbalized and clearly set up as the point of departure and framework for the therapeutic venture. In general this will include a conscious mutual agreement between the patient and therapist regarding the goals of their work, since if they are working towards different goals treatment will become much more difficult. The therapeutic contract also involves questions of time, money, absences and other reality factors.

A. Fee

One of the important elements in the therapeutic contract is the matter of a fee, and the setting of an appropriate fee may have a variety of meanings for the patient as well as the therapist. Many patients ask about fees at the time of their initial call to make the diagnostic appointment. In general, it is not wise to set a definite fee for treatment without first having seen the patient and having had an opportunity to evaluate the type of therapy that will be indicated, as well as the nature and extent of the patient's resources. On the other hand, the patient may need to know the charge for the diagnostic visit. A useful compromise is to set a definite fee for diagnostic appraisal, but to indicate that the fee for ongoing treatment will be set after the patient has been evaluated and conclusions have been reached as to the type of treatment necessary and the other factors involved.

One group of considerations in setting an appropriate fee is the frequency of therapeutic visits and the probable overall duration of the treatment. When the visits are to be relatively frequent, the patient may be unable to afford the same fee per session as he could afford if the visits were less frequent. The same concept holds for anticipated long-term therapeutic work, as compared with relatively brief treatment.

Other factors which must be considered regarding the issue of a fee relate both to the patient, and to the therapist. Ideally, for the patient the fee should represent a significant expenditure. If the fee is set too low, the patient may use this as a symbol to depreciate the therapy and not take it seriously. The patient may also have to feel grateful to the therapist for the low fee, which in turn may mobilize feelings of guilt and the feeling that he is getting something unfairly. This also means that if the patient develops feelings of anger towards the therapist, and the therapist has been so generous, he may feel greater guilt for expressing such angry feelings. For many patients, paying too low a fee may lend reality to transference ideas that the therapist is really not interested in them, and that if they were paying a higher fee therapy would somehow be better or less distressing. In an opposite direction, other patients may interpret too low a fee as a sign of excessive personal interest in them, or may then fantasy that the therapist will make other non-financial demands upon them in compensation. A low fee may be a source of difficulty in patients for whom manipulation of objects has been an important element in their pathology. In such a situation, a low fee may become a symbol of positive triumph over the therapist and thus from the outset influence the therapeutic relationship in a variety of ways.

On the other hand, setting too high a fee may preclude therapy for the patient, or may realistically jeopardize the financial resources of the patient or family to such an extent that it places a significant added burden on the therapy. In such situations, the patient may also have expectations of a magical cure and have the feeling that since he is paying so much, it is the therapist's obligation to perform the treatment and that he has no further need to participate. At times it may encourage the fantasy of being the therapist's favourite patient by virtue of paying more than other patients (and at times this becomes a reality and not a fantasy).

Setting a high fee may also at times be used by the patient as an aggressive act against the other relatives by forcing them to make sacrifices, and hence the therapist may unwittingly participate in this form of acting-out against the family, to the ultimate detriment of the treatment. In an opposite direction, too high a fee may intensify feelings of guilt in the patient, and likewise may incur the anger of the family against the patient. For some masochistic patients, the setting of too high a fee may provide continuing masochistic gratification, with the therapist then becoming the persecuting or sadistic object of interaction.

From the standpoint of the therapist, the issue of fee will also have a variety of meanings. For some therapists, a wish to be liked, kind, giving and not to seem demanding may motivate them in the direction of setting too low a fee. Some therapists may also feel guilty about accepting money for their services, which again may lead them in this direction. A fee which is too low may stimulate conscious or unconscious anger at the patient and his demands, and may lead to a variety of negative counter-transference reactions, particularly if the patient proves to be unrewarding in other aspects as well. The therapist may also feel that since he is giving his time for a low fee, the patient should be grateful and appreciative, and should like the therapist, and negative transference reactions in the patient may be more difficult to tolerate.

There may also be a variety of reactions to setting too high a fee. These may include a positive preference for this patient, a feeling of guilt, or a sense of pressure to do more for this particular patient to compensate for the higher fee. If the therapy proves unsuccessful, guilt feelings for having charged the higher fee may be compounded.

Each therapist must consciously work out this problem for himself and set what he considers to be a reasonable assessment of the value of his time, or a scale with upper and lower limits of such value, commensurate with his training and experience. In setting this scale, the therapist must also be guided to some extent by the fee range existent in his particular community for the type of therapy he is providing. Then if the patient can afford this upper limit reasonably, the therapist can feel comfortable at charging it; likewise if the patient can only afford the lower limits. If, for other reasons, the therapist decides to see a patient at more or less than his usual fee limits, he must work through for himself whatever counter-transference feelings he may have about this, since otherwise counter-transference distortions may interfere with therapy.

The therapist should try to arrange the therapeutic contract in such a way that the significant dynamic interactions over money can be most effectively used in keeping with the overall strategy and goals of the therapeutic process. In insight-directed therapy, where it is anticipated that there will be a mobilization of conflict, the development of a transference relationship, and ultimate ego maturation, it is advisable that the patient himself actively participate in setting the fee. This brings the issue of money and payment for the therapist's services into sharper focus for the patient. The patient may prefer to by-pass this and have the therapist discuss the fee with someone else, and may plead ignorance of financial matters or attempt to evade the issue in some other way. By expecting the patient to be an active participant in this issue, the therapist is tacitly favouring a more mature ego attitude towards money and the various interactions around it, and also is presenting the patient with a conflict situation which then must be resolved.

The therapist may also anticipate that as treatment progresses, many unconscious attitudes, reactions, impulses and defences may emerge through the way in which the financial transaction is handled. Therefore, in insight-directed treatment, the therapeutic situation may be set up in such a way that the issue of the fee remains active throughout the treatment. Billing is usually done directly to the patient, even though some other family member may be the financially responsible individual. The more that problems over money and financial matters are part of the neurotic symptom complex, the more would the therapist want to present the patient personally with the bill at the end of each month, and ask that the cheque be brought to the session. This means that money actually changes hands regularly between patient and therapist, and then the patient's feelings regarding money or any deviations from the usual pattern can be more readily observed and dealt with in the treatment situation. Even the way in which the patient accepts the bill or renders the cheque can offer significant material for therapeutic work (i.e. whether or not he looks at the therapist, whether or not he and the therapist touch the cheque at the same moment, whether or not this act mobilizes anxiety, etc.). If the bill is mailed to the patient and he returns the cheque by mail, it becomes much easier to evade this entire issue with a variety of rationalizations.

When treatment is supportive in nature, the therapist is more flexible and makes dynamically varying uses of the issues of setting and collecting the fee. At times these interactions may be used to gratify drive-derivatives, and at other times to strengthen defences, in accordance with the specific supportive strategy which is being attempted.

For example, in passive-dependent individuals if strategy calls for the gratification of dependency wishes, it may be reasonable to discuss the fee with someone other than the patient, and to by-pass the patient in the billing and collecting of the fee. The therapeutic contract is thus set up in such a way that the patient is not directly reminded each month that the therapist's interest, attention and effort are being paid for in money. However, if a patient's reaction-formation against dependency is intense, and an effort is being made to strengthen this defence, it would be more appropriate to discuss fees directly with the patient and to send the monthly statement directly to him. This permits him more easily to maintain the defence of not accepting anything passively from anybody. One chronic schizophrenic patient had such great anxiety at the prospect of owing anyone anything that she wanted to pay her bill in cash after each session rather than feel that she owed the therapist money for even a month. In order to reduce anxiety over this conflict, this arrangement was made, and one sign of improvement was her gradual ability to allow the bill to go unpaid for the month. In patients who are depressed, particularly when there is significant morbid guilt present, it is again often wiser to arrange for fees through a relative in order not to intensify the patient's guilt at the financial burden that the illness causes the family.

Unfortunately, in many clinics and agencies the setting and collecting of the fee is done by a person other than the therapist, and the therapist pays little or no attention to financial matters. While this may improve the efficiency of clinic operations, it may detract from the therapeutic interaction, and opportunities to observe this important part of the interpersonal relationship may be lost. The issues described above regarding too low a fee must be kept in mind in clinic settings, and where feasible, even a token fee may be important. It may help in reducing shame and guilt regarding charity, in increasing the patient's investment of himself in the therapy, in permitting affective discharge, etc.

There is no single way in which setting and collecting of the fee should be done, but it is essential for the therapist to recognize at varying depths of consciousness the multiple meanings of money and the transactions surrounding it.

B. Time

The same dynamic approach and recognition of the significance to the patient must be considered in regard to factors of time, which is one of the other keystones in the therapeutic contract. This includes the total length of therapy, frequency of visits and duration of each session.

It is usually not possible to predict precisely how long a patient is likely to require for his treatment, but in accord with the strategic goals, upper and lower limits can usually be reasonably estimated. Generally speaking, insight-directed treatment requires a significant and continuing investment of time, and the greater the degree of change desired, the longer the overall duration of treatment will be.

In discussing the duration of insight-treatment, therefore, it is important that the therapist be candid, and neither too optimistic nor pessimistic. At the same time it is wiser that he not be too definite, since a precise statement may help to entrench in the patient the fantasy that if he only 'puts in this amount of time' the cure will take place automatically. Likewise, if he has been given a specific time, changes or reactions that may occur sooner may be discredited and discounted by the patient. And if the treatment takes longer than anticipated, other transference complications may occur.

The total duration of supportive therapy varies between even wider limits than in insight-therapy. At times it may be very brief, and the patient may have a prompt therapeutic response after only a few sessions. At other times it may have to be on-going for indefinite periods, sometimes for many years, as in the case of some chronic psychotic or borderline patients where continuing the treatment allows them to be maintained outside of a hospital. In other instances treatment may become intermittent rather than continuous, and the therapeutic task may be to support the patient during acute symptomatic exacerbations or at times of crisis, and then to discontinue the sessions until another such exacerbation or crisis recurs. Therefore, in supportive therapy it is frequently more useful to leave the time factor purposely vague for the patient by using concepts like 'as long as it seems necessary', thus permitting maximum flexibility.

Another issue is the frequency of sessions. Although there are no absolutes and the optimal frequency will vary from patient to patient, an insight-directed approach generally requires that sessions be sufficiently frequent for the patient to develop a significant emotional investment in the therapist and in the therapy, and ultimately to develop a transference relationship. The therapist should be alert to a commonly occurring fantasy that the more frequent the sessions, the more severe is the illness, and he should be ready to make suitable explanations in this regard. There should optimally be some degree of continuity from one session to the next, and sessions should be on a regular scheduled basis rather than varied in accordance with the patient's exacerbations or remissions of symptoms. At times when resistance is high, the patient may prefer not to come or may have the feeling that he has nothing to say, whereas at other times he may have a wish to come more frequently. The establishment of a regular schedule of appointments in insight-directed treatment facilitates the development and management of a transference relationship, and the patient's wishes for a departure from the usual scheduling can more readily be seen in their transference meanings.

In supportive psychotherapy where one of the main goals is the immediate attention to and relief of symptoms and anxiety, and where the relationship is to be kept primarily at the level of conscious rapport, the therapist has a greater latitude and flexibility in the scheduling of sessions. Variations in frequency based on symptomatic exacerbations or remissions are encouraged, and at times of increasing symptomatology or stress, the therapist may readily suggest or concur with the idea of extra or more frequent sessions, without interpreting the underlying transference meanings. Similarly, if the patient manifests more intense resistance and wants to come less frequently, or in situations where the immediate tactical goal is to dilute the therapeutic relationship, interviews might be spaced out in order to achieve a more comfortable conscious rapport, without stimulating more intense unconscious transference manifestations.

Another factor is the length of each session. In insight therapy, the reduction of resistance and defences, and establishment of a transference relationship requires that there be a relatively constant therapeutic situation. As part of this constancy, sessions of fixed length are generally advisable. A frequent model is 45 or 50 minutes, but with some patients effective therapy can occur using 30 minute sessions. If the therapist shortens or lengthens the duration of the session in accordance with the nature of the patient's material or symptoms, this in effect involves a manipulation by the therapist, as the result of which resistance and transference manifestations are more difficult to demonstrate. Patients quickly become aware of the judgmental and critical attitudes implied by such manipulation, and they in turn may use these to manipulate the therapist further.

After the transference relationship has been established, giving extra time when symptoms are more severe, and not giving it when symptoms are lessened, tends to reinforce regression and symptom formation. If the patient is given an extra 5 or 10 minutes when talking about a particular topic, whereas the interview is stopped on time or early when he talks about other things, the focus of the therapist's interest quickly becomes apparent. Sometimes patients will 'save up' the most significant material until the end of the session, in hopes thereby of obtaining further time, which becomes more difficult to manage the more that the therapist has participated in such a pattern. Likewise if a patient 'runs out of things to say' part-way through a session, the implied pressure to fill the rest of the session serves as a force on the patient to produce more material, and to bring to his mind things he has attempted to maintain at preconscious or unconscious levels. In this way, even though the patient may have conscious wishes to leave and to avoid the therapeutic situation, such resistances can be dealt with and interpreted in the framework of the transference relationship and the ongoing therapeutic process.

In supportive psychotherapy, where the aim is to maintain defences and resistances and at times to gratify unconscious drive-derivatives, tactics regarding the length of sessions are quite different. The strategic need to avoid stimulation of preconscious or unconscious material may at times suggest that interviews be limited to 10, 20 or 30 minutes, so that emphasis can be on 'conscious reporting' by the patient. The same would hold if the emphasis is on drug therapy, or if a patient has intense conflict over close emotional involvement in an interpersonal relationship. An extreme example is a chronic schizophrenic on maintenance dosage of Thorazine who was incapacitated by anxiety in a personal interview situation. Effective therapeutic contact was maintained by a 5-minute telephone conversation every 6–8 weeks.

If a patient 'runs out' of material to discuss in a particular session, the tactical goal might be to avoid the vacuum of the remainder of the session. Hence the therapist might appropriately terminate the interview on these lines 'Perhaps that is as much as you have to say today'. Contrariwise, in some situations the patient may need the encouragement, gratification and reinforcement of an extra few minutes at the end of the session. This may be required as a sign of interest by the therapist, or a sign of reassurance regarding the material that the patient has been discussing, and such 'gifts' may readily be made, keeping in mind the overall dynamic understanding of the patient's conflicts.

C. Absences

The same technical differentiation occurs in regard to the question of absences and ideally should be discussed while establishing the therapeutic contract. It can be anticipated that in a state of heightened resistance in insight-directed treatment, a patient may at times wish to avoid the therapeutic session altogether, and may then use various rationalizations for the absence. The therapeutic task, however, requires that the patient attend his sessions anyhow, in order that these resistances may become more clearly apparent to him. Therefore, the tactical goal is to do everything possible to insure that the patient attends the sessions.

One effective aid is to indicate that the patient is financially responsible for all scheduled sessions, whether he attends or not. The prospect of having to pay for the session even if he does not come will at times enhance such a patient's conscious motivation to attend, and thus will tend to decrease this form of acting-out. Furthermore, as transference manifestations increase, some patients may use this form of behaviour as a means of expressing negative or hostile feelings towards the therapist, and of 'getting even with him' for transference frustrations. If the therapist is to be paid for the session anyhow, the patient will be less likely to use this ultimately self-defeating mechanism.

A further factor in this regard is the counter-transference. If the therapist loses income by virtue of the patient's resistance to treatment, he may develop counter-transference feelings of aggression, or he may feel under increased pressure to manipulate the situation in order that the patient should not skip sessions.

If the absence is planned and announced well in advance, the dynamics of the situation are different, and the therapist might react accordingly. He must be aware, however, that patients may consciously or unconsciously manipulate their external life situation in such a way as to avoid therapeutic sessions (i.e. planning a business conference for the time of the session when another time would do just as well).

In situations of unavoidable absence such as illness, other arrangements may be necessary, although even this may not be as simple as it appears. For example, when is a cold severe enough to warrant avoiding a session, or when is a headache bad enough to make it reasonable for the patient to stay at home? The therapist must be careful about placing himself in a judgmental role by charging for some of these absences and not for others, thereby implying that one instance was not justified while the other instance was.

In supportive therapy where the strategy is to permit such defences as avoidance, the usual arrangement is not to charge the patient for absences, and to accept the financial loss without necessarily focusing on the patient's motivations. Even in a supportive situation, however, if a patient manifests significant anxiety or guilt over such absences, it may be therapeutically helpful to charge for the absence, thus minimizing such responses.

D. Confidentiality

The therapist must remember that no matter how common the various fantasies, feelings, memories, or relationships are in his experience, to the individual patient they are highly personal, meaningful, and often a source of fear, guilt, or shame. All patients are therefore concerned about the confidentiality of their communications, and the therapist frequently needs to clarify this matter to the patient. If the therapist is to interview significant persons in the patient's life, this concern about confidentiality is increased.

The therapist must respect the patient's confidence even more carefully than the general physician, since the effectiveness of his treatment may be seriously jeopardized by failures to do so. Leaks of information, overheard conversations, openly available records, identifiable anecdotes, etc., may severely hamper the patient's trust. This is particularly difficult in relationship to the patient's other physicians, nurses, ancillary personnel, lawyers, employers, etc., all of whom may have a professional interest in the patient and his progress. However well intentioned their remarks or reports to the patient regarding conversations with the therapist, the patient frequently will suspect and wonder if highly confidential material has also been divulged, and this may inhibit his freedom of communication in subsequent therapy sessions. Each therapist must develop his own practices regarding these issues, but all must be aware of their importance.

E. Other Factors

A variety of other factors impinge upon the therapeutic situation and must be considered for their dynamic significance. For example, the physical setting of the therapeutic session should provide a comfortable and quiet situation, and attention must be paid to the problem of sound transmission. If the patient can hear noise outside of the consultation room, he will also anticipate that what he says can be overheard, which will tend to inhibit the material. Privacy is particularly important to some patients when coming to or leaving their sessions, regardless of the form of therapy.

If the therapist takes notes during the treatment session, some patients feel that they are not receiving his full attention. Likewise, they may be influenced by those things which they see the therapist writing, and those things they think the therapist does not bother to note, which in turn leads to a form of editing. If the therapist does not take notes, however, some patients may have the feeling that he is not interested or is not paying attention. In either case, the therapist must set his own style but be dynamically aware of the possibility of the patient reacting to it in a variety of ways.

The same is true for interruptions, such as telephone calls during a therapeutic session. The patient may have a variety of reactions to the fact of the interruption itself, particularly as the transference relationship intensifies. Also, he may overhear the therapist in contact with someone else, which may lead to a variety of distortions and comparisons based on transference, but displaced to the reality situation. The significance of such observation of the therapist in contact with someone other than himself will vary for the patient, depending on whether strategy calls for a transference or a reality oriented relationship.

Summary

In summary, the details of the structuring of the therapeutic situation and agreement should vary as a function of the total therapeutic strategy. Their dynamic implications should be recognized in order that they may be most effectively used to further the patient's progress towards the specific chosen therapeutic goal.

SUGGESTED READING

CHODOFF, PAUL (1964) Psychoanalysis and fees. *Compr. Psychiat.* **5**, 137

FINGERT, HYMAN H. (1952) Comments on the psychoanalytic significance of the fee. *Bull. Menninger Clin.* **16**, 98

G.A.P. Report 45 (1960) Confidentiality and Privileged Communication in the Practice of Psychiatry

HAAK, NILS (1957) Comments on the analytical situation. *Int. J. Psycho-Anal.* **38**, 183

HOLLENDER, MARC (1960) The psychiatrist and the release of patient information. *Am. J. Psychiat.* **116**, 828

KUBIE, LAWRENCE S. (1957) *Practical and Theoretical Aspects of Psychoanalysis.* International Universities Press Inc, New York

KUBIE, LAWRENCE S. (1964) The changing economics of psychotherapeutic practice. *J. nerv. ment. Dis.* **139**, 311

LIEVANO, JAIME (1967) Observations about payment of psychotherapy fees. *Psychiat. Quart.* **41**, 324

LORAND, SANDOR & CONSOLE, WILLIAM A. (1958) Therapeutic results in psychoanalytic treatment without fee. *Int. J. Psycho-Anal.* **39**, 59

SLOVENKO, RALPH & USDIN, GENE L. (1961) The psychiatrist and privileged communication. *Arch. gen. Psychiat.* **4**, 431

WIENER, DANIAL N. & RATHS, OTTO N. (1960) Cultural factors in payment for psychoanalytic therapy. *Am. J. Psychoanal.* **20**, 66

CHAPTER X

The Therapeutic Process: The Patient's Role

Introduction

Psychotherapy can be defined as a psychological process occurring between two (or more) individuals in which one (the therapist), by virtue of his position and training, seeks systematically to apply psychological knowledge and interventions in an attempt to understand, influence and ultimately modify the psychic experience, mental function and behaviour of the other (the patient). This form of interaction is distinguished from other relationships between two people by the formality of a therapeutic agreement (whether explicit or implicit), the specific training, skill and experience of the therapist, and the fact that the patient (either voluntarily or by coercion) has come to the therapist seeking professional therapeutic help.

The bartender, teacher, pastor, lawyer, friend or relative may also successfully modify the behaviour of another person, often in a beneficial fashion. However, the lack of a formal therapeutic agreement, as well as the usual lack of training, and the unsystematic way in which the interactions are carried out, preclude these relationships from being considered psychotherapeutic, although some of what is to follow in this discusson may apply to them.

Therapeutic Atmosphere

Psychotherapy takes place in an interpersonal relationship between therapist and patient, regardless of whether the goal of treatment is to be supportive or insight-directed. As mentioned earlier, it involves a therapeutic alliance between the therapist and those consciously co-operative and sustaining aspects of the patient's ego, pitted against the conscious and unconscious conflictual elements in the patient's mental and emotional life. The initiation of therapy therefore requires the establishment of a suitable two-way relationship between patient and therapist in which both will continue their various efforts and tasks in attempting to reach the goals that have been set.

One of the first steps in the establishment of this relationship is that the therapist provide a therapeutic atmosphere in which both can work. This is difficult to define, but includes the therapist, through verbal and non-verbal behaviour, indicating his therapeutic intent and willingness to work towards the goal of helping the patient within the limits of his capacities. The general emphasis is on the therapeutic needs of the patient and on the fact that the chief function of their meeting together is ultimately the patient's treatment and welfare. The therapist must also *feel*, (and thereby non-verbally impart to the patient), a sense of respect for the patient as an individual, in spite of his illness or symptoms, and must take the patient and the patient's complaints seriously, regardless of the degree of disability, their nature or their irrationality. This is often at variance with the attitude the patient has met in other people, who frequently may depreciate, ridicule or show little interest in the patient, once the diagnosis of an emotional illness has been made. To be most effective, the therapist must himself accept the idea that the patient's difficulties stem from an emotional or psychological disturbance beyond his full conscious control, and must recognize that such symptoms and disabilities are none the less distressing and disabling.

Another important factor in establishing such a therapeutic atmosphere is that the therapist have sufficient understanding and flexibility in his approach to be capable of meeting and accepting the patient at the patient's own level of psychic functioning at the moment. Frequently the patient already feels inferior, ashamed or guilty for his neurotic illness, and explicit or implicit demands by the therapist that the patient relate to him in a rigidly set pattern dictated by the therapist or his preconceived ideas, will generally further alienate the patient and make him feel that he is not being understood.

For example, a patient with an acute schizophrenic reaction who speaks in terms of the primary process and symbolic reasoning, is by virtue of his disturbance incapable of secondary process logic and rational thought. Repeated questions or demands by the therapist that the patient express himself more clearly and more logically may make him feel less understood and, therefore, make it more difficult to relate himself to the therapist. It is more effective for the therapist to attempt in part to communicate with such a patient at the level of the patient's current thought-processes, thereby attempting to establish a human contact and bridge by which the patient may feel somewhat more understood.

The same concept holds for a passive, dependent, whining patient, who by virtue of his disturbances will be incapable of tolerating significant frustrations. Even though these ego attitudes may be unpleasant for the therapist, it is necessary that he accept them as symptomatic for this particular patient. The same would be true of patients in whom acting-out has been a major mode of adaptation, or patients whose symptoms or behaviour are personally or morally offensive to the therapist. The therapist must learn to be capable of accepting and tolerating this, particularly in his initial contacts with the patient, if he hopes to establish a treatment relationship.

Such behavioural attitudes or reactions must be seen as having an unconscious meaning, and they are in a sense dynamically equivalent to more classical neurotic symptoms. The demand that the patient in essence control or give up the symptom (i.e. acting-out, or phobia) before entering treatment is not only doomed to failure, but also alienates the patient further from establishing the necessary therapeutic relationship.

The greater the patient's ego strength and the more that therapy is planned for an insight-directed approach, the more reasonable is it for the therapist to maintain a more neutral and expectant therapeutic attitude, based on the assumption that if the patient is a suitable case for insight-directed therapy, he should be capable of tolerating this. If the patient is incapable of tolerating such a neutral therapeutic atmosphere, but insight-treatment is still the therapy of choice, a variety of parameters may have to be introduced. It must be recognized, however, that these may have varying later consequences for the therapeutic process.

Therapeutic Relationship

As will be elaborated in Chapter XII on Transference, a large and important part of the relationship between patient and therapist is based on unconscious forces within the patient which, through displacement and projection, significantly influence and modify the patient's reactions in the therapeutic situation. In spite of the major importance of the unconscious transference components, however, they do not represent the totality of the therapeutic relationship.

The treatment relationship also involves conscious reactions to the therapist which are reality-oriented. In addition to his transference roles, the therapist is also a real person, and his reality-oriented current behaviour in the treatment setting will influence the patient's capacity to develop a useful therapeutic relationship.

The way in which the therapist behaves and reacts, his knowledge and capacity for sensitive understanding of the patient's productions and behaviour, his own personal habits or idiosyncrasies, his tactfulness and capacity to express himself and the inevitable variations in his day-to-day performance may all influence the therapy, positively or negatively, regardless of whether the treatment goal is insight-directed, or supportive.

For example, if a therapist behaves coldly or indifferently, or if he is critical and makes moralistic judgments of the patient, or if he is inattentive and forgetful of what the patient tells him, the patient will have a variety of reactions to the therapist. In such a situation, there would be a reality stimulus to the patient's reaction but the final behavioural response will also be partly determined by unconscious intra-psychic factors. It is these latter factors that determine whether or not the patient responds with anger, depression, guilt, masochistic submission, withdrawal, acting-out, or realistic confrontation, etc.

Education of the Patient

Keeping these factors in mind, the way in which the therapist introduces the patient to his part in the therapeutic procedure has considerable significance for the promptness and effectiveness with which the treatment process begins. Although he may have explained the patient's role during the establishment of the therapeutic contract, generalized verbalization is seldom enough, even for relatively sophisticated patients. It is the nature of the therapist's interventions and his attitude when making them that help the patient to an emotional understanding and acceptance of the previous verbal explanations of what psychotherapy involves.

From casual inspection, the therapeutic situation often appears to be random, and to lack organization. Closer observation, however, permits a view of therapy as a relationship with a definitely established structure, the various elements of which are logically derived from basic theory and strategy.

A. Patient Participation

One element is that as much as is possible, the patient should maintain an on-going participation in the therapeutic process itself, through continuing to talk, express himself, respond and interact with the therapist. In an insight-directed treatment situation, the more active that the patient is in working out the discovery and understanding of his conflicts, the more genuine and effective will be the insight which develops. The more that the therapist takes the initiative in explaining, interpreting or talking in the treatment situation, the more likely it is that the patient will acquire only a limited or intellectualized understanding. He may accept the therapist's ideas as coming from an authoritarian source much like those he might read in a book, but thereby he misses the experience of personal conviction and emotional impact that self-developed insight can bring.

To this end, the therapist encourages the patient's efforts at self-exploration, even if these are hesitant, fumbling or initially unsuccessful. Until the pattern of patient participation is well established, the therapist should focus much of his attention in this area. To make early explanations of the content of conflicts is to foster passivity in the patient.

Even in supportive treatment, it is important to emphasize the patient's ongoing role in the therapeutic process, since the more that the patient verbalizes his conscious mental processes and reactions, the more effective can be the therapist's subsequent intervention. The usual strategy in supportive therapy is to help the patient elaborate and express those mental processes which are currently conscious, but in such a way as *not* to encourage the return to consciousness of previously unconscious material.

For example, if a patient says 'I think I am going crazy', and says very little further, it becomes difficult for the therapist effectively to reassure the patient on this matter since as yet the patient has not mentioned why he thinks this. And support or reassurance given before the patient has expressed some of his conscious thoughts on the matter will tend to leave him unconvinced. If the therapist can encourage the patient's elaboration of his conscious fears and of the thoughts which lead him to think of himself as going crazy (i.e. conscious fantasies of killing his children) the intervention which is then offered can then be more effectively accepted by the patient.

In other words, after the patient has expressed what is consciously on his mind, then the therapist has an opportunity to offer interventions designed to help the patient suppress, repress, isolate or in other ways deal with the disturbing fantasy or impulse. By comparison, in an insight-directed treatment approach, after the patient has verbalized such a consciously disturbing fantasy, strategy then dictates that he should be helped to explore further the determinants and meanings behind the fantasy. The patient's wishes to be satisfied with mere conscious expression of the fantasy would be understood as resistances against further exploration, uncovering and understanding.

B. *Verbalization*

It is particularly essential in insight-directed treatment that the immediate tactical goal be to help the patient speak as freely and frankly as possible, and try not to hold back thoughts even if they are distressing, embarrassing, unclear or at times irrational or unconnected.

In this context, the term 'Free Association' may occur in the mind of the therapist as well as in the mind of the patient. This is a specific technique and device usually reserved for the classical analytic situation, and is seldom attempted in the situation of face-to-face psychotherapy. The classical analytic situation has a number of built-in factors and forces which promote a more intense regression in the service of the ego than is desirable or manageable in the type of insight-directed psychotherapy under discussion here. Even in the classical analytic situation, free association develops only slowly and gradually after significant earlier therapeutic work has been done.

In early psychotherapy sessions it is important that the therapist recognize the patient's need to hold back aspects of consciously distressing and disturbing material, to say nothing of the less-readily available preconscious and repressed unconscious material. It is unreasonable to expect the patient immediately to drop all of his usual defences and social guardedness, and to express himself without restraints, but the ultimate aim in the therapeutic strategy of an insight-directed approach is to help the patient speak with a minimum of inhibition.

Therefore, in the early sessions the therapist's tactical aim is to provide an atmosphere in which the patient can speak freely, and to encourage frankness, and from time to time deal with the more obvious manifestations of withholding as a resistance. In this connection, it is important that the therapist does not immediately challenge the patient on material he brings up, nor emphasize irrationalities, nor make distressing or unpleasant interpretations of such material. If the therapist asks a patient to speak freely without conscious editing but then promptly points out that the material is irrational, unrealistic, contradictory, or fragmented, etc., the patient is put into a double bind. Such interventions will tend to make the patient more cautious about what he says, which will be ultimately contrary to the therapeutic strategy. Particularly in the beginning of therapy, it is the way in which the therapist responds to the patient's material that sets the stage as to whether or not the patient will go on to increasing frankness, or whether he will feel himself to be 'held responsible' for all he says and, therefore, be more cautious and concealing in the material that he produces.

Likewise, another tactical aim is to emphasize to the patient that the major burden of talking is his, and that it is the material which is currently in the patient's mind which will be the primary focus of attention. Therefore, the therapist tends to remain more passive and to intervene primarily in the direction of keeping the patient's material flowing through the use of an open-ended, generalized type of questioning or intervention. For example, early in the course of treatment the patient may begin a session with questions as to what he should talk about. The therapist's response would generally be in the direction of helping the patient become accustomed to initiating thoughts and ideas, with such interventions as 'Let's begin with whatever has been on your mind since you were last here', or, 'Let's start with what is on your mind right now'. At times it may be necessary to help the patient see that he has an uncertainty or anxiety about beginning or taking the initiative, and to try to help him understand the specific meaning of such an inhibition.

In other words, early in therapy the chief focus tends to be on the process of communication itself rather than on the content of existing conflicts. This may involve reminding the patient of 'the basic rule', explaining again the needs for open communication, acknowledging the difficulties in self-expression, or interpreting the specific resistances against exposure and exploration of mental life. The therapist's task is to present this concept to the patient in ways that he can grasp and use. Often an analogy of some kind can be helpful (i.e. 'when a dentist works on an abscessed tooth it will cause temporary pain, but it would do no good to work on some other tooth instead'; 'when a hairdresser is to set your hair he can't do the job you want if you keep your hat on'; etc.). One must also keep in mind that in these early sessions the patient often is testing the situation and the therapist in regard to his patience, willingness to listen, non-judgmental attitude, ability not to react in a moralizing way, etc.

In setting this early therapeutic atmosphere, the therapist's non-verbal attitudes and responses of acceptance of the patient and his material are equally as important as the specific verbal interventions he makes. It is often tempting to make interpretations to the patient of the meaning behind his communications, in hopes of speeding up the therapeutic process. In the long run, however, therapy is expedited most by promoting the development of an optimal therapeutic situation and relationship in the beginning phases, rather than by focusing on the content of psychic conflict.

The more that treatment is supportively oriented, the greater is the need to emphasize secondary process rational and logical reasoning, and hence the less will the therapist emphasize to the patient that he should express thoughts as they come to his mind, even if irrational. Likewise, the therapist will be more active in focusing the material, or suggesting topics for consideration, and asking direct or specific questions. The therapist is also less likely to emphasize the patient's responsibilities for producing therapeutically useful material in the treatment, and although he listens to whatever spontaneous material the patient produces, he encourages the patient to maintain conscious reasoning and editing. The emphasis tends to be on reporting by the patient of consciously perceived events and reactions, and the therapist does not encourage reporting of introspective exploration.

C. Self-observation

Another function which the therapist encourages in this early phase, particularly in insight-directed psychotherapy, is the patient's capacity for self-observation. This involves fostering a split in ego functioning between emotional reaction, and intellectual reflection. After permitting the expression of an emotional experience in an increasingly regressive way, the patient is encouraged to stand off, take emotional distance from himself and observe and reflect upon that which he has just experienced and expressed.

Pure emotional abreaction or expression of conflict is only a means towards the ultimate goal of treatment, which is a healthy integration and more effective control of such mental processes. Therefore, after the patient has experienced or expressed something in an emotional or regressive fashion, the therapist might intervene by asking the patient how to evaluate with conscious secondary process reasoning what he has just expressed, or to consider what his further thoughts are concerning the material he has just brought up. In this way, the attempt is to foster an ebb and flow between regressive self-expression of conflict and affect, and progressive self-observation and reflection upon that which has been expressed.

There are some patients, however, whose major defence involves the use of intellectualization and isolation to an advanced degree, and who at times use self-observation to the point that they respond in treatment as if they were talking about someone other than themselves. In such a situation the therapist would not foster further self-observation, but would instead interpret this as a manifestation of anxiety and defence.

In the supportive therapy situation, the therapist must be aware that some patients may need a prolonged and uninterrupted opportunity for emotional expression. Therefore, he must at times be more hesitant in challenging these responses. By virtue of their illness, some patients cannot take effective emotional distance from their problems. The therapist in such cases may have to accept prolonged periods of catharsis and abreaction.

When the patient is encouraged towards self-observation, it is usually done in the framework of 'common sense', and the emphasis is on pointing out irrationalities in order that the patient may exert more effective conscious efforts at control.

D. Details

Another area of education for the patient is in the matter of the expression of the details of thoughts, experiences and feelings. This is particularly the case in insight-directed treatment, where the specific details of a thought-process or its associations may be the crucial factor which gives the patient and therapist insight into the underlying disturbances and conflicts, and in such situations the use of generalizations or the avoidance of detail may serve in the function of defence. Asking the patient to fill in the details of a particular series of associations is often the first step towards awareness of that which has been repressed, and hence eventually towards insight.

For this reason, in a supportive relationship the therapist often does not press the patient for details, since to do so may challenge defences and result in a beginning undoing of repression.

However, some patients, particularly those with obsessive-compulsive defences, may devote a large proportion of their therapeutic time to the recital of minutiae, which again may serve in the function of resistance. In such a situation, the therapist's role would be to help the patient see how he obscures material by *indiscriminate* emphasis on *all* detail.

The supportive approach to such a pattern of interaction would be to permit it for a longer time as a means of defence, or at times as a method of expression of an unconscious drive-derivative (i.e. the patient who feels that he must force the listener to give his attention, or the wish to bore and irritate the listener, or the wish to make the listener wait).

E. Affect

Another area where the education of the patient is necessary is in the matter of expression of affect in the therapeutic situation. For some patients it is necessary to interpret the defences against expression of affect and actively to inquire about feelings, particularly where isolation or intellectualization are prominent defences. In other situations, the patient may have expressed affect quite freely and then be ashamed and apologize for having given way to his feelings.

It is essential that the therapist be capable of accepting the patient's expression of affect without impatience or anxiety, and if necessary that an explanation be offered to the patient indicating that an important part of psychotherapy is not only the thought content, but also the feelings which accompany it. No attempt is made to provoke or entice the patient into expressing his feelings, but it is important that the patient clearly understands that the expression of feelings is also a part of his treatment, and that the therapist can tolerate such expression comfortably.

In supportive therapy it may in some cases be indicated to permit the patient the continuing use of isolation and the avoiding of intense affect as part of the maintenance of the system of defence. At the other extreme, if the patient is intensely involved with the expression of affect, it may be necessary to help him regain control of his feelings, particularly towards the end of the session, through the encouragement of isolation, or emphasis on conscious control and suppression. But the emphasis in supportive therapy is on the expression of those affects which are consciously perceived by the patient, and the strategy is to avoid mobilization of unconscious affects.

F. No Quick Answers

It is important in these early sessions that the therapist's interventions also get across to the patient the awareness that there are no immediate answers as to what lies behind a particular experience or thought, and that the mutual therapeutic task is to begin a search for them. To accomplish this it is essential that the therapist avoid any attitude of smug knowledge or superiority, or give the impression that he already knows the answers and is withholding them from the patient. Early in the treatment process, the patient is not yet able to appreciate the importance of his discovering insights for himself, and a feeling that the therapist is 'holding out' will frequently mobilize hostility and negativism.

In this connection, the therapist should be aware of the impact of the question 'Why ?' in this phase of the treatment. Such a question will generally force the patient to rationalize his motivations and thoughts, and will also suggest that there is an immediate or known answer which the patient is expected to have at his command. It may also encourage the patient to 'guess at the right answer', particularly if the therapist has a specific idea in mind and hopes that the patient will arrive at the same idea himself.

A more useful approach is to phrase such questions in a more general way (i.e. 'What are your thoughts . . .', or, 'What comes to your mind . . .'), without implying that there is a specific or immediately available answer. The tactical goal is to help the patient to a recognition of the fact that he and the therapist together are searching for an understanding which will come only gradually, but that there are probably other thoughts, associations or fantasies behind the particular behaviour or mental contents, and the patient should now begin to direct his attention and exploration to these.

In supportive therapy, the situation tends to be far more flexible in this regard, and the therapist's interventions are more variable and are made in light of the overall strategy. For example, where strategy calls for an emphasis on the therapist as an omniscient and authoritarian figure, the tactic might be to give prompt and definitely phrased 'answers'. If strategy calls for emphasis on current conscious problems and avoidance of the past, the tactic may be actively to de-emphasize the significance of 'finding answers' and to stress conscious control instead. Where strategy calls for a de-emphasis of the role of the therapist, the tactic might be to avoid positive interpretations and to reinforce the patient's own attempts to find 'the answers' quickly.

G. Regression

In insight-directed therapy, another early educational aspect is to encourage the patient to a therapeutic regression in the service of the ego by suspending his conscious editing and critical judgment in presenting his thoughts and feelings until after the material has been expressed. The strategy behind this is that through the regression there will ultimately be a partial return of previously repressed conflict which can then be subjected to conscious scrutiny.

In other words, in insight-directed therapy, the attitude of the patient should come to be 'speak first and think later', thereby fostering movement away from rigid adherence to the rules of the secondary process. In order to encourage this, it is essential that the therapist does not immediately expect the patient to be responsible for what he has said, or expect that it should be sensible and consistent, or fit into a specific predetermined pattern. If the therapist asks the patient freely to express whatever comes to his mind, and then immediately points out logical inconsistencies in what the patient has said, he directly contradicts what he has asked the patient to do, and thus makes it more difficult for the patient freely to express himself in the future lest he again run into criticism and feel himself to be 'shown up'.

In the early phases of an insight-directed treatment approach, if the patient does undergo a significant ego regression during the treatment session, it is important that the therapist help him to reverse such a regression towards the end of the session. The therapist must remember that the experience of regression itself may mobilize considerable anxiety, which may make it difficult for the patient to permit himself such a regression in subsequent therapeutic sessions. Helping the patient to reverse the regression provides a control of the degree of regression that will occur, and emphasizes to the patient that this is a reversible process and one which the therapist will not permit to get out of hand.

Such a reversal can be fostered by an intervention which focuses on the integrative and self-observing ego processes, or which asks the patient to summarize what has occurred in the session, or which merely points out that the session is nearing an end, thereby alerting the patient to the necessity of reinstituting his ego controls.

As therapy proceeds and the patient has had the repeated experience of undergoing such reversible ego regressions, such interventions become less necessary since the patient himself can now more effectively control the duration of the regressive process.

On the other hand, in supportive treatment strategy calls for the avoidance of further regression. Therefore, the therapist encourages the patient to an attitude expressed in the idea 'think first and then speak', whereby he encourages the maintenance of the secondary process and strengthens the effectiveness of the ego defences. In situations in which the patient has already manifested a significant ego regression in terms of directly expressing primary process material, the immediate tactics are to listen to such material, but as soon as possible after its expression to help the patient towards a more advanced and secondary process appraisal and evaluation of what he has said, or to focus the content of discussion into other areas.

In the attempt to avoid further regression, or if it occurs to reverse it, the therapist may interpose himself in a more reality-oriented intervention by giving the patient reassurance or direct interpersonal contact, and he prepares to close the session well in advance by focusing on the more progressive aspects of the material presented by the patient. This may also include going beyond the allotted time, or actively encouraging the patient to pull himself together, or inviting the patient to sit in another room until he feels more composed and ready to go home.

H. Social Amenities

Another area where education of the patient is necessary, particularly in insight-directed treatment, is in regard to the usual social amenities of an interpersonal situation. As will be elaborated in Chapter XII on Transference, insight-directed treatment involves the establishment of a therapeutic relationship in which there is a displacement of unconscious internal conflicts into the therapeutic situation, so that they may become more fully conscious and then be subjected to ego assessment and integration. To this end, the therapist deliberately diminishes the reality nature of the relationship since the greater the reality elements, the more difficult will it be to develop and demonstrate transference distortions. The therapist also attempts to carry out the treatment in a situation of relative transference frustration, thereby to intensify drive-derivatives in order that they may more readily become conscious.

As a result, the usual social amenities which are part of realistic non-therapeutic interpersonal relationships are generaly suspended in an insight-directed treatment situation. The therapist attempts to avoid interchanges in the nature of social chit-chat at the beginning or end of the sessions, and during the course of the therapeutic contact such things as helping the patient to pick up something which has been dropped, offering or receiving cigarettes, helping the patient off or on with a coat, casual comments or conversation, etc., are deliberately avoided. As therapy proceeds, such behaviours may become the vehicle for expression of various unconscious transference wishes or defences, and unthinkingly gratifying such derivatives may be contradictory to the overall strategy.

However, a patient unacquainted with the techniques of insight-directed therapy may experience this type of response as an insult, or as a manifestation of coldness or lack of interest by the therapist. Also, early in the course of a therapeutic contact such activities do not have the transference implications that they may come to have as the relationship develops further, and hence the patient will be less able to understand the therapist's behaviour and approach in these matters. Some type of explanation is therefore often necessary, in order that the patient can become aware that this is a part of the structure of the therapeutic situation.

One helpful way of dealing with this is to focus the patient's attention on to such behavioural manifestations from the beginning, while at times permitting their gratification. For example, a patient may ask the therapist for a cigarette which in the course of a normal social relationship would be offered without comment. In an insight-directed treatment situation, however, this may have a variety of different meanings and hence early in the course of treatment the therapist may give the cigarette but then ask the patient for further thoughts and associations in connection with this interchange. It may not be possible as yet to interpret its specific meaning since this may either be unknown to the therapist, or the patient may not yet be ready to accept such an interpretation, but the implicit suggestion that this behaviour may have other hidden meanings which should be explored is important in the education of the patient.

For the sake of the ultimate development of the transference relationship, it is important that such manifestations not be immediately over-interpreted before the patient has had the necessary experence and understanding to accept and integrate such an interpretation in a meaningful way. On the other hand, to let such behaviour continue without comment may encourage further acting-out and demands for drive-derivative gratification. It can most effectively be used in illustrating for the patient the way in which the process of psychotherapy is structured and proceeds. In other words, it begins to focus the patient into the necessity for observing the meaning and significance of the various interactions that he feels and experiences towards the therapist.

Paradoxically, the more that the therapist responds behaviourally to the patient's provocations, manipulations or seductions, the more 'dangerous' the therapeutic situation becomes for the patient. He may already feel an inability to control his own impulses except through massive neurotic defence mechanisms, and the more the patient feels that he is the stronger, and that he cannot rely on the therapist for the control of the relationship between them, the greater will be his anxiety. And if the patient can manipulate or control the behaviour of the therapist in minor ways, he may have interfering doubts and fears about the therapist's control in response to major provocations that may emerge later as the transference deepens. In this way, in the early therapeutic sessions, the patient frequently tests the therapist to see where the limits are and how far he can go. The therapist's attitude most helpfully is that in the therapeutic situation the patient is free to think and express in verbal form any and all thoughts, feelings, fantasies or impulses. However, the patient is not free to act upon them. One way in which such limits are established without the therapist taking a critical or prohibiting position is to focus the patient's attention on the acting and behavioural manifestations and, where possible, to interpret their meaning. This encourages the patient to abstain from action and instead to verbalize the impulse behind the act.

The patient may also be testing at this time to see whether the therapist is comfortable in his role, and whether or not he can tolerate the patient's feelings, or whether he can be frightened by the threat of action. In an insight-directed treatment approach, if the therapist permits the patient to act on his impulses without comment, the patient may be blocked from further regressive awareness of more primitive impulses by virtue of his anxiety that they may overwhelm his controls and likewise be expressed in behaviour.

The main point to be emphasized by the therapist and his attitude in these early sessions is not a moralistic or critical judgment of the patient's behaviour, but rather that it is in the best interests of the therapy if the patient can attempt to control the behaviour itself while verbalizing the feelings that stimulated it.

As will be elaborated in Chapter XII, the strategy of a supportive therapeutic approach involves the attempt to minimize transference distortions and frustrations, and to emphasize a therapeutic relationship based an conscious rapport and in keeping with the patient's ego structure and defences. With such a strategy, the tactics are to encourage the reality elements of the treatment relationship. Therefore the therapist is more likely to observe the social amenities, and to interact with the patient around them, more in keeping with his attitudes and behaviour in a non-therapeutic realistic interpersonal relationship. In supportive treatment, such realistic responses and gratifications by the therapist will usually not produce the effects described in the insight-treatment situation, since the rest of the treatment strategy is designed to avoid further regression and the uncovering of unconscious transference distortions. Hence the social amenities and interactions around them tend to be experienced by the patient in their realistic context, and regressive transference distortions are less likely.

However, in this context the therapist must follow the lead of the patient, recognizing that for some patients emotional distance is a requirement by virtue of their conflicts and defences, and that, therefore, a 'chummy' and personal relationship may mobilize greater anxiety and hence be contra-indicated. But in situations where this type of emotional distance has previously been maintained by the patient, it is particularly important for the therapist to respond positively to any overtures which the patient may make.

In such a setting, the response should be enough to meet the patient in his first venture towards a closer relationship, but not be so intense that it frightens or overwhelms him.

I. Patient's Efforts at Change

Another aspect of the patient's role is that he continue in his active attempts to modify his overall behaviour and reactions outside the therapeutic situation, on the basis of what is learned or experienced in the treatment setting. In both supportive and insight-directed psycho-therapy, mere verbalization of thoughts or feelings in the treatment setting is of little use alone, unless it results in some change of behaviour outside of the treatment sessions. It becomes important for the patient to recognize the continuity of his own mental life, and the fact that what he talks about or learns in the treatment setting is applicable and related to his present life outside of treatment, and that what occurs in his life outside the treatment session is also related to some of the intra-psychic emotional reactions and symptoms of which he complains.

Therefore, in both types of treatment the patient is eventually encouraged to face the symptom-producing situations or relationships, and to apply the lessons of his therapy to his current life. In the supportive situation, the therapist actively uses suggestion, reinforcement, approval, disapproval, or whatever interventions are appropriate to produce the desired behavioural change. In insight therapy the patient is expected to try new modes of adaptation on his own in order that he may become more independent and less reliant on the continuing activity of the therapist.

In other words, the patient's task includes continuing attempts at new modes of adaptation in interpersonal relationships, work, sexuality and generalized reactions in his current life outside the treatment. And these attempted new mechanisms or modes of integration should reflect the progress of the material and work going on in the process of treatment.

In this regard, one of the differences between supportive and insight-directed treatment is that in supportive therapy, the therapist focuses the patient's attention primarily on *conscious* ego mechanisms and attitudes, and emphasizes the role that they play in the patient's overall adaptation. In insight-directed treatment, on the other hand, the therapist also emphasizes and helps the patient to become aware of the *unconscious* conflicts, mechanisms and methods of adaptation, and as the patient becomes increasingly aware of these unconscious forces, he must then attempt to put this *now conscious* awareness to active use.

SUGGESTED READING

COLEMAN, JULES V. (1949) The initial phase of psychotherapy. *Bull. Menninger Clin.* 13, 189

DEUTSCH, FELIX (1949) *Applied Psychoanalysis*. Grune & Stratton, New York
GILL, MERTON, NEWMAN, RICHARD & REDLICH, FREDERICK C. (1954) *The Initial Interview in Psychiatric Practice*. International Universities Press Inc, New York
WOLBERG, LEWIS R. (1967) *The Technique of Psychotherapy*, Second edition. Grune Stratton Inc, & New York

CHAPTER XI

The Therapeutic Process:
The Therapist's Role

The role and activity of the therapist in the treatment process is dictated by the overall strategy and treatment goal, although individual tactics are influenced by the vicissitudes of the specific treatment relationship. The range of the therapist's activity runs in a spectrum from quiet listening at one end, to vigorous and forceful intervention and control of the patient's overt behaviour at the other.

All ranges of activity in various admixtures may occur in both insight-directed and supportive treatment. Varying shifts in the nature and level of the therapist's activity may occur during a single session; similarly, more lasting and general shifts in activity may occur during the various phases of treatment, or in response to specific vicissitudes of the treatment in progress.

In considering this spectrum of activity, it is helpful to describe the various forms, beginning with the least active. But it should be recognized that in the natural therapeutic setting such a division of activity into categories is not a static one, nor is it sharply circumscribed.

Listening

The first category to consider is that of quiet listening to the patient and giving him an opportunity to talk. The therapist provides a situation in which the patient may feel free to talk to another human being and be sure of that other person's interest, attention and concern, without any demand that he (the patient) return the favour. In this way the therapist is offering the patient a unique experience which in itself may have major significance and value.

Most non-therapeutic relationships occur on a give-and-take basis in which each participant is expected to be interested in the welfare and concerns of the other, and neither is permitted for long to exploit or claim exclusive attention to his own problems or desires. The psychotherapeutic situation, however, is different in that by mutual agreement, reached in the establishment of the therapeutic contract and relationship, the major (if not exclusive) area of interest is the patient and his difficulties and problems, and aside from the financial obligation, the therapist does not make personal requests or demands of his own on the patient. The luxury of having some-one listen to all that is said and treat it with regard, respect and interest is in itself a relatively unique phenomenon, and provides a significant gratification to the patient which is rarely offered in other human relation-ships.

However, the therapist's activity in listening involves a good deal more than the mere passive reception and recording of material verbalized by the patient. He also must make observations of the patient's non-verbal behaviour, thereby expanding his understanding of the latent meaning behind what the patient is saying. Such things as facial expression, tone of voice, posture, manifestations of affect such as anxiety, depression or guilt, the clenching of fists or jaws, etc., all add to the therapist's more precise understanding of the meaning of the patient's experience. The method and manner in which the patient presents, discusses or describes his thoughts and feelings will influence the ultimate understanding by the therapist, and such things as hesitation, embarrassment, shame, blocking, glibness, pleasure, etc., must be noted.

In keeping with the concept of psychic determinism, the pattern and sequence of the patient's material will likewise be of significance and should be noted, since ideas occurring in temporal juxtaposition frequently have other associative connections.

Another group of observations that should be made are those concerning material which has been omitted by the patient. If a particular area, relationship, reaction or body of material which might normally be anticipated as important in the patient's emotional or mental life has not been mentioned, such an omission may be significant in various ways.

Another body of data which the therapist must observe while listening is his own personal reactions to the patient and to the patient's material. The therapist uses himself as an exploring instrument, on the basis that his own personal reactions to the patient may indicate some of the effects which the patient produces in other people with whom he interacts. This may give the therapist a better understanding of the patient's inter-relationship to his environment outside the treatment setting.

At the same time as he is observing the various components of the primary data presented by the patient, the therapist's attitude in this listening process is one of 'free-floating attention'.

The therapist does not limit himself to the specific ideas, thoughts or feelings produced by the patient at that particular moment, but instead he considers the full range of possible meanings, implications and connections that the patient's material brings to his mind. He permits his own thoughts and associations to range freely over this material, without rigidly preconceived ideas as to its meaning and significance, and he looks for connections or associations of which the patient may or may not have been conscious.

As the therapist listens and observes, he may be reminded at times of similar phenomena, behaviour or experiences in general human living, or in particular other people. This may suggest possible meanings or implications for what the patient is saying. The therapist also may be reminded of events, experiences or reactions previously described by the patient in another context, which may or may not have bearing on the current material.

Another element in the listening process is the therapist's capacity for sensitive empathy with the patient as the patient presents his thoughts or describes his experience. Such empathy involves the therapist making a partial and transient identification with the patient, through which he attempts in a controlled fashion in part to experience those things the patient is describing. He puts himself into the patient's shoes, and tries to respond within himself as if, for the moment, he were the patient undergoing the particular experience or reaction. At that moment, the therapist tries to think and feel as if he were the patient, and not himself, and thereby tries to gain access into the inner emotional life and experience of the patient who is facing him.

In other words, the therapist uses himself as a recording and exploring instrument. He attempts to induce in himself a state of regression in the service of the ego, the ultimate goal of which is an attempt to understand the latent or unconscious meaning behind the total expression of the patient's material.

This process requires of the therapist that he be capable of giving up his own immediate identity and ego boundaries, and in a regressive fashion, attempt partially to identify with the image of the patient as it has evolved during the therapeutic contacts, and attempt to experience whatever the patient is describing as if he, the therapist, were the patient.

The therapist in this process will also have access to his own personal associations, experience, and reactions, and he can use them as a guide or point of comparison in evaluating possible omissions, exaggerations, or distortions in the patient's material. However, although he, the therapist, might have reacted or responded in a particular way to a certain set of circumstances, he must recognize that the patient, with a different background, experience, and intra-psychic organization, may respond differently.

As in other regressions in the service of the ego, such a regression within the therapist must be controlled, and be reversible at his conscious will. The partial identification and empathic understanding must alternate with a reversal of the regressive process, and a return to the secondary ego processes appropriate to an individual who bears the responsibilities and obligations of a therapist from whom the patient is seeking a specific form of help. In other words, after the therapist has attempted to develop an empathic emotional understanding of the patient's reactions, he must return psychologically to his own identity as therapist, and then evaluate this understanding from his own intellectual and theoretical frame of reference, and from his general knowledge of human phenomena and psychopathology. Only then is the therapist able to appreciate the overall significance of the material produced, and its part in the total psychic experience and functioning of the patient.

In the framework of general theory, and of the specific material previously produced by the patient, the therapist must assess whether or not the empathic understanding he has obtained is accurate, or whether it reflects some type of personal distortion. He must also look for other specific evidence supporting or negating such an understanding, and organize it in the context of his formulations regarding the patient and the patient's problems.

In addition, the therapist must decide how this bit of understanding fits into the overall strategy of therapy, and also how it is influenced by the immediate tactical situation. At times the therapist may gain a significant understanding of the meaning of a particular symptom or disturbance, but overall strategy may be such that this will never directly be presented to the patient. Not infrequently the therapist may gain a significant insight and an awareness into the underlying dynamic meaning behind particular conflicts or symptoms, but it may be a number of months or longer before the patient will be ready to work out and understand such a meaning. In subjecting his new insight to the secondary process, the therapist may also find it necessary to prepare the patient by various intermediate steps to arrive at this same understanding.

The therapist must also be aware of the immediate therapeutic situation as it influences his decision whether or not to present what he has understood to the patient. For example, if the therapeutic session is almost over, it may be tactically wiser to wait for another time, recognizing that the end of a session is usually not the best time to present the patient with a new idea.

The intensity of intermittent regression in the service of the ego and empathic identification with the patient must be controlled at optimal levels by the therapist. If it becomes fixed, or if reversal of the regressive process becomes difficult, the therapist loses much of his effectiveness by virtue of such an over-identification. He thus becomes less objective, and casts himself in the role of a friend or real object in the patient's life. However, if the therapist is incapable of such regression and empathy with the patient, and if he cannot experience or understand the patient's material except from his own level of development and emotional experience, he is to that extent a less therapeutically sensitive individual, and is therefore also hampered in the treatment process.

In summary, listening in a therapeutic sense involves an extremely active process occurring silently within the therapist, by which he permits himself the full range of observations of the total behaviour of the patient, and of his own associations and emotional responses to the material presented by the patient. He induces in himself a partial regression in the service of the ego, thereby searching for connections, associations, meanings and an empathic understanding through a partial and reversible identification with the patient. Having arrived at such an understanding, the therapist then reverses his own regressive ego processes, and returns to the objective position and secondary process thought of a therapist interacting with a patient. He then evaluates and organizes the understanding so achieved in the light of his overall theoretical and clinical knowledge, and also in the light of the strategy and immediate tactics of the particular treatment process. How such understanding and awareness are used by the therapist is a function of the therapeutic strategy and goals.

Clarification

The next most active form of intervention by the therapist may be considered under the concept of clarification, the immediate tactical goal of which is further to elaborate or clarify some aspect of the patient's experience, behaviour or thoughts.

Ideas, thoughts, feelings or memories which are partial, vague or ill-formed, are more difficult for the patient consciously to integrate. The more that such issues have been verbalized clearly, the more readily may they be subjected to the secondary process.

Clarification is focused on conscious and preconscious mental processes, and such interventions presume that the patient has access to the material, although he may not as yet have expressed it for himself or been fully aware of it. Clarification cannot be effective in instances where the material is unconscious, since those processes are not available easily to the patient's conscious attention.

The purpose of clarification may be to give the therapist a more clear or focused idea of what is being presented. However, at other times the therapist may have a reasonably complete understanding of the process but feel that the patient needs more clearly to recognize what he is expressing. Sometimes this involves rephrasing what the patient has already said but from a slightly different point of view in order that it may become more clear or precise. At other times it may involve asking the patient himself to rephrase some idea, so that in the process of doing this the patient becomes more explicitly aware of what has been going on in his own mind. Such interventions by the therapist may also include the request for greater detail, for further elaboration or for the patient to fill in with material that has been omitted or only partially expressed.

Confrontation

The next most active form of intervention is confrontation, by which the therapist directs the patient's attention to something conscious or pre-conscious which has already been expressed, but to which the patient's attention is not focused at the moment. At times this involves pointing out similarities or differences in certain bodies of material, or showing the patient repetitive patterns derived from the experiences, feelings and thoughts already presented. It may involve calling the patient's attention to behaviour or responses of which he can easily become conscious, or it may at times involve reminding the patient of previously expressed material or experience.

In essence, confrontation involves directing the patient's attention to elements of experience or behaviour observed in him by the therapist, but without drawing any inferences as to the possible meanings behind them.

Interpretation

Clarification and confrontation are often considered as preparations for interpretation, which is the next most active type of intervention by the therapist.

The therapist's role in listening and observation has already been described, and as these processes occur he continues to draw for himself a variety of inferences as to the latent meaning of the patient's communications and behaviour. He subjects such inferences to critical scrutiny to assess their accuracy and validity, and to marshall the supporting evidence for them. When the therapist communicates some element or aspect of these inferences to the patient, this is known as an interpretation.

The tactical goal of an interpretation is to help the patient become consciously aware of the meaning of some element in his own mental life. Strategically this involves the patient recognizing mental contents that were previously unconscious and defended against and, therefore, interpretation is a tool chiefly in an insight-directed treatment situation, and it is less commonly used in supportive treatment. The technique and details of the art of interpretation are an extensive and complex subject which cannot be fully elaborated in this discussion. Only some of the highlights will be described here, recognizing that interpretation is a skill which is developed only gradually with the therapist's increasing clinical experience and sophistication.

Interpretations can be classified as involving content, or resistance. When the topographical hypothesis served as the basis of therapy, the therapeutic task was seen as 'making the Unconscious Conscious'. As a result, the therapist was extremely active and direct in making interpretations of the content of unconscious drives, and if the patient could not accept or understand the interpretation, it was thought to be a reflection of the patient being in a state of resistance, and lacking co-operation.

The development of the structural hypothesis and the elaboration of ego psychology have resulted in a shift of therapeutic technique, and a recognition that unconscious resistances and defences against awareness must first be reduced in order that an interpretation of the content of the drives can be fully effective. Mere interpretation of such content, without regard for the resistances maintained against this awareness, will result in minimal or no therapeutic change.

In Chapter IV the basic concept in psychopathology was developed that defence mechanisms are methods by which the ego avoids the experience of anxiety which occurs when there is a threatened return to consciousness of an unacceptable drive or drive-derivative. The reduction of a defence by interpretation modifies the dynamic steady state in the direction of permitting the drive-derivative closer access to consciousness. The theoretical prediction would therefore be that successful interpretation of a resistance or defence will tend temporarily to increase the patient's anxiety. In clinical practice, this is generally true.

When an unconscious drive-derivative becomes fully conscious, it can be subjected to the secondary process and can be more readily integrated and mastered by the ego. The theoretical prediction would be that correct interpretations of the content of the drive-derivatives will reduce the intensity of anxiety. In general, this proves to be correct in clinical practice.

Thus, the usual procedure in insight treatment is first to interpret resistances to the patient, since if they are conscious, the patient's ego can attempt to reduce the intensity of their use. This is generally followed by an interpretation of the content of the drives which had been defended against by the resistances.

One characteristic of effective interpretation is the need to work from the surface of the mind towards the depths. In other words, interpretations should start with some mental process which is conscious to the patient, and proceed towards a further exploration of material which is not as yet conscious but relatively close to consciousness. The process of interpretation involves a step-wise and sequential deepening of the patient's awareness. As this awareness increases, the conscious point of departure for further interpretation is likewise deepened. Interpretations which make long jumps between the patient's conscious awareness and the inference drawn by the therapist will tend to be less specific and less accurate by virtue of the level of inference and leap that have been made by the therapist. They also leave the patient without a sense of personal experience and conviction, and this generally leads to intellectualized understanding.

Another factor in the technique of interpretation is the correct timing of when to impart to the patient the inference which has been drawn. An interpretation which is made before the patient's resistances have been reduced, or prior to the time the patient's ego processes are capable of integrating the material to be interpreted, may have one of several effects. In some instances, it may fall on completely deaf ears, and have little or no meaning for the patient. At other times, premature interpretations, particularly if correct, may mobilize more anxiety and conflict than the patient is capable of tolerating, or may evoke further regression. Such premature interpretation may also result in mobilizing new resistances against the material that has been interpreted, thereby delaying the treatment process.

An interpretation which is made too late (after the patient himself has already become conscious of the material being interpreted) has little therapeutic impact, and means that the therapist has missed an opportunity to have speeded up the therapeutic process by having made this interpretation sooner.

A correctly timed interpretation of content is one which is given at a time when the patient's resistances have been sufficiently lowered that the material to be interpreted is relatively close to the patient's consciousness, although he has not yet verbalized or conceptualized it. The same general principle holds for the interpretation of the resistances themselves. When the particular defence or resistance in question is extremely intense, or when it still serves a major psychic function, an interpretation of its existence will in all likelihood be relatively ineffective. The most effective time to interpret such a resistance is when there is evidence that its importance or use is beginning to diminish, or that the drive-derivatives against which this resistance was maintained are coming closer to consciousness.

In other words, the correct time for an interpretation involves a judgment by the therapist of the patient's readiness to accept and understand that which is being interpreted.

Another issue regarding the timing of an interpretation is the more focal one of the point in the session, or in the treatment schedule. For example, if the therapist arrives at an inference towards the end of a treatment session, it may be wiser to postpone making the interpretation to another time, particularly if it is likely to evoke considerable anxiety. To make the interpretation at that time would leave the patient to struggle with the material, and the anxiety mobilized, by himself rather than to have the therapist's support and help in the immediate interval after the material has been made conscious. It might also encourage the patient to solidify old resistances, or to develop new ones, in the interval until the next session. The same would be true in situations where the therapist anticipates a cancelled session, holiday or vacation. These interrupt the regular therapeutic continuity and hence it may be wiser not to confront the patient with a lot of new or distressing material to deal with during the separation.

Another aspect of interpretation is the factor of dosage, or the amount to be interpreted at any one time. A full or complete interpretation would include the current drive-derivatives as well as the defences against them, and the genetic origins of both. It would also include the manifestations of the conflict in the transference interactions with the therapist, and a recapitulation from this to other current attitudes and relationships. Even in insight-directed treatment most interpretations are incomplete and partial, and are made with the intention of elaborating or completing them at a later time. It is important not to overwhelm the patient with material, or with the interpretation of large number of resistances simultaneously, or with an interpretation which is likely to mobilize more anxiety or conflict than the patient can tolerate. The immediate tactical aim is to help the patient gain a particular piece of understanding, and to fill out more of the complete interpretation after the first part has been dealt with and accepted.

In supportive treatment, the therapist may be particularly inclined to give partial or even partially incorrect interpretations in an attempt to achieve a specific symptomatic response. In this way he may be offering the patient an opportunity to use mechanisms of displacement or rationalization, and to continue the repression by focusing the patient's attention to an aspect of the problem which is less anxiety-provoking, and more acceptable. The same might be true in the use of interpretation to reinforce intellectualization by providing the patient with an explanation of the content of a conflict while strengthening defences against its emotional impact and fostering the use of further isolation of affect.

Another aspect of interpretation is tact and phrasing. The therapist is trying to show the patient some aspect of his own mental processes which unconsciously he does not wish to recognize or understand. It is therefore essential that this be presented in a tactful way, and that the therapist avoid making the interpretation a form of direct or veiled criticism. This concept of tact often involves emphasizing to the patient that the unpleasant aspect of the material is not the patient's total reaction or wish, but that he is in a state of conflict between two opposing tendencies. For example, if the therapist wants to interpret a patient's unconscious hostility towards his children, it is important to point out that although he is involved with unconscious hostile or aggressive impulses, he also has conscious attitudes of warmth, love and desire for the children's safety. In this way, the patient can more readily begin to explore the unconscious hostility since this is not presented as his *only* attitude or wish, and the therapist is also recognizing his attempts to struggle against such impulses.

In terms of phrasing an interpretation, it is helpful to use the patient's own idiom and vocabulary, and there are times when the therapist and patient develop a personal and specifically private vocabulary between them. In this connection, it is helpful to avoid the use of technical or theoretical terms, particularly in insight-directed treatment, in order that the interpretation will have a personal and emotional impact, rather than a purely intellectual one. In supportive treatment, on the contrary, if isolation and intellectualization are being reinforced, the use of technical terms might be highly appropriate. At times it may be necessary to modify the phrasing of an interpretation, using different words or a somewhat different perspective or emphasis, in an attempt to make the material as meaningful as possible for the particular patient, and in this connection, it is helpful to stay away from stereotypes.

In terms of tact and phrasing, it is also important that the therapist maintain the therapeutic atmosphere while making interpretations. If his attitude is one of condescension, smugness, superiority, criticism, or a feeling of triumph over the patient when presenting him with an inference regarding his behaviour, this will significantly interfere with the patient's capacity effectively to tolerate and integrate the new insight. It is helpful to keep in mind that without the patient's co-operation and efforts, such an insight or inference would be impossible for the therapist, and therefore the success belongs just as much to the patient as to the therapist.

Such a sobering attitude in the therapist is helpful in minimizing the patient's responses to the interpretation as an attack. In spite of this, however, there are patients who respond to all interpretations as an attack, or criticism. When the therapist becomes aware of this, it is important to deal with such generalized reactions to interpretations before making further similar interventions.

After each interpretation made to the patient, it is important that the therapist assess whether or not it was correct.

A variety of reactions may occur in response to a correct interpretation. There may be the production of further material by the patient which confirms the content of the interpretation offered. It may also bring a change in the patient's behaviour in the treatment session, or in his life outside. The interpretation of a resistance may result in an intensification of the patient's anxiety, and the correct interpretation of content will frequently be followed by a reduction of anxiety. At other times the patient will have a subjective feeling 'that's right', or may indicate a feeling that the interpretation now seems obvious, and may even have some chagrin that he was unable to recognize it himself.

Another response to a correct interpretation may be laughter without recognizing the source. This results from a change in the dynamics of the psychic economy at that particular moment, where the psychic energy previously used in the defence against the material just interpreted is suddenly released as excess since the defence is no longer so necessary. The sudden laughter is similar to the dynamics of humour and wit.

Another frequent indication of a correct interpretation is a highly emotional, vigorous and immediate denial, sometimes followed by a subsequent direct or indirect confirmation. The dynamics of this response involve the breaching of a defence which is immediately reinstituted. If the interpretation were not correct and did not influence the patient in an affective way, there would be no need for the violent or emotional denial and instead there would result a more controlled or considered opinion by the patient.

As mentioned before, when an interpretation is correct in content, but poorly timed in the sense of being premature, there may be a sharp intensification of anxiety. At other times, there may result an intellectual, but non-affective acceptance by the patient, and sometimes it may result in a temporary change of the relationship between therapist and patient.

If an interpretation is incorrect, many times there is no particular response in the patient, and no evidence that it has resulted in a further forward movement in the treatment. With particularly passive and dependent patients whose major aim is to please the therapist by accepting whatever is offered, there is often a glib positive response which lacks the emotional impact of a correct interpretation. At other times the patient may ignore the interpretation, and continue as if it had not been made, or avoid the subject completely. Frequently the patient may disagree in a quiet, controlled fashion, quite different qualitatively from the intense emotional negation that may follow a correct interpretation.

The assessment of the correctness of an interpretation is facilitated if, before he makes it, the therapist predicts to himself what effect he expects the interpretation to have. He then can compare, at least in general terms, the patient's response with his own prediction. Then if the prediction proves to have been incorrect, he is in a position to examine the total situation again to try to find the cause of the error.

Suggestion and Prohibition

The next most active form of intervention by the therapist is the introduction of definite positive or negative suggestions, instructions or prohibitions into the therapeutic relationship, in an attempt directly and immediately to influence the patient's thoughts, feelings or behaviour. Since such interventions involve considerable activity by the therapist and a departure from the neutral participant-observer role, they are more common and indicated in cases seen in supportive therapy. The therapist can readily make use of his position in the patient's current life and psychic economy, emphasizing his own reactions to the patient's behaviour and not infrequently suggesting the particular change on the basis of his personal interest in the patient and the patient's welfare.

In other words, by virtue of the dynamics implicit in the therapeutic relationship, the therapist uses himself and the patient's wish to please him as a motivating force. Having attempted or successfully accomplished the task set by the therapist, the patient will anticipate and expect some sign of recognition or reward for his efforts. Thus it becomes important that the therapist find ways of gratifying such demands, but he must choose a reward which will be appropriate to this particular patient, considering his specific psychodynamics and psychopathology.

By such interventions the therapist actively intercedes in the patient's dynamic equilibrium, at times in regard to the intrapsychic components, and at times in regard to the patient's interactions with his environment.

Such activity may be directed towards strengthening the patient's conscious controls or his unconscious ego defences. Examples of this would include such things as: 'Put such thoughts out of your mind, and think of something nice instead'; 'Learn to think more and count to 10 before you speak or act'; 'If you're afraid to be alone, arrange to have someone go with you'; 'When you feel that way, go outside until you can control it', etc.

At other times, such interventions may be designed to gratify some component of the unconscious drives or drive-derivatives. Examples of this would include such things as: 'You should try to date more'; 'Take a vacation and get away from your troubles for a while'; 'Feelings of anger are normal, so when you feel that way, express it and don't hold your feelings in so tightly'; 'As long as it is agreeable to both partners, anything you want to do sexually is all right'; 'Learn to be more selfish', etc.

Where possible the therapist may actively attempt to help the patient find a more effective and stable compromise which permits expression of drive-derivatives as well as defences. This might include encouraging the patient to find an appropriate hobby, or an interest in athletics, or in outside service and activity, or suggesting socially approved ways of expressing unacceptable drives.

The therapist may also give specific advice on how to behave or react in various reality situations, or how to handle or resolve particular external problems.

In using all these various active interventions, it is generally wiser to wait until the treatment and therapeutic relationship is sufficiently well established that there is a reasonable likelihood the patient will be able and willing to co-operate with the therapist's suggestion. Such interventions are also more effective if given at a time when the transference and thera-peutic relationship is chiefly positive, since the patient will then be in a more receptive mood. If the suggestion is made at a time when the relation-ship is negative and the patient is consciously or unconsciously hostile to the therapist, there will be a tendency for the patient to reject and refuse the intervention, and hence it is unlikely to be successful.

If such interventions are presented to the patient as absolute requirements or demands, and for one reason or another the patient is unable to fulfil them, he may be left with a feeling of loss of face, guilt or shame, and a feeling that the therapist will be angry or disappointed. Making such an absolute demand may also challenge some patients to defy the therapist.

It is therefore wiser to phrase this type of intervention in a tentative way, stressing such ideas as 'To the best of your ability', or, 'It would help if you would try this'. It is also wise first to attempt to do this with symptoms or behaviour patterns which are the least entrenched, and least anxiety-provoking, since in that group there is a greater likelihood of immediate success from the intervention. Such success with relatively minor symptoms or disturbances will enhance the patient's confidence as well as the therapist's prestige. This will make it more likely that subsequent suggestions will likewise lead to successful change.

Although these forms of active intervention are most common in supportive treatment, there are also occasions during the course of insight-directed therapy where they become necessary in order to further the therapeutic movement. Uusually they are introduced after other less active forms of intervention by the therapist have proved unsuccessful.

This is particularly the case when extensive discussion of the pre-conscious and unconscious meanings behind a particular symptom or disturbance has not produced significant change, and a static state has persisted for some time. Such interventions are then presented from the standpoint that it would help the ultimate therapeutic progress and understanding if the patient would consciously try to modify or control the particular pattern involved, and then permit himself to be aware of the thoughts and feelings that occur as the symptom is being consciously changed.

In other words, in supportive psychotherapy, the therapist uses himself and his own wishes as a motivating instrument during these interventions. In insight-directed treatment, the emphasis is on the need to provide new material for discussion on the basis that if the patient is able, through conscious effort, to modify the symptom or behaviour, then the feelings and thoughts hidden behind it may more readily come to consciousness, and be subjected to therapeutic work.

Such interventions are thus placed in the framework of the patient doing what is best for himself and his treatment. From that point of view, the patient's expectation or request for a direct reward can then be dealt with as a manifestation of transference by helping him see that his motivation is more the wish for transference gratification than the wish to do what is in his own best interest. Also, if the patient refuses or avoids the requested change, this likewise may be dealt with as a manifestation of resistance or of other transference implications.

Even with such active interventions in an insight-directed treatment situation, the therapist attempts to maintain the neutral participant-observer role, and to de-emphasize his own personal involvement in the suggestion.

Active Control

The most active form of intervention by the therapist is that in which he assumes a surrogate-ego function for the patient and carries out (either himself or through designated helpers) ego functions which the patient himself is not capable of maintaining at that time. Such interventions range from interceding on the patient's behalf with relatives, employers or social agencies, etc., to controlling the patient in a hospital setting with all the regulations of the patient's behaviour that this entails. This may go so far as providing for physical restraint or seclusion or the forcible administration of somatic or drug therapy. Any such active control or manipulation will have a psychological impact on the patient, over and above any chemical or physiological effects that may also occur.

Such forms of intervention constitute ways in which the patient increasingly becomes a passive object of the therapist's active efforts or manipulations, and they occur almost exclusively in a supportive treatment relationship where the patient has manifested such intense ego regression that for the moment he is incapable of autonomous function.

It is important that the therapist be alert to indications of a reversal of this regression. As the patient himself becomes capable of increased ego participation and activity, the therapist to that degree should be ready to relinquish the surrogate-ego role, and to reinforce and encourage the patient's efforts to assume control of his own behaviour and problems.

There are instances during the course of an insight-directed treatment relationship where, in response to an acute conflict or crisis, such an intervention by the therapist becomes necessary (i.e. the patient developing an acute psychotic reaction, or becoming a serious suicidal risk). It must be recognized, however, that such interventions are contradictory to the overall strategy of an insight-directed therapeutic approach, and the necessity for them may constitute a reason for changing the goals of the treatment in a more supportive direction. Even if the decision is made to continue towards the goals of insight-directed treatment, the impact and repercussions of such interventions on the treatment relationship must be anticipated. The fact of their occurrence will have various effects on the transference relationship as it is subsequently evolved and ultimately resolved.

The Therapeutic Position

At all levels of activity, it is necessary that the therapist be simultaneously aware of the nature and impact of all the various forces involved in the dynamic equilibrium. To do this, he must take an observational position equidistant from id, ego, super-ego and environmental processes.

In this regard, the 'ontogenetic development' of the individual therapist to some extent recapitulates the 'phylogenetic development' of psychoanalysis. Freud and the early workers were at first particularly preoccupied with the various dramatic, insistent and compelling manifestations of the drives and their derivatives. It was only after continuing and more sophisticated clinical experience that their attention was increasingly focused on the other components of mental life. It was this shift which resulted in the development of the structural hypothesis and an increasing emphasis on ego and super-ego psychology.

This same evolution occurs during the training and development of most dynamic psychiatrists. Initially their attention and interest is directed towards verifying the presence of the unconscious drives and their various manifest derivatives. It is only after increased clinical experience that they develop a corresponding interest in ego and super-ego functions, and recognize their importance as determinants of psychopathology. It is only after this personal evolution occurs in the therapist that he is able to take the ideal observational position described above.

The importance of taking this position stems from the fact that psychotherapy is a highly selective process, and that the therapist plays an active part in influencing and focusing the material under discussion. Consciously and unconsciously the patient is acutely sensitive to the interventions made by the therapist, and it has been repeatedly demonstrated that indications of the therapist's interest and attention will significantly influence the subsequent material produced by the patient.

By paying more attention or intervening in response to certain communications and not to others, the therapist helps to determine the material brought up, even though he may follow the patient's lead. And the less that the therapist usually says, the greater will be the impact on the selection process when he eventually does take some particular element of the patient's communication as a focus of interest or intervention.

Regardless of the type of treatment, the therapist must be interested in all the different aspects of the patient's mental life. In any particular session or group of sessions, he may focus upon one of the groups of mental functions. But if some other group of mental processes is repeatedly omitted from the therapeutic work, it is important that the therapist recognize this and try to understand the reasons for the omission.

The therapist's ability to take this equidistant therapeutic position is an important factor in permitting the patient to present his material with minimal external contamination or distortion.

In summary, the role and range of activity on the part of the therapist is a considerable one, both within the single therapeutic session, and over the total duration of treatment. However, if the therapist has a clear idea of the basic strategy, and of the goals of treatment, then the tactics of the various interventions he makes can be internally consistent and logically structured in keeping with the basic theory.

SUGGESTED READING

FELDMAN, SANDOR (1958) Blanket interpretations. *Psychoanal. Quart.* **27**, 205

FENICHEL, OTTO (1941) *Problems of Psychoanalytic Technique.* The Psychoanalytic Quart. Inc

FINESINGER, JACOB E. (1948) Psychiatric interviewing: Some principles and procedures in insight therapy. *Am. J. Psychiat.* **105**, 187

GLOVER, EDWARD (1931) The therapeutic effect of inexact interpretation. *Int. J. Psycho-Anal.* **12**, 397

KRIS, ERNST (1951) Ego psychology and interpretation in psychoanalytic therapy. *Psychoanal. Quart.* **20**, 15

LOWENSTIEN, RUDOLPH M. (1951) The problem of interpretation. *Psychoanal. Quart.* **20**, 1

PARAD, HOWARD J. (1958) *Ego Psychology and Dynamic Casework.* Family Service Assn of America

PAUL, LOUIS P. (1963) *Psychoanalytic Clinical Interpretation.* Free Press of Glencoe, New York

CHAPTER XII

Transference

Introduction

Some of the elements in the therapeutic relationship have been described in Chapter IX, where it was pointed out that a significant component occurs at the level of a reality agreement and interaction between patient and therapist. However, a far larger component of the patient's relationship and reactions to the therapist stems from unconscious forces and factors within the patient. These unconscious forces have also been alluded to in several earlier chapters under the term Transference, and this concept will now be elaborated.

In Chapter V the point was made of the way in which the ego scans the external reality situation, seeking objects on which to displace and express the unconscious infantile or childhood drives and fantasies, or the various defences against such drives. The genetic hypothesis emphasizes that at any particular point in time, an individual's reactions are influenced by the sum total of his experiences and relationships up to that point, and that the earliest parental object relationships serve as the prototypes of subsequent relationships. As conceptualized by the repetition compulsion, unconscious drives (and the defences against them) remain active and continue to press for discharge and gratification from objects as closely identical to the original ones as possible.

With these concepts as background, transference may be understood as a form of displacement in which the individual unconsciously displaces on to a current object those drives, defences, attitudes, feelings and responses which were experienced or developed in relationships with earlier objects in the individual's life. Since the prototype of all object relationships are the earliest relationships to the parents, these serve as the ultimate core and origin of the psychic experiences being transferred to the current object. However, transference may also involve displacement of later experiences and relationships with objects other than the parents. This diplacement occurs unconsciously, and thereby leads the individual to experience reactions towards the current object which are derived not from the reality of the present situation and interaction, but rather from his own unconscious internal psychic life.

Such displacements are ubiquitous and occur to some extent in all people. They are manifested by reactions to an object which are not in keeping with, or which are out of proportion to, the reality aspects of the current relationship. These may be expressed by a generalized pattern of reaction and expectation regarding other people, or by highly specific reactions to a particular person. In the latter, there is some characteristic of the person or the relationship which is unconsciously associated to the individual's relationship with an earlier object.

There is no sharp dividing line between a realistic response to a current object and a response in which displacement is a factor. The displacement may involve only a selection of reality factors for conscious attention, by which an individual is aware of those aspects of a current object or relationship that fit in with the displacement, and in a selective fashion denies or ignores other attributes. The more that an object relationship is involved in distortion, or based on unconscious displacement of intra-psychic forces, the more neurotic is the relationship. The more that an individual is involved in unconscious infantile or childhood conflicts (the more severe the neurotic disturbance), the greater will be the likelihood of interactions in the current sphere being based on displacement, and the greater will be the potentiality for such displacement when new relationships are formed.

Transference Development

When such displacements occur in the therapeutic situation they are known as transference reactions. In a transference response, the patient displaces to the therapist and to the therapeutic relationship the drives, affects, moral values, defences, and integrative mechanisms previously experienced in relationships to other important objects in his life. These unconscious transference reactions constitute a significant part of the patient-therapist relationship, and must be distinguished from the non-transference aspects which are the patient's appropriate responses to the reality interactions between himself and the therapist.

When the patient first comes to therapy, he may bring with him a variety of pre-formed transference reactions, by virtue of his unconscious displacements to others in his environment. These may range from positive, expectant and trusting attitudes, to negative, cynical and suspicious ones. Even the patient who comes to an initial interview and refuses to talk on the basis that he doesn't trust the therapist is manifesting a transference relationship, since by his behaviour he is saying, 'People are untrustworthy, and you are like everybody else, and I cannot trust you'. There may be a variety of fantasies and conflicts behind such an attitude, but the patient is not responding to the reality of the therapist's attitude or role, but rather on the basis of an expectation displaced on to the therapist and based on the patient's previous fantasies or experiences with other objects.

Regardless of the intensity or extent of the patient's pre-formed transference attitudes, a number of factors in the structure and development of the therapeutic situation predispose him towards the further development of more intense transference reactions than he would experience in a non-therapeutic reality relationship. Thus the term 'transference' is usually reserved for the unconscious components of the patient's relationship to the therapist in the treatment situation. And as will be elaborated, this unconscious transference relationship becomes an important therapeutic tool, the use of which is different in insight-directed versus supportive therapy.

A. Regression

In the process of symptom-formation, the patient has already undergone a significant degree of regression with a reawakening and further intensification of infantile or childhood conflict. As a result, the potentiality for the displacement of this earlier conflict in the form of a transference reaction will be greater than it was prior to the onset of the illness or disturbance; and the more regressed the individual, the greater can the distortions be in the transfer of feelings from past objects on to the therapist.

Parenthetically, this difference in the depth of regression in part accounts for the difference in transference reactions in cases of psychosis as compared with neurosis. A psychotic individual, by virtue of his greater regression, is likely to develop intense, but volatile and unstable transference reactions, which are not as readily offset by the awareness in the patient that the feelings or fantasies expressed are not realistically appropriate. The psychotic patient's inability to recognize that such reactions are based on transference, and the thought or expectation that such a relationship is or should be a real one, may make the therapy of psychotic patients considerably more difficult and complex.

B. Position of the Therapist

Another factor is that the therapist, by virtue of his position, skill and training, becomes endowed by the patient with the power of an authority figure to whom the patient now turns with a request for help in his distress. In other words, the patient comes for treatment because he has been unable himself to deal with the symptoms or problems that beset him, and he now appeals to someone whom he hopes will have the necessary skill and power to provide the benefits and help he is seeking.

In this way, there is an immediate creation of an unequal situation in which the patient's needs for the therapist are greater than those of the therapist for the patient, and the patient finds himself in a situation of appealing to an authority figure whom he may also endow with a variety of magical powers and other expectations. Thus there is recreated in the treatment setting the situation of a relatively weaker and helpless child relating to a relatively stronger authority and parental object who is perceived as holding the needed power, help, and sources of satisfaction.

In addition, there is the factor of the common cultural role of the physician or therapist, which stems also from infantile and childhood feelings and further reinforces the magical expectations of the patient.

C. Repetition Compulsion

Another factor leading to intensified transference reactions in the treatment situation involves the effects of the repetition compulsion. The patient seeks to repeat previous experiences of psychic importance, either to achieve again the pleasure of those infantile and childhood drives which were gratified, or to re-experience previously frustrating situations with the goal of achieving gratification this time.

In either event, the continuing wish for satisfaction and the continuing attempts at drive discharge, in the setting of other transference forces, leads to the use of the therapist as the anticipated object of such gratification. The therapist then becomes the object of displacement of the drives, and the projected source of super-ego values, prohibitions, and punishments, particularly since the therapist deliberately presents himself as an object for the patient's fantasies. The ego must integrate these conflicting forces developing in the relationship to the therapist, and the tendency is to use the same mechanisms as those used in the earlier conflict situation.

In a general way, the more repetitively and frequently that the patient and therapist meet, the more does the therapist become the object of the drives, the super-ego, and the defences.

D. Absence of Reality Information

Another factor in the therapeutic situation that leads to the intensification of transference reactions is that the patient must express to the therapist a large amount of personal information, while the therapist, on the other hand, responds with relatively few personal cues or confidences concerning himself. And the patient has relatively few modes of access to information about the therapist as a real person. In other non-therapeutic relationships, when the patient interacts with an object, he receives a far larger number of returning external reality responses to which, in turn, he can react, thereby keeping the relationship more reality oriented. In the treatment setting, and in conjunction with the other factors in the treatment process, the less that the patient knows about the therapist, the more likely is he to displace and project to this neutral object the drives and defences which emanate from unconscious intra-psychic processes.

This same principle is used in projective psychological testing, where the subject is called upon to respond to a non-specific stimulus. Since no realistically specific or 'right' response is possible, whatever reactions the subject has to the stimulus must be a reflection of processes within himself rather than related directly to the stimulus object.

Furthermore, in the treatment situation, if the therapist does not immediately correct such transference distortions, or confront the patient with the reality of the situation, and if he is not depreciatory or critical of the patient's transference reactions, there will be further fostering of transference development.

E. Regression in the Service of the Ego

The development of regression in the service of the ego during insight-directed treatment was described in Chapter X and will be elaborated in Chapter XIII. As with spontaneous regressions, this will intensify the patient's tendency towards the displacement of conflict. Regression in the service of the ego occurs chiefly during the therapeutic session, and since the therapist is present at that moment, he tends to become the object of the drives and super-ego, and hence of the defences as well.

F. Transference Frustration

Another factor bearing on the development of the transference is the frustration of the patient's displaced wishes as they arise, and the carrying out of treatment in a situation of relative abstinence of drive gratification by the therapist. Such abstinence tends to intensify the pressure of the unconscious transference drives seeking discharge, and to bring them closer to consciousness. This in turn permits both the patient and therapist more easily to recognize the nature of the unconscious wish, and of the accompanying fantasy of danger if the wish is expressed. On the other hand, gratification of the unconscious derivatives of a drive tends at least temporarily to reduce drive tension, thereby decreasing the pressures toward conscious awareness. Thus the rule of abstinence applies chiefly to insight-directed treatment, where it is coupled with the therapist's interpretations of the transference relationship.

G. Fantasy Nature of the Relationship

Different from other reality interactions and situations, the therapeutic relationship remains primarily one of fantasy rather than reality for the patient. Since the expression of transference drives or fantasies by the patient will not result in a response by the therapist at the level of reality, the patient becomes free to experience and express drives and wishes which would ordinarily be withheld in situations where the object would tend to respond directly.

For example, if a person in real life expresses sexual attraction for someone else, an overt sexual response or relationship may be forthcoming. In the treatment situation, the patient's knowledge that expression of such feeling will not result in a sexual response by the therapist or lead to overt sexual activity, permits him to become conscious of such wishes, and to express them directly. Similarly, in a reality relationship, if an individual expresses hostility towards someone else, there is a likelihood that there will be a retaliation, or a significant change in the total relationship. The fact that this does not occur in the treatment situation, and that the therapist neither retaliates nor withdraws, permits the patient more freely to develop such transference feelings.

On the one hand, this absence of a response in the therapist becomes a source of frustration for the patient, in that the drive-derivatives become increasingly manifest and conscious, but cannot be satisfied. At the same time, however, this lack of responsiveness is a source of reassurance, in that it permits the patient an opportunity to express the feelings and fantasies previously warded off, without having to take immediate responsibility for them, or to be afraid that they will lead to some type of immediate act.

If the therapist becomes involved in a realistic social or emotional relationship with the patient, or if he gratifies derivative transference wishes in the treatment sessions, the patient will have difficulty in permitting the emergence into consciousness of more regressive transference manifestations, lest these also produce action and gratification contrary to the rest of the patient's mental life. Some patients find it necessary to test the therapist repeatedly in this regard before they can emotionally accept reassurance of his therapeutic intention.

H. The Therapist's Activity

The development and intensity of transference reactions is also significantly influenced by the therapist's behaviour and interventions. By keeping himself and the therapeutic situation relatively constant, he establishes a setting in which changes in the patient's responses to him can be more easily recognized as resulting from shifts in intra-psychic forces within the patient. By maintaining transference abstinence he aids the intensification of drive pressures, as described earlier. By accepting the patient's expression of transference distortions without criticism, defensiveness, personally hurt feelings, or premature reality explanations he fosters the further expression of transference manifestations. By confrontations or interpretations of transference manifestations (regarding the drive or super-ego components, or the ego defences against them) he promotes further verbal expression and elaboration of these reactions, and indicates his interest in them as well as his willingness to deal with them openly as with any other psychic processes. And by demonstrating the relevance and significance of transference phenomena, he places the whole subject in a reasonable and useful perspective for the patient's self-observing and therapeutic ego functions.

In a therapeutic situation where strategy calls for minimal conscious awareness in the patient of transference elements, the therapist responds differently regarding these tactical manoeuvres. The therapist's intention is to emphasize only the conscious components of the relationship, and he responds so as *not* to foster the emergence of unconscious transference responses.

Manifestations

The manifestations of transference are extremely varied and no catalogue or listing would be possible. As in all psychic experience, they reflect the interplay of id, ego and super-ego forces as these are increasingly focused upon the therapist, and reflect the specific details of the patient's past history and experience, as well as the vicissitudes of his current life and the treatment situation itself. Within the individual patient, manifestations will also vary in relationship to the patient's progress in his therapy.

In a general way, transference reactions may be classified as positive or negative. The positive transference refers to all drives and drive-derivatives relating to the libidinal impulses, both those directly eroticized and those which have been neutralized in forms of non-sexual love, while the negative transference refers to all of the various derivatives of the aggressive drives. The transferring of both positive and negative drive-derivatives may originate from conflicts or fixation points at any or all levels of psychosexual development, and the specifically transferred wishes, expectations, and defences will be organized in forms appropriate to the level of conflict currently activated. They will frequently involve precise repetitions of conflicts or experiences with significant earlier objects which occurred at those levels.

For example, positive transference derivatives may be oral and may involve wishes for passivity, dependency, maternal protection, unqualified love, etc.; they may be anal and involve wishes for praise, compliance, control, penetration, homosexuality, anal pleasure, etc.; or they may be phallic-oedipal wishes for praise, exhibitionism, admiration, genital sexuality, pregnancy, etc. Similarly, the negative transference wishes may stem from oral conflicts over basic mistrust, rejection, destructive sadistic or hostile devouring wishes, etc.; from anal conflict involving defiance, anal sadism, mastery, obstinacy, etc.; or from phallic-oedipal wishes involving competition, power, castration complexes, potency, etc.

The transference manifestations may also be mixed, and show various simultaneous combinations of both positive and negative qualities, as well as considerable fluctuation in their intensity and variability in their pattern, depending on the specific nature of the predominating drive or drive-derivative at any particular moment.

In both positive and negative transferences, the ultimate manifestations will also be a function of the various ego defences and integrative measures against such drives, and the super-ego prohibitions and threats of punishment for their expression. Therefore, the transference phenomena as they are experienced or expressed in the treatment situation may at one time show a greater preponderance of the drives, and at other times greater preponderances of the defences or fears of punishment.

In general, the more frequently a patient is seen and the longer the total duration of contact, the more intense will be the transference relationship, other things being equal. However, patients who are accustomed to establishing intense, volatile and affective object relationships may at times

15

develop significant transference reactions very quickly, even if therapeutic interviews occur relatively infrequently. Contrariwise, there are patients who keep emotional distance from objects, and who utilize a variety of defence mechanisms against the affective experience of object relationships and maintain rigid defences against regressions. Such patients, even if seen frequently and over an extended period of time, may experience and express only the defences against developing a transference relationship, and never become conscious of the drives.

A positive transference reaction ranges in intensity and directness from an allusion to the therapist through expressing positive attitudes towards other people in a similar position (i.e. teacher, doctor); to more directly positive references to the therapist or his possessions; to an increasingly personal curiosity about the therapist and his reactions and other interests; and at the other extreme, to the direct expression of a genital or pregenital wish or fantasy towards the therapist. There is variability regarding how much of this is experienced or expressed away from the session itself, or in the presence of the therapist, but not infrequently, a patient may even become conscious of sexual arousal during a therapeutic session.

Similarly, the negative transference may be experienced in a spectrum of reactions, ranging from indirect allusions of hostility towards other objects; all the way through an increasingly less displaced and more affective experience of anger directed against the therapist; to the extreme of violent wishes to express hostility and aggression directly against the therapist. The most extreme form would be a physical attack on the therapist by the patient (usually only occurring in borderline or psychotic patients), but the same feelings and fantasies may exist in a less regressed patient who is capable of impulse control, and who expresses them only through verbalization.

Conflict in the Transference

As the therapist increasingly becomes the object of the patient's positive and negative drives and drive-derivatives, a new situation of danger and conflict will develop. The same forces which initially led to the development of the neurotic disturbance are now being mobilized in the therapeutic setting, and the therapist has now become the forbidden or dangerous object, and the treatment situation itself is increasingly involved in the patient's conflict. In other words, in the treatment setting, the patient now experiences drives and drive-derivatives parallel to those he experienced outside of the treatment situation. He will attempt to utilize the same integrative, adaptive and defence mechanisms in dealing with the conflicts related to treatment and the therapist as he has used in the past with other similar conflict situations outside of therapy.

In this fashion, the conflicts in the patient's relationship to the therapist become copies of his conflicts in relationships with others in his current life, and also are copies of earlier conflicts in accordance with the genetic hypothesis. In fact, in the therapeutic transference, precise repetitions of earlier experiences, attitudes and relationships may be re-experienced in current form with the therapist. From a study of these transference reactions, reconstructions of the earlier experiences can at times be drawn.

The full-blown and overt manifestations of transference reactions can usually be easily recognized. It is the earlier and more subtle manifestations which are in some ways more significant for the therapist, since the strategy and tactics of the management of the transference rests more on them. Therefore, the early recognition of their significance is important.

Indications of Transference

Some of the many indicators that an increasingly positive transference relationship is developing include such things as the patient beginning to come early for his sessions; or beginning to pay more attention to his appearance, and trying to dress more attractively; or making peripheral remarks about such things as the pleasantness of the office, the comfort of the chair, or attractiveness of a picture; or reporting direct or indirect references to the therapist in the manifest content of a dream; or reporting his own or others' positive statements, experiences or references to psychiatry and psychotherapy; or showing increasing interest and thought about treatment, either during or before therapeutic sessions. This list could be extended indefinitely, but it serves to illustrate the types of indicators to which the therapist must be alert.

Similarly, more subtle evidences of developing negative transference may include such things as complaints about the inconvenience or sacrifices required for the therapy; reports of unsuccessful medical or surgical treatment; expressions of dislike for the physical surroundings in the office; reports of other people's criticisms of psychiatry or of the therapist; references to failures of psychotherapy; argumentativeness regarding psychiatry or psychiatric theory; delays in paying the bill; reporting of dreams in which the content suggests fights or disagreements; reports of increasing irritability and negative interactions with others outside of the therapeutic situation.

In listening to such material, the therapist may at times be able to recognize the transference meaning behind the communication if he keeps in mind the question, 'Why is the patient bringing this up at this time?' In this connection he must also keep in mind that one feeling may disguise or be used as a defence against the expression of some other more disturbing feeling.

For example, a patient expressing hostility and anger may be warding off awareness of an increasingly positive involvement with the therapist, the latter being more anxiety-provoking than the former. Vice versa, the patient who repeatedly expresses exaggerated feelings of admiration, attraction or dependency on the therapist, may be warding-off intense underlying hostility. The conflict which evokes the greatest stress or anxiety will be the one the patient is least likely spontaneously to express. If a patient expresses a particular feeling or attitude in consciousness, without significant manifestation of anxiety or difficulty in verbalization, the likelihood is that at that moment such an expression is serving more in the process of defence, and that it hides or disguises a still more anxiety-provoking underlying conflict.

Some behavioural manifestations of the patient may be indications only of the occurrence of a transference reaction, without being specifically identifiable as either positive or negative. Examples of this include such things as coming late to the therapy sessions; or avoiding therapeutic sessions without significant reasons; or having few or no spontaneous associations or thoughts after an initial period of relatively spontaneous communication; or experiencing increasing anxiety or tension in regard to the treatment itself; or the development of specific symptoms (i.e. headache, nausea, pain, etc.) in the treatment situation. The therapist may recognize these as general manifestations of a transference reaction but must then look for more specific evidence of its precise nature.

Strategy of Management: Insight-directed Therapy

The strategy involved in the development and utilization of the transference relationship is a function of the overall therapeutic strategy and goals. In insight-directed therapy, the transference relationship and the repetition with the therapist of reactions and responses to earlier key figures in the patient's life is used as one tool in the previously described mobilization of conflict. Its specific effect is the presentation to the patient of a *currently meaningful and affective conflict situation* in the therapeutic relationship, which recapitulates some of the earlier conflicts that originally led to neurotic symptom formation. In other words, transference in insight-directed treatment is used as one of the means by which previously unconscious conflict is again mobilized and brought to the patient's awareness.

Another advantage in studying such responses in the transference relationship, as compared with other relationships in the patient's current life, is that the treatment situation is more controlled since the therapist does not respond emotionally to the patient's interactions. Furthermore, the therapist is aware of the totality of the situation, which he cannot be when the patient gives a biased or incomplete report in treatment concerning an experience that occurred outside. Generally speaking, the therapist can also use the patient's responses in the transference situation to show him how similar experiences outside of treatment are being managed and dealt with, thereby imparting insight to the patient in regard to his current dynamic interactions with objects in his present life.

In the development and subsequent elaboration of the transference relationship in insight-directed therapy, there is a remobilization of intrapsychic conflict displaced to the current interpersonal relationship between patient and therapist. As the patient becomes increasingly aware of his drives and defences in relationship to the therapist, the older conflicts are consciously re-experienced in an emotionally meaningful and immediate form. The patient then is in a position to use this edition of his conflict as a means of recall, through association, of earlier pathogenic experiences of adolescence, latency or childhood.

The patient is then confronted in the therapeutic situation with the same active conflicts he originally warded off. But in the current edition, the patient has a more fully developed ego, as well as wider opportunities for finding more reasonable solutions to the conflicts. He also has the aid and alliance of the therapist, and the benefits of his own subsequent life experience, all of which make resolution of these conflicts more likely in the present setting. After the patient has faced and found solutions for the current therapeutic edition of his conflicts, such solutions may also be usefully applied in the various conflict situations outside the treatment setting.

After the development of a transference relationship, there may be an improvement of function outside the treatment situation, along with an intensification of symptom formation or discomfort in the treatment itself. This results from the fact that the therapist has now become an important object of the patient's drives, and hence the therapeutic setting now becomes the situation in which much of the conflict over unacceptable drives and drive-derivatives is mobilized and focused.

During the course of formal psychoanalysis, one of the major tactical goals is the further development of this trend in the transference, to the point that the analyst becomes the chief object of the patient's increasingly regressive drives and defences. This results in the analytic situation becoming the major, if not exclusive, source of conflict stimulation, which is known as the *transference neurosis*. It is through the exploration and analysis of this regressive transference neurosis that the infantile and earlier childhood experiences and conflicts can return to the patient's conscious awareness.

In the forms of insight-directed psychotherapy being discussed here, the intensity and extent of the regression in the transference is much more limited. The therapeutic situation does not lend itself as completely to regression. Furthermore, one tactical goal is to avoid deeply regressive transference experiences, since it is less likely that they can be successfully resolved in this type of treatment. Unless a patient is ultimately able effectively to resolve the transference relationship, the total impact may be harmful rather than helpful.

The optimal level of transference in face-to-face insight-directed psychotherapy is one in which the patient experiences emotional conflicts in relationship to the therapist, but which does not evoke so much anxiety or distress that the patient is unable to continue in the therapeutic task. Through this he repeats in a controlled fashion some of the same conflicts experienced in his everyday adult life situation with others outside of treatment. By such a treatment approach, it also becomes possible for the patient to gain a general awareness of the adolescent and latency editions of some of his current conflicts and patterns of response, but the detailed exploration of infantile and early childhood conflicts is more sharply limited. Although the therapist may recognize the transference repetitions of infantile and early childhood experience and conflict, the major focus as far as the patient's interactions are concerned should be on the current forms in which these conflicts are manifested.

In insight-directed treatment this strategy applies not only to the positive transference, but also to the negative transference and the ways in which the patient deals with hostile or aggressive drives and drive-derivatives.

Tactics of Management: Insight-directed Therapy

A number of techniques are available to the therapist in his attempts to regulate the intensity of the transference, and maintain it at an optimal level for insight-directed treatment.

The first of these is for the therapist to maintain the structure of the therapeutic situation in a relatively constant and consistent form, and try to minimize departures from it. As a result of this, variations in the patient's reactions to the therapist can more easily be demonstrated as resulting from shifts within the patient's own intra-psychic organization, rather than being responses to external manipulations, or to changes in the therapist or the therapeutic situation.

However, the therapist must be alert to the transference component in the patient's responses to the inevitable vicissitudes of the treatment situation. Such things as absences, holidays, vacations, lateness or subtle differences in the therapist's feelings or behaviour may evoke a variety of realistic *and* transference reactions which must be evaluated in the context of the total treatment situation.

For example, early in treatment before the patient has developed a significant transference relationship, if the therapist should be 5 minutes late, the patient may not respond to this, nor need it be a manifestation of resistance if he does not mention a reaction to the lateness. At this point, the patient may be used to being kept waiting by doctors for an hour or more, and he may see the 5-minute lateness as a relative accommodation and pay no particular attention to it. However, once the transference relationship has been established, the patient may respond to a similar 5-minute wait with feelings of rejection, depression or anger, and he may fantasy that this is a sign of the therapist's lack of concern or interest in him.

In an insight-directed treatment approach, the therapist usually avoids detailed explanations or apologies for the various vicissitudes in the treatment relationship, thereby permitting the patient to use them as a stimulus for transference feelings and fantasy. The elaboration of such reactions will be more readily possible if the patient is not restricted in advance by the reality explanation of the event. Frequently, after such transference feeling and fantasy has been expressed, the therapist may then give the realistic explanation to the patient, thereby helping the patient to see the intensity of the distortion created by his own intra-psychic reactions. When thus confronting the patient with reality following his expression of a transference distortion, it is important that the intervention be presented from a constructive and therapeutic point of view, and the patient not be made to feel foolish or criticized for the distortion.

The technique of intensifying transference wishes through frustration of drive-derivatives has been mentioned earlier, along with the theoretical rationale of increasing the patient's awareness of the unconscious drives, and simultaneously giving reassurance regarding overt behaviour. This maintenance of a state of relative transference abstinence occurs automatically if the therapist keeps to his neutral participant-observer role in the face of demands or provocations by the patient to abandon it. Such provocations may be aimed at drawing the therapist into a more personal and emotional interaction, either positive or negative, during the treatment session, or they may involve a demand that the therapist interact at a realistic level in the patient's life or relationships outside of treatment.

When the therapist maintains his neutrality, and does not react to the provocations, the transference is intensified since the patient will respond on the basis of intra-psychic forces, rather than in reaction to the therapist's behaviour, or changes in the therapeutic situation. At times the patient may experience this as a humiliation, and feel resentment on the basis that he is expressing intense emotional reactions, while the therapist manifests none. Patients often complain that the situation is an unequal and unfair one. The therapist's own attitude must be that this relationship was not established to be equal or fair, but rather to be therapeutic. He should continue to interpret the patient's defences against the relationship and the resistances against the feelings which the patient has already developed and experienced, but is unwilling to express.

The therapist does not specifically change his behaviour in order actively and deliberately to frustrate a particular transference wish, since this in itself represents a form of manipulation of the patient and the relationship, and thus the constancy of the situation would be lost. Nor can the therapist always avoid some transference gratification. For example, a patient may derive exhibitionistic pleasure from talking to the therapist about himself, but directly to frustrate this would preclude further progress. Or a masochistic patient may be gratified by interpreting the therapist's interventions as criticisms and attacks, but to continue the treatment the therapist must still make his interventions.

The main point is for the therapist to recognize that in insight-directed treatment any departure from the neutral participant-observer role should be carefully considered beforehand, with recognition of the impact that such a departure is likely to have.

Interpretation is the most effective technique for control of the intensity of transference in insight-directed treatment. Although the patient may have an understanding of the basic rule to speak freely about whatever is in his mind, he nevertheless may continue to carry a reservation against this in regard to 'personal things' about the therapist and the therapeutic relationship. This must be overcome by confrontation and interpretation if the transference is to develop. The mobilization of conflict and anxiety in the transference relationship has been described, and will result in continuing attempts at defence against awareness of the transference phenomena, and attempts to avoid intensifying them. At times when resistance to the development and expression of the transference is high, the therapist's task is the interpretation of these resistances, in an attempt to intensify the conscious awareness of transference.

However, when transference conflicts have mobilized greater anxiety than is therapeutically optimal, interpretation of the content of the transference wishes themselves, whether positive or negative, will tend to reduce the immediate intensity of anxiety. This may be accompanied by an explanation of how such transference reactions are representative of similar responses in other current or past relationships. In this way the immediate intensity of the transference is diluted by focusing the patient's attention away from the current transference phenomena, and by extending the conscious sphere of the ego. By such interpretations of content, the therapist can most effectively deal with and control the patient's previously described transference provocations, without abandoning the participant-observer role. In other words, the interpretation of transference follows general principles of interpretation described in Chapter XI.

In some instances, after a significant transference relationship has been established in the course of insight-directed therapy, it may produce a resistance to further progress in the treatment, and the patient's uncon scious wish to maintain the transference relationship takes precedence over his conscious wish to be cured. This is known as the *transference resistance*. This occurs because the underlying neurotic disturbance consists in part of a wish for gratification of infantile or childhood drives by the infantile or childhood objects. In the developed transference relationship, the therapist has become an important object of these drives. The wish for their gratification may motivate the patient to give up the search for reality-oriented objects and satisfactions, and instead cling to the therapist and the therapy with the fantasy of eventual gratification by him. In such a situation the patient may stop his attempts to find conflict solutions, and may manifest increasingly regressive reactions and behaviour in hopes thereby of forcing the therapist to provide the sought-after gratification. This may also involve an unconscious wish to evoke guilt in the therapist, with the hope that the greater the guilt or anxiety produced in the therapist, the more likely it is that he will ultimately gratify the transference wishes. This type of reaction is particularly frequent during the termination phase, and will be discussed further in Chapter XVII on Termination.

A clinical illustration of transference resistance is a young woman seen in once-a-week psychotherapy with significant improvement and increasing understanding of some of her severe and disturbing problems. She missed one session for a realistic reason, and the next day found she was able to go downtown without her usual severe phobic anxiety. That night she had sexual intercourse with her husband and for the first time in her life experienced a vaginal orgasm with great pleasure and satisfaction. The next day, while reflecting on the course of events, she had the sudden thought 'I'm just about well and I will soon have to stop going to see the doctor'. She was aware of her wish to continue the relationship with the therapist, and of her mixed feelings regarding her improvement. This was followed almost immediately by depression and anxiety and a later recurrence of the sexual frigidity. The return of symptoms at that time represented her unconscious wish to remain sick in order to continue the transference relationship.

The occurrence of the transference resistance is another reason for relative abstinence regarding drive-derivative gratification in insight-directed therapy. Gratifying the transference wishes tends to intensify this resistance, and give support to the fantasy of ultimate transference gratification. In the state of abstinence, there is less reinforcement of these regressive expectations.

In insight-directed treatment such a resistance is managed by increasing the patient's awareness of it through interpretation and by confronting him with the recognition that his ultimate welfare will be greater if he gives up this resistance in the transference, and goes on to optimal self-development.

Part of the insight-directed therapeutic process is the resolution of the established transference relationship after it has been used to help the patient to become consciously more aware of the various elements in his conflicts. Ideally, the patient comes gradually to accept the frustration of his transference drive-derivatives, in keeping with the reality principle, by utilizing mechanisms of conscious repudiation and sublimation, rather than the previous unconscious ego defences which resulted in neurotic symptom formation.

By virtue of ego and super-ego change, the patient should gradually come to accept without guilt the fact that his wishes in the transference were part of the process of therapy, just as in their original form they were once part of the process of growth. Accepting the frustration of transference wishes makes it possible for him now to find more realistically satisfying and age-appropriate objects and gratifications.

One of the major therapeutic hazards of face-to-face therapy occurs when the therapist is overly ambitious, and tries to explore the deepest genetic layers of the personality and is reluctant to accept the limitations of the treatment method. Such attempts to deal with infantile and early childhood conflicts by fostering a deeply regressive transference neurosis in the setting of a limited insight-directed therapy, generally result in long or interminable treatment with little genuine therapeutic change. It may at times result in serious disorganization of personality, or at best in intellectualized insight.

In other words, in psychotherapy the therapist looks for generalized patterns and reconstructions of reactions, and may offer these to the patient as an explanation of the origins of his behaviour, but he focuses most of his attention on the manifestations of the current derivative conflicts. He tends to utilize the patient's transference reactions as illustrations of his adaptation to current conflicts, and to seek parallels between the patient's behaviour in the transference and his behaviour in the outside environment. A significant degree of structural personality change can frequently be achieved with such a more limited focus. As the patient resolves the transference conflicts, and begins to respond differently in the therapeutic relationship, and as he develops increased awareness of current patterns of defence and integration, he is then more capable of modifying his responses, at least to some degree, in relationships outside the treatment situation.

Strategy of Management: Supportive Therapy

The patient who is being treated supportively has the same potential for the development of a transference relationship as does the patient in insight-directed therapy. In fact, the spontaneous occurrence of more intense regression in many of the patients treated supportively may increase their transference potentials.

It is therefore essential to keep in mind the factors in the therapeutic situation which foster transference development, as discussed earlier, but to use them in ways designed to be supportive of the patient in keeping with the overall strategy previously described.

In a supportive treatment situation, the transference strategy calls for the maintenance of a generally positive relationship in which the patient is aware primarily of the element of conscious rapport. While many of the deeper and unconscious transference conflicts and phenomena may be present, they are not intensified, or interpreted, and they are deliberately allowed to remain repressed and unconscious.

The use of the transference relationship as a vehicle for mobilization of conflict in insight-directed treatment has been described. The strategy of its use in supportive treatment is part of the overall plan to maintain or strengthen defences, avoid the mobilization of conflict and in all ways possible reduce the adaptive burden placed on the patient's ego.

To this end, the therapist makes use of the patient's unconscious transference potential as a guide in selecting or carrying out his interventions. Although these will be based on the patient's unconscious transference wishes, drive-derivatives and defences, the therapist's activity and interventions are chosen so that the patient's reaction to them can be significantly related to the reality of the therapist's behaviour, thereby minimizing the degree of transference distortion. For example if the patient's transference wish is to depend upon an authoritarian figure, the therapist might react in such a way as to create the maximum authoritarian image. The patient's response may then be at least partially on the basis of how the therapist has presented himself in the therapeutic situation.

By providing gratification for transference drive-derivatives within the realistic framework of the supportive therapeutic setting and in ways appropriate to the interactions of a treatment relationship, the therapist helps the patient to reduce the immediate intensity of the drive which is seeking discharge. This in turn reduces the intensity of the conflict experienced by the ego, and hence the stress to which the ego must adapt.

The situation is analogous to that of an individual who is aware of mild hunger. The longer he must wait before eating a meal, the more intense becomes the hunger and the more conscious he is of the drive to satisfy it. However, if he were to eat a snack when he first becomes aware of the mild hunger, the awareness of hunger would again subside, and if he were to continue eating small snacks, he would have very little appetite by the time dinner is ready.

By offering gratifications of transference need-derivatives within the limitations of the supportive treatment situation, the therapist is providing the patient with an important conscious and reality object relationship. At the same time, the transference components (ultimately stemming from the parental objects as described earlier) give it the unconscious significance to the patient of a parent-child relationship.

As the patient-therapist interaction in supportive therapy comes increasingly to represent a positive and child-parent relationship, the therapist is in a position to use this relationship to stimulate specific responses in the patient. It can be used as a force to promote ego and super-ego identifications with the therapist, and also to influence specific ego mechanisms of defence and adaptation. As in the original version, if used appropriately it can also, at unconscious levels, help to stimulate whatever potential the patient has for further emotional maturation.

Tactics of Management: Supportive Therapy

The tactics of therapeutic management of the transference in supportive treatment can be logically evolved from these basic concepts of strategy, and will differ considerably from those described for insight therapy.

The therapist permits and encourages the patient to maintain defences against conscious awareness of transference phenomena, and does not interpret these as resistances. He also supports the patient's defences against regression, and to the extent that this is successful, reduces the intensity of transference distortions.

By actively giving his own opinions and judgments, and by giving appropriate personal information about himself, the therapist provides the patient with a reality-bound awareness of himself as a real person. This also serves to reduce the likelihood of fantasied transference distortions, and increases the reality of the interactions.

The therapist also makes use of manipulations of the therapeutic situation to control the intensity of the transference relationship. For example, if the transference is becoming more intense than optimal, it is possible to space out the frequency of the interviews, thereby reducing the intensity of the relationship. This should be done in such a way that the patient does not experience it as a rejection, but rather as a positive sign of movement and improvement, with appropriate reinforcement given by the therapist.

Another way of reducing transference intensity is to shorten the interviews, particularly if the patient has finished 'reporting' on his current life situation and experiences. If the patient is made to stay for the additional allotted time, the contributions from his own intra-psychic experience will be increased, and there will be a greater likelihood of mobilization of unconscious and more regressive transference reactions.

Such manipulations of the duration and frequency of interviews must occur before transference feelings become intense or conscious, since if they are undertaken after the patient is aware of a significant transference relationship, he is likely to have a reaction of rejection or anger. This is another reason for the therapist to be alert to the early indicators of developing transference, and to carry out such manipulations in a prophylactic way before the relationship becomes too intense.

In spite of the therapist's intention to maintain the positive transference reactions at unconscious levels, some patients may still become consciously aware of transference feelings or fantasies. Another technique for controlling the impact of this is the early interpretation of their content. In this way, the transference wishes are attentuated and more effectively controlled by the patient's ego. Such interpretations of content are generally accompanied by an explanation to the patient that 'such feelings towards the therapist are part of treatment', or that 'many people in treatment have such temporary feelings, and when the treatment is over, these feelings will again subside'. In more sophisticated patients this can be accompanied by statements such as 'You've heard about patients who depend on or fall in love with their therapist during the treatment, and that's what this is'. Such interventions help to reduce anxiety and to improve defences against further emerging transference wishes.

Another tactical goal is the attempt to maintain rapport and the transference relationship on a positive level, and to avoid mobilizing unconscious negative transference reactions or feelings of rejection. Therefore, in situations where the stimulation of such feelings can be anticipated, the therapist intervenes in ways designed to avoid this.

For example, the therapist would be likely to make a careful factual explanation to the patient as to the reason why a session had to be cancelled, and he might suggest a substitute appointment. This would confront the patient with the reality of the event, reduce the frustration or rejection experienced by the patient, give a positive reinforcement of the therapist's therapeutic intent and desire to be of service, and thereby reduce the extent of the regressive negative transference distortions.

In spite of such efforts, consciously negative transference reactions may still occur. As with positive feelings, the early interpretation of their content tends to reduce their intensity, and to reassure the patient of the therapist's acceptance in spite of such feelings.

In instances where the patient needs to ventilate hostility and anger, this is not opposed. But the attempt is made to keep from intensifying the transference elements by focusing the hostile reaction at the level of the current realistic situation in treatment, or to patient's external object relationships, rather than considering these as manifestations of resistance and displacement of transference as might occur in an insight-directed treatment approach.

There are also instances where the patient's relationship is predominantly negative at the conscious level, with repeated expressions of hostility, resentment, rejection or disappointment. Even in this situation, the attempt is made to maintain the interactions at the level of the current relationship to the therapist and the treatment and as a form of reality-oriented response. In such a relationship, if the transference were purely a negative one, the patient generally would not come back. The fact that the patient returns for regular therapeutic visits is an indication that, in spite of the apparently negative relationship, there must be some type of positive attachment behind it. Such a situation often reflects the patient's defensive need to mask or hide such underlying positive feelings, and the therapist may merely accept the patient's consciously negative attitude.

The therapist also makes tactical use of his parental authority resulting from the transference to help the patient modify his super-ego forces and attitudes. Such interventions as active value judgments, giving reassurance about the normality of various thoughts or feelings, and encouraging and giving permission for various forms of behaviour may have a significant mollifying effect on the patient's feelings of guilt or fears of punishment. In the opposite direction, setting limits, making prohibitions, or offering appropriate criticism may help provide the patient with guides to establishing more effective controls in instances where super-ego development is lacking.

In these various ways the therapist is providing the patient with external conscious super-ego functions which, in either direction, are more in keeping with the reality principle than are those of the patient. The use of such external standards may help the patient to a more stable equilibrium and reduce the stress of conflict. And to the extent that the patient ultimately identifies himself unconsciously with the therapist, such externalized standards may be eventually internalized.

Another tactic is to foster and encourage the patient's transference wish to identify himself with the therapist. This represents another reason for the therapist to offer the patient appropriate realistic information about himself, and about his interests or activities as a real person, since the more that the patient knows of these facets, the greater is the opportunity of finding ways of making such identifications. For example, such things as an interest in sports, music, art, hobbies, community activities, etc., may offer the patient constructive ways of expressing such identifications, and this may also provide the nucleus for the subsequent development of effective sublimations. This is in contrast to insight-directed treatment, where such unconscious identifications would more likely be dealt with as resistances against self-development.

Situations in which the transference becomes a resistance also occur in supportive treatment, although they are not as frequent as in insight-directed therapy. If this should occur, the therapist might tell the patient directly that he will continue seeing him as long as the patient wishes, and that illness or symptoms are not a prerequisite for coming to see the therapist. In this way, the patient can accept the remission of symptoms without giving up the transference relationship. In this connection, the therapist must keep in mind that the treatment relationship may come to have a very important conscious and unconscious meaning in the life of the patient, and in some extreme instances, it may represent the only emotionally significant contact that the patient has.

For this reason, ultimate resolution of the transference relationship is not a tactical goal in supportive treatment as it is in insight-directed therapy. In fact, if the relationship has been a positive and successful one, the therapist may interact in ways designed to help the patient maintain it indefinitely. Sometimes this involves maintaining periodic contact with the patient, even though the frequency of interviews may be sharply reduced (i.e. once every 3 or 6 months). At other times it may require only emphasizing to the patient that the therapist is always available to him if needed, or requesting that the patient send a card once a year to let the therapist know how he is faring.

The immediate tactical goal is to help the patient maintain a relationship in which he is consciously aware of the element of positive rapport, while deeper unconscious transference meanings persist but are not elaborated in consciousness. This type of dilute transference relationship may be of significant help to the patient in maintaining and solidifying the gains achieved in the active treatment. Also, if there should be a subsequent recurrence of symptoms, or an emotional crisis, or the occurrence of a significant conflict which the patient is unable to manage, he can then return to the therapist with an established and ongoing relationship of positive rapport and transference, which will tend to shorten the time necessary for a subsequent therapeutic contact.

For this reason, when patients are seen in an institutional or clinic setting where the particular therapist may not be permanently available, it is often useful to intervene in ways designed to help the patient develop his continuing transference to the institution or clinic, rather than to the therapist himself.

Clinical Illustrations

These differences in the strategy and tactics of the utilization of the transference relationship in insight-directed and in supportive therapy can be highlighted by illustrations using several characteristic clinical situations.

In planning for supportive treatment of a patient whose major transference wishes are overtly passive and dependent, the therapist might accept the authoritarian role, offer active advice and guidance, indicate openly his expectations of the patient's behaviour, and reinforce through signs of approval any progress which the patient makes. He would try to present an openly friendly, warm, and personal attitude toward the patient, and consider offering medication for its symbolic and transference-gratifying values.

In insight-directed treatment of such a patient, the therapist would tend to remain more neutral and less gratifying in order that the extent and intensity of the dependent wishes become more conscious, and that the patient's reliance on external rewards and approval can be more easily demonstrated. Through such a transference relationship the patient is given an opportunity to learn that he is capable of directing and planning his own behaviour, that such independence does not mean a loss or change in the therapeutic relationship, that as an adult he now has the capabilities for increased freedom, and that mature mastery and independence can in themselves be pleasurable.

In supporting a patient with a characteristic reaction formation against his own passive-dependent yearnings, the therapist would minimize his own role, encourage the patient's independence and initiative, reduce the frequency of interviews as promptly as possible, and indicate his confidence in the patient's own abilities. He would avoid making the patient aware of the underlying dependent longings.

However, in the insight-directed treatment of such a patient the therapist would oppose the various distancing manoeuvres, gradually focus on the exaggerated independence as a character defence, mobilize the patient's anxiety over his own unconscious dependent yearnings, and through the transference reactions help the patient become aware of the origins and distortions regarding his dependent conflicts.

Frequently in the early phases of a therapeutic relationship, as the unconscious positive transference is developing, there may occur a marked and apparently spontaneous symptomatic improvement known as a 'transference cure'. This results from the rapid establishment of a transference relationship in which the patient unconsciously hopes to achieve the gratification of love from the therapist. Recognizing that the therapist wants him to get well, the patient may give up his symptoms and complaints in an attempt to be 'a good patient' and do what the therapist wants, thereby unconsciously hoping ultimately to receive the desired infantile satisfaction and care.

16

In a supportive relationship, the tactical goal would be to maintain this transference improvement and reduction of symptoms, and therefore the therapist would reinforce such improvement with appropriate interventions, or overt signs of approval and recognition. He would also try to reduce the intensity or frequency of sessions, thereby diluting the developing transference relationship. This would be done in order that it can remain persistently positive, and in order to reduce the likelihood of ultimate transference frustration. If transference wishes become more clearly conscious and are then frustrated, there will be a loss of the positive transference and its replacement by an overtly mixed or negative one, in which case the symptomatic remission is likely to disappear.

Such a 'transference cure' may also occur during the course of insight-directed treatment. But since the goal of treatment is the development of insight and definitive resolution of conflict, the therapist would not alter the structure of therapy in response to the current remission of symptoms. If the patient expresses a wish to reduce the frequency of visits, or a fantasy that the illness had been cured, the therapist would interpret these as wishes to avoid the uncovering and understanding of his basic problems. The therapist would emphasize that this is only a temporary remission since an understanding of the psychopathology has not yet occurred and, therefore, the conflicts which evoked the symptoms are still present.

Another illustration of the differences in management of the transference would be in the treatment of patients with a masochistic character disorder who have an unconscious need for punishment or suffering. In a supportive transference relationship, the therapist might adopt a demanding, critical, scolding, and slightly punitive attitude towards the patient, thereby gratifying the unconscious masochistic need to suffer in a controlled fashion within the therapeutic situation. As a result, there will be less need for the patient to seek similar gratification in his real life outside of the treatment, and the patient will also have an opportunity consciously to complain, and to externalize his unconscious aggression against the therapist. If the therapist is kind, giving, encouraging or sorry for such a patient, his unconscious sense of guilt and needs for punishment will be intensified, and the patient will then be more prone to seek this type of masochistic suffering in his life outside.

Two brief examples may illustrate this. A middle-aged woman presented herself with symptoms of anxiety and depression, and recited a long tale of woe and mistreatment at the hands of her husband. The therapist maintained a stern and critical attitude, openly scolded and blamed the patient herself for most of her difficulties, finally telling her to stop feeling so sorry for herself. The patient's response was, 'Doctor, you're absolutely right. I feel much better already'.

A middle-aged professional man with a masochistic character disorder was treated in a psychiatric hospital for almost a year by a therapist who was openly warm, encouraging, sympathetic and kind. During this time his symptoms of anxiety and depression persisted unchanged, and he remained passive and regressed in his ward behaviour. He was then transferred to a new therapist who was deliberately and consistently cold, critical and authoritarian, and who demanded that the patient participate in ward responsibilities and activities in spite of his suffering. The patient complained bitterly and persistently about the new therapist, and his 'lack of understanding'. But within 2 months his symptoms and behaviour had improved to the point that he could be discharged to his home in a distant city. During the next year or more, the second therapist received a letter from the patient every few months describing his continued improvement. Each letter contained a long section of bitter complaint and criticism against the second therapist, and praise for the first one. The therapist's answering letters were again deliberately brief, cold and critical of some point in the patient's report.

In an insight directed treatment approach, the patient's wish for masochistic suffering and punishment in the transference would be frustrated by the therapist's neutral and non-punitive attitude. This will help to intensify the transference wish to the point that the patient can become aware of his unconscious need for this type of angry attack or punishment, and of his behaviour which provokes such attacks from the environment. Such conscious awareness in the transference is a first step towards the ultimate definitive resolution of the conflicts behind the masochism.

Another common clinical situation which illustrates the differences in management of the transference occurs in the treatment of patients for whom conflicts over latent homosexuality are intense. The therapist can anticipate that as treatment progresses and a transference relationship is developed, the latent homosexual drives will be an increasingly prominent element and the therapist will be their object. The strategy of supportive therapy suggests that such latent homosexual conflicts should remain unconscious, and that efforts should be directed towards strengthening the defences against them.

Therefore, in supportive treatment it is often helpful, if the unconscious homosexual conflicts have been recognized during the diagnostic period, to arrange for therapy with a therapist of opposite sex from the patient. The developing transference phenomena may then *appear* to be heterosexual, and thus more acceptable to the patient, and repression of the latent homosexuality can be more easily maintained.

However, for a variety of reasons, such a manipulation of therapists may not be feasible, and the therapist and patient may be of the same sex. In that case, it is particularly important that in structuring the therapeutic situation, the therapist be careful to avoid interventions which the patient might consciously or unconsciously interpret as seductive.

Thus the therapist would emphasize the formality of the situation, arrange that the patient himself receive the bill, avoid being too warm or friendly, avoid calling the patient by his first name, avoid giving the patient unnecessary extra time or attention, and in general, act in ways which will avoid stimulating conscious awareness of positive transference responses. The therapist also would consider the necessity to dilute the transference when arranging such things as the optimal frequency and duration of therapeutic sessions. And, in choosing which elements of personal information about himself to give the patient, the therapist would try to avoid any which might potentiate the homosexual transference.

As the treatment progresses, the therapist would be particularly careful to permit or encourage the patient's various defences against awareness of the homosexual components in the transference. However, if positive transference manifestations become conscious to the patient in spite of efforts to maintain repression, the therapist's interventions would be aimed at emphasizing the elements of dependency, and de-emphasizing the elements of love or sexuality.

The strategy of insight-directed therapy suggests that the patient should ultimately become consciously aware of his latent homosexual conflicts as the first step to resolving them. To this end, the therapist would make use of the patient's transference potential in such a way as to promote the patient's gradually increasing awareness of his homosexual conflicts in the controlled situation of the transference relationship. The tactics for doing this are those described earlier in the section on the general management of transference reactions in insight-directed therapy.

Summary

Such illustrations of the differences in managing the transference relationship in supportive as compared with insight-directed treatment could be continued indefinitely. However, they would serve only to emphasize the basic differentiation of strategy.

In supportive treatment, strategy calls for the use of the transference as a tool for the immediate reduction of conflict and strengthening of defences, thereby as quickly as possible re-establishing a stable dynamic equilibrium. In insight-directed treatment, strategy calls for the use of the transference as a tool for the mobilization of previously unconscious conflicts, and their ultimate conscious resolution to whatever degree possible.

In supportive treatment, the transference is used to achieve an immediate goal, while in insight-directed treatment, transference is used to achieve a delayed, long-term, but potentially more stable and effective goal.

SUGGESTED READING

BALINT, MICHAEL (1953) On transference of emotions. In: *Primary Love and Psychoanalytic Technique*. Liveright Publ. Corp.
BENEDEK, THERESA (1946) Control of the transference relationship. In: *Psychoanalytic Therapy*, ALEXANDER, F. & FRENCH T.M. Ronald Press
BRODY, MORRIS W. (1955) Transference and counter-transference. In: *Psychotherapy. Psychoanal. Rev.* **42**, 88
GREENACRE, PHYLLIS (1954) The role of transference: practical considerations in relation to psychoanalytic therapy. *J. Am. Psychoanal. Ass.* **2**, 671
GREENSON, RALPH R. (1967) *The Technique and Practice of Psychoanalysis*. International Universities Press Inc, New York
HARRISON, SAUL I. & CAREK, DONALD J. (1966) *A Guide to Psychotherapy*. Little Brown Company, Boston
HOFFER, WILLY (1956) Transference and transference neurosis. *Int. J. Psycho-Anal.* **37**, 377
NUNBERG, HERMAN (1938) Psychological interrelation between physician and patient. *Psychoanal. Rev.* **25**, 297
RADO, SANDOR (1942) The relationship of patient to therapist. *Am. J. Orthopsychiat.* **12**, 3
SAUL, LEON J. (1951) A note on the telephone as a technical aid. *Psychoanal. Quart.* **20**, 287
SPITZ, RENÉ A. (1956) Transference: The analytical setting and its prototype. *Int. J. Psycho-Anal.* **37**, 380

CHAPTER XIII

The Therapeutic Process:
Resistance, Regression and Conflict

Introduction

The concept of resistance in psychotherapy has been mentioned in earlier chapters and must now be explored and developed further. The resistances are those psychic functions within the patient which are actively opposed to the therapeutic task of bringing unconscious material to conscious awareness, and of modifying old behaviour patterns in favour of newer and more appropriate patterns of integration. In the narrow sense, resistances represent the continuing operation and function of the patient's ego defences as they emerge and are manifest in the therapeutic situation. However, any component psychic process beyond the specific ego defence mechanisms may be used by the patient in the function of resistance.

Three major sources of resistance have been mentioned before. First is the need to maintain repression of unconscious conflicts and thereby avoid the anxiety, guilt or other unpleasurable affect (and ultimately the unconscious 'danger' situation itself) which would occur with the sudden emergence of such conflicts into consciousness. Particularly in the insight-directed therapeutic situation, forces are developed which encourage the patient to lift the repression, but these involve experiencing initial unpleasure and hence the patient also has a wish to oppose the demands of the therapeutic process.

A second major source of resistance is the repetition compulsion and the patient's continuing wish for gratification of infantile and childhood drives and drive-derivatives. Insight-directed therapy involves helping the patient ultimately accept the frustration of these wishes. The continuing wishes for gratification result in forces within the mental apparatus opposed to this frustration, and hence, resistant to a therapeutic process aimed at increasing maturation.

The third major source of resistance is the fear, anxiety and uncertainty experienced by the patient when attempting to develop new adaptive modes and mechanisms, and the discomfort involved in trying out new and possibly unsuccessful patterns of behaviour. This results in further internal forces opposing the therapeutic process.

In the earlier theory of therapy based upon the topographical hypo-thesis, the concept of resistance was equated with the patient being 'unco-operative', and resistances were seen as something bad, to be removed as soon as possible so that treatment could continue. The recognition that resistances chiefly occur unconsciously was one of the major pieces of clinical data which forced the reorganization of psychoanalytic theory, and the development of the structural hypothesis. The development of ego psychology led to the further realization that resistances are an essential part of psychic function even in the therapeutic situation, and that only through elaboration and understanding of these resistances could many unconscious aspects of ego function and of psychic life be made conscious. In fact, as described in Chapter VIII, one of the important criteria of suitability for an insight-directed therapeutic approach is the existence and maintenance of defences and resistances. The absence or sharp reduction of defences and resistances is an indication of relative ego failure and decompensation.

Resistance

Resistances during psychotherapy occur at varying levels of consciousness, similar to the levels of consciousness in the operation of ego defence mechanisms generally, as described in Chapter II. In some instances the patient may be fully conscious of the existence of the resistance and even of the conflict which is being avoided. For example, a patient may delib-erately choose to avoid discussing particular conflicts, and may consciously withhold material or lie to the therapist.

At other times the patient may not be spontaneously aware of the existence or manifestations of a resistance, but may easily become aware of this when his attention is focused upon it by the therapist. For example, a patient may be vaguely aware of 'beating around the bush', or of a feeling that somehow something is blocking him. After the therapist points out the material being avoided, the patient may readily see it, and acknowledge that there had previously been a wish to avoid discussing this material or conflict.

The most therapeutically significant and difficult type of resistance may occur completely unconsciously, where the patient is unaware of the material being avoided, and also of his efforts at maintaining the defence. For example, a patient may consciously try to co-operate and work hard in the therapeutic process, but nevertheless use unconscious ego defence mechanisms such as displacement, isolation, or projection, without being aware of the existence of these mechanisms or of the effect they have on the material he produces.

This distinction between conscious, preconscious and unconscious resistance may be illustrated by the common phenomenon of a patient who fails to show up for a therapeutic session. At times this may be a conscious choice made by the patient on the basis of a reluctance to come for his session. At other times the patient may have a conscious wish to come, but find a plausible rationalization which he follows in not coming for the session (i.e. 'I was tied up at work'). When the therapist points out that there may have been a wish to avoid the session that day, the patient often recalls having had such feelings or thoughts, or having had a feeling of relief at not coming. At other times a patient may have a conscious wish to come to the session and may in fact have reminded himself of it earlier in the day, and then find that he has 'completely forgotten about it' until after the time of the session.

As mentioned in Chapter II, any psychological function or experience may be utilized by the ego in the service of defence, and it is therefore impossible completely to catalogue all of the manifestations. Likewise, in the therapeutic process, any psychic experience, function or external event may be used in the service of resistance, depending on how the patient's ego integrates and adapts to it. Some resistances may be fixed and persistent, while others may be transient or intermittent. Some resistances occur commonly among large numbers of patients, while others may be quite specific to the individual. Within a given individual, a particular bit of behaviour may at times serve the function of resistance, whereas at other times the same behaviour may have a different significance.

For example, with some patients the subject of sexuality is repeatedly avoided, or quickly concealed behind simple generalizations. Other patients may discuss it extensively and in detail, on the assumption that this is what the therapist wants to hear. In both instances the patient's behaviour is a function of his resistance. Some patients repetitively discuss only the details of current realistic situations, and are unable or unwilling to discuss past life experience. However, other patients dwell extensively on past and early childhood experience, as an attempt to avoid a more pressing, immediate and anxiety-provoking current conflict. Some patients never mention dreams, while others bring so much dream material that there is hardly time for anything else. In between therapeutic sessions, some patients may never think about the treatment; other patients may discuss it in detail with various people; and both extremes may be manifestations of resistance. Other forms that resistance might take include such things as externalization of problems and blaming of others; a continuing focus on description of symptoms without attempting an introspective search for the factors behind them; behaviours designed to enlist the therapist's sympathy or approval; editing of material which the patient expects would cause the therapist's disapproval; internal reservations regarding the validity of psychological data while outwardly concurring with the therapist; withholding of information or associations; 'acting-out' of conflicts with others outside the treatment; various actions within the therapeutic situation which replace verbalization; reservations in regard to accepting the role of a patient, etc. The list of possible manifestations of resistance is an endless one.

Resistances continue throughout the course of therapy regardless of the type of treatment undertaken. They vary considerably in terms of the degree to which they are conscious, as well as in terms of the nature and pattern of the particular resistances which are active at any one time. There is also variation in the intensity with which they are utilized by the patient.

The therapist's task is to recognize their presence, their intensity, and their significance in the patient's current psychic functioning, and to identify the conflict which is being kept from consciousness by their use. The way in which the therapist then manages or deals with these resistances will be a function of the type of therapy being undertaken and the overall strategy of the therapeutic process.

Strategy and Tactics: Insight Therapy

In insight-directed treatment, strategy calls for a gradual reduction of the intensity of the resistances in order that conflicts previously defended against through these mechanisms may now emerge into consciousness and thereby be subjected to conscious ego integration. The first step is to help the patient recognize that a resistance is being manifested, and to delineate its nature and specific function. The next step is to help the patient recognize the psychic material or conflict against which the resistance was erected and maintained.

The chief therapeutic tool for this is the interpretation of resistance, which follows the general rules of interpretation described in Chapter XI. This includes interpreting from the surface of the patient's consciousness, rather than from the depths. In other words, the therapist usually starts with resistances of which the patient himself may be aware, or resistances whose manifestations are recognized by him as ego-alien, rather than ego-syntonic. Those aspects of mental life which the patient sees as strange, or not in accord with his conscious wishes, can more readily be perceived by him as manifestations of a neurotic process than such things as ego-syntonic character traits.

For example, suddenly stopping in his conversation, or forgetting something which he was about to say, or the wish repetitively to avoid certain topics, or the experience of anxiety when coming to the therapeutic session can be recognized by the patient as forces in opposition to his avowed wish of seeking therapy. However, character traits such as punctuality, or careful logical thought, or an elaborate vocabulary, or the avoidance of expression of unpleasant feelings, may also serve as resistances. But early in the course of treatment, these will not appear strange to the patient and, therefore, it will be far more difficult to enlist his co-operation in reducing such resistances. Such manifestations of resistance are usually best interpreted later in the course of treatment.

In instances where a particular resistance is extremely important to the patient's total psychic function and where it is used intensively, early interpretation is likely to be unsuccessful, since the patient does not yet feel ready to give up such mechanisms lest he be overwhelmed by anxiety.

Tact in phrasing interpretations of resistance involves helping the patient to see this as another mental phenomenon to be examined and studied, rather than to accuse the patient of being unco-operative or to suggest that it is a sign of stubbornness or wilful opposition to treatment. The patient must be helped to see that in spite of his conscious attempts to help himself, there is another unconscious portion of his mind opposing this through the various defence mechanisms he is using. It is through these interpretations of resistance that the patient becomes increasingly aware of the operation of his own unconscious ego processes.

Resistances are usually not interpreted the first time they occur, but rather the therapist tends to wait until patterns of resistance begin to crystallize and become more apparent. Then the therapist tends to focus on those which most immediately interfere with the process and progress of treatment, rather than indiscriminately to interpret all resistance at any time it occurs. Furthermore, there must be a recognition that a single interpretation of resistance may not result in its elimination, but that it may have to be repeated subsequently. Here the question of tact is important, in order that the patient may not feel he is being 'nagged' by the therapist.

If the conflict which is being warded off by the resistance were acceptable to the patient without anxiety, it would have been permitted access to consciousness spontaneously. Therefore, the interpretation of a resistance will tend to mobilize anxiety. Not infrequently, this in turn may result in a flurry of other intensified resistances as the patient may attempt to fill the immediate defensive gap.

This may be illustrated by a common reaction occurring with a slip of the tongue. From the logical point of view of the patient's own conscious therapeutic desire, he should be pleased to have made such a slip, since it represents a momentary breach of defence, and hence may give a cue as to an unconscious underlying conflict. But if the therapist suggests that the slip had a meaning, the patient often will deny this vigorously, or present various alternative rationalizations, or depreciate and deride the therapist's attention to such 'insignificant detail'.

The interpretation of a resistance will generally not be complete at any single time. A complete interpretation would involve not only the existence of the resistance, but also the conflict which is being excluded, as well as the origins of this particular mode of defence and its role in the total psychic economy of the patient. It would also include its existence in other forms in the therapeutic situation and in the patient's current external life.

For example, if the resistance which has been recognized is that the patient plans ahead of time what he will discuss during his treatment hours, a series of interpretations might run as follows. First, the therapist might point this out as a repetitive pattern. 'It seems that you have a need to plan what you are going to say here before you come.' The next step might be to interpret the reason behind this. 'You do this planning because of your fear of being spontaneous while you are here.' A further step might indicate to the patient what his fear of spontaneity represents. 'You're afraid to be spontaneous here because you think I will disapprove of what you might say.' Next this interpretation might be linked to earlier genetic material. 'You think I will respond this way because this is what happened with your parents.' Another step in this process might be to show the patient the occurrence of the same mechanism outside the therapy situation. 'This is a factor in your shyness and difficulty in talking in a social situation.' This series of interpretations does not exhaust the particular resistance in question, but it is being used only as an illustration of how interpretations of resistance may be made sequentially and with varying degrees of completeness at any one time.

Strategy and Tactics: Supportive Therapy

The strategy of supportive psychotherapy includes the maintenance of repression against unconscious conflict, and the strengthening of ego defences in an attempt to re-establish a more stable dynamic equilibrium. When such an equilibrium occurs, anxiety will be reduced, and hence the need for secondary defence mechanisms and further symptom formation will be lessened.

With this in mind, the therapist surveys the patterns of defence and resistance utilized by the patient, searching for those which can most readily be reinforced and encouraged by appropriate interventions. Rather than interpret the patient's resistances, the therapist permits the patient to maintain his defences unchallenged, and in many instances may actually encourage them by offering the patient various rationalizations or other interventions to strengthen them.

Examples of such tactics include the following: when phobic patients rationalize the source of their anxiety, the therapist might accept the patient's reasoning and suggest further ways to help the patient live more comfortably within the limitations of the phobia; when patients manifest guilt for hostile feelings towards a loved object, the therapist might explain the ubiquitous character of such feelings and suggest acceptable ways of expressing them; for patients who insist their illness has a physical cause, the therapist might minimize the psychological components and offer a reasonable physiological explanation for specific symptoms; if a patient insists he can never take a vacation, the therapist might accept the explanation, and not try to expose the possible conflicts over pleasure, family relationships, dependency, etc., that cause the symptom; where patients manifest undue concern over sexual assault, the therapist might accept the patient's projections to the environment and leave the unconscious sexual wishes repressed; for patients with latent homosexual conflicts, the therapist might accept heterosexual promiscuous behaviour without trying to interpret its defensive function. These few examples could be extended indefinitely but they serve to illustrate the principles involved. The challenge in this type of supportive therapy is to develop the ability to assess the defensive dynamics quickly and accurately, and on the basis of such assessment, to intervene with imagination and skill.

The exception to this is the situation in which a particular resistance or defence threatens the existence of the treatment relationship, or places the patient in a situation of jeopardy outside the therapeutic situation. Examples include such things as serious suicidal risks, refusal to take necessary medication, breaking off of therapeutic contact, development of disruptive delusional thinking, etc. Here the therapist would attempt to interpret the defence to the patient, accompanied by the type of active intervention and suggestion described in Chapter XI. The therapist might at the same time try to institute or strengthen some other compatible defence to take the place of the one he is asking the patient to abandon.

Clinical Illustrations

This difference in approach between insight-directed and supportive treatment can best be described through the use of representative clinical examples. In insight-directed treatment, if a patient has been using isolation and intellectualization in an attempt to ward off intense affect, the tactical goals might be the interpretation of this defence against affective experience, the avoidance of further interpretations of intellectual content, the avoidance of technical terminology and theoretical constructs, and the emphasis on the patient's immediate emotional experience. In supportive treatment, if a patient manifests the capacity for intellectualization and isolation of affect, interventions might be designed to strengthen this defence through providing the patient with further intellectual and theoretical understanding of concepts and constructs, and the utilization of technical and 'scientific' language. The therapist might also refrain from encouraging the expression of intense affect.

During the course of insight-directed treatment, if the patient were to become restless part way through a session and suggest that he wished to leave, the immediate tactical manoeuvre might be an attempt to oppose his leaving through an interpretation of the wish to leave as a resistance. During the course of a supportive treatment relationship, if the same thing were to occur, the therapist would not oppose the patient's wish to leave as firmly, and might even support it by an intervention such as, 'If there is nothing else that you feel like talking about today, perhaps we should stop early'.

In insight-directed treatment, if a patient were to quote statistics concerning the incidence of sexual frigidity in women, and then maintain that her own frigidity is not unusual, the tactical goal would be an attempt to help her recognize this as a resistance and reluctance to facing and exploring the specific issues involved in her own sexual frigidity. In supportive psychotherapy, if a woman were to express undue concern or shame over her sexual frigidity, or to indicate her guilt because of her husband's complaints, the therapist might quote statistics to her on the overall incidence of sexual frigidity in women, thereby attempting to allay her feelings of shame and differentness. He might further try to emphasize her other positive assets as a wife which compensate for her lack of sexual responsiveness.

In insight-directed treatment, if a patient with compulsive hand-washing or other rituals related to cleanliness attempts to justify these on the basis of protection against infection or the simple wish to be neat and clean, the therapist might attempt to help him recognize this as a rationalization, and to help him see that he is reluctant to explore the irrational aspects of such a symptom, or the latent meanings behind it. In the supportive treatment of such a patient, the therapist might accept the rationalizations at their face value, and might even offer medical or commonsense explanations as a means of further justification for them. If the ritual were one which seriously impaired the patient's capacity to function, the therapist might try to find some other type of substitute but less disabling compulsive ritual to encourage instead.

During the course of insight-directed treatment, if a patient asks the therapist for direct advice or instructions on how to deal with a particular situation, the tactical goal would be to attempt eventually to interpret this as a manifestation of resistance against the development of his own capacity to make such a decision. In a supportive treatment situation, the therapist might accept the patient's expressed idea that as his therapist he is in a better position to know what is best for the patient, and might provide such advice or instruction, thus permitting the continuing resistance against conflicts over the development of independent judgment and decisiveness.

Patients in insight-directed therapy may at times verbalize conscious guilt over specific sexual practices. The therapist would generally refrain from active reassurance, and instead would use such material to further the exploration of the patient's sexual conflicts. He might also focus on the patient's inhibition in regard to developing his own sexual education, or setting his own sexual values. In supportive therapy, however, the therapist might actively provide reassurance, education, or moral judgment regarding the particular practice, leaving the deeper sexual conflicts untouched.

Such clinical examples could be continued indefinitely, but the ones already given serve to illustrate the variations in the tactical approach to resistances based on the difference of strategy between insight and supportive psychotherapy.

The Mobilization of Conflict

In earlier chapters, the differences in strategy regarding the mobilization of conflict and its resolution were briefly described. In insight-directed therapy, the immediate tactical goal of an interpretation of defence or resistance is to help the patient's self-observing and integrating ego functions become aware of the existence of such mechanisms, and thereby to encourage a decrease in the intensity of their use. Such a reduction in the defensive forces, through the conscious co-operation of the patient, results in a temporary disruption of the dynamic equilibrium as the material previously defended against comes closer to conscious awareness and expression. This partial return of the previously repressed material evokes again the signal of anxiety, against which the neurotic symptom was established in the first place. Therefore, if interpretations of defence and resistance are successful, there will result an intensification of anxiety and conflict, deliberately induced by the therapist in his attempt to help the patient become increasingly aware of the conflicts which were previously warded off and repressed.

Contrariwise, when the patient becomes fully aware of the previously unconscious conflict, he can subject it to secondary process ego control and integration. He can then establish a new level of dynamic equilibrium in which the previously unconscious material has now been integrated as part of conscious ego functioning, and the signal of anxiety will again subside. When correctly timed and effectively understood by the patient, interpretation of the content of conflicts will result in a reduction of anxiety.

In the process of insight-directed therapy, it is therefore necessary to mobilize conflict and anxiety through the interpretation of resistances and defences. This is then followed by a partial resolution of the conflict and reduction of the mobilized anxiety through increased conscious ego awareness and control after the interpretation of content. One of the problems for the therapist is the regulation of the intensity of such anxiety and conflict, and its maintenance at an optimal level for therapeutic progress.

If resistances are reduced too rapidly and too extensively, the patient may be flooded by very intense anxiety, as a result of which he may be incapable of further effective participation in the therapeutic work at the moment. He may then either withdraw, or find the anxiety intolerable, or be unable to take sufficiently effective distance from himself and his symptoms to make further progress. However, if the patient maintains a comfortable state of equilibrium for prolonged periods of time, and there is no mobilization of anxiety and conflict, then progress towards the ultimate goal of self-awareness and understanding of unconscious conflicts has been temporarily suspended.

Tactically, therefore, when the patient is already manifesting a significant degree of anxiety, the therapist will tend to focus his interventions towards interpreting the content of the conflicts which were previously repressed and thus bring to the patient's conscious awareness the danger situation signalled by the anxiety. The immediate aim is that of reducing the level of anxiety. During intervals when the patient is relatively free of anxiety, the therapist will tend to focus his interventions on the interpretations of resistance and defence, in order that there should be a mobilization of conflict as the first step towards conscious recognition, insight and ultimate further integration.

The process of insight-directed psychotherapy thus involves the intermittent mobilization of conflict and anxiety in amounts that are tolerable and will not overwhelm the patient. This is followed by interpretations of content, designed to help the patient's conscious ego integrate that quantum of the previously unconscious conflict. This produces a repetitive cycle in which the patient temporarily 'feels worse', followed by conscious ego resolution or integration and 'feeling better again'. As the patient struggles with his conscious and unconscious conflicts, his ultimate psychological development, maturity and self-confidence in the face of stress are enhanced.

It is advisable that there be occasional 'breathing spells' in order that the patient may consolidate his insight and awareness, gain emotional distance and perspective about himself and his problems, and develop increasing confidence in his improvement and in the therapeutic process itself. However, if the patient continues for prolonged periods to feel comfortable and to talk easily and glibly, or feel that he is enjoying his therapeutic experience, the therapist must recognize this as a state of resistance against the goal of ultimate insight.

The strategy of supportive therapy has been described previously and includes the attempt at reduction of the intensity of overall stress to which the patient's ego must adapt. Therefore, one tactical goal is to avoid the further mobilization of anxiety and of unconscious conflict. The therapist also tries by whatever means are appropriate to reduce the intensity and impact of conflicts which are already conscious to the patient. He tends to focus the patient's attention to such conscious conflicts as exist and may at times actively participate in resolving or containing them. A variety of methods for doing this has already been mentioned in previous sections, and anything which tends to reduce the intensity of internal and/or external stress and conflict is appropriate. This includes such things as appropriate use of the unconscious transference relationship, derivative drive satisfaction, provision of an external but benign super-ego, active participation in problem solving, active education in areas of confusion or doubt, interceding with the important people in the patient's environment, etc. At times the therapist must encourage the patient to discuss his *conscious* conflicts, or interpret the avoidance of such conflicts, but it should be done in ways which permit the patient to maintain or strengthen defences against the unconscious components of his illness.

The tactical goal is the immediate reduction of stress placed on the ego's integrative capacity. The fact that this may result in an increased dependency, or feelings of helplessness, or fantasies of the therapist's omnipotence and control is of secondary importance at the moment.

The importance and utilization of the therapeutic and transference relationship in keeping with overall strategy regarding conflict was discussed in Chapter XII.

Regression: Insight Therapy

One of the tactical devices used in the mobilization of conflict during insight-directed psychotherapy is the promotion of a regression in the service of the ego, in order that conflicts stemming from earlier experience may again be activated and experienced in an emotionally meaningful way.

In some patients, regression in the service of the ego occurs relatively easily, particularly in those with creative or artistic talent who have made previous use of such regression in their artistic and creative activities. For other patients, however, the experience of a regressive pull may be anxiety-provoking, particularly in patients with rigidly fixed character structure, or patients who focus on external reality as a prominent defence.

A variety of factors other than the patient's innate capacity influence this process of regression. The patient is asked to suspend his more advanced secondary process thinking and logical concepts, and to permit an increasing return of earlier modes of thought and fantasy more in keeping with the primary process. This is further fostered by the therapeutic atmosphere in which the patient is not held immediately accountable in logical fashion for the material that he produces. The therapist furthermore encourages the patient to experience in an emotional way whatever is occurring in his mind, and he interprets the patient's defences against such affect, even if it is appropriate only to an earlier phase of the patient's life. The therapist also repetitively interprets defences against earlier unconscious conflicts, thereby further fostering the regressive process. The regressive effect on the transference resulting from the therapist's withholding reality cues about himself, and maintaining the relative transference abstinence were discussed in Chapter XII.

17

Another important factor is the therapist's own attitude towards the regressive process. During such regression, the patient may make unreasonable or irrational demands, and with the reversion towards primary process thought and fantasy, he may express ideas similar to those which occur in patients with more serious pathology. If the therapist responds to this with anxiety, or a major change in his interactions, the patient may also experience increasing anxiety and have difficulty permitting further regression. On the other hand, if the therapist responds by offering greater activity and reassurance, the net effect may be a reinforcement of the regressive process. This in turn may result in more fixed and deeper regression, now motivated by the wish for the gratifications which were withheld when the patient was not in a regressed state. If the therapist has confidence in himself and his capacity to deal with the patient's regression, and if the regression is truly one in the service of the ego, the therapist's calm acceptance of the regressive manifestations makes it possible for the patient to undergo the experience more comfortably and confidently.

The distinction lies in the reversibility of the regression, rather than in the regressive process itself. If the regression is primarily restricted to the treatment situation, and is reversible at the end of the therapeutic session, and the patient returns to his life outside of treatment with minimal contamination of his reality-oriented behaviour, then it is one in the service of ego. If the regression is fixed and not readily reversible, or the patient is undergoing regression in his life outside of treatment, then the therapist must evaluate the possibility of more severe psychopathology and possibly incipient psychological decompensation.

Regression during the course of treatment is not an end in itself, but only a tactical means towards the end of helping the patient achieve emotional awareness of the nature of his conflicts. There must follow a reversal of the regression, in order for the patient to reintegrate or resolve the experienced conflicts in a more mature and healthy fashion from the standpoint of the secondary process and the reality principle.

This means that another aspect of the therapist's task is to help the patient control the rate and intensity of the regressive experience. Techniques for this include confrontations aimed at fostering the patient's secondary process self-observing ego functions. At times the patient may do this for himself, as when a patient in the midst of a regressive experience begins himself to question why he is reacting in such an emotional fashion. The therapist's interpretations of content relating to such experiences enhance the patient's conscious ego awareness and hence his ability to deal with the conflict and thereby to recover from the immediate regression.

If a patient spontaneously enters a regressive experience, the therapist would not interpret further resistances against deeper regression, as he would in the situation where resistances against regression are relatively intense. Other ways of controlling the degree of regression include asking specific factual questions, and focusing the patient away from the regressive material being experienced.

Another technique is to intervene towards the end of a therapeutic session in a way designed to help the patient prepare for his departure. This includes such things as helping the patient to summarize the material that has been expressed during that session, or in other ways warning the patient that the end of the session is near. In this way the therapist allies himself with the healthy and the more maturely integrative ego functions, thereby avoiding the situation in which the regression carries over into the patient's life outside of treatment.

For example, a woman may spend considerable time during her session ventilating hostility and anger towards her children, but it is necessary for her to be able to return home and give them the appropriate maternal care which they need and which her conscious adult ego wishes to provide. Or a professional man may have expressed his wishes to be passively dependent and taken care of, but at the end of the session he must be prepared to assume his mature worldly and family responsibilities.

In the ideal insight-directed therapeutic situation, such regressive re-experiencing of conflict in an emotional form alternates with periods of more mature progressive secondary process and reality-oriented integrative attempts to resolve these conflicts by the non-experiencing ego.

Regression: Supportive Therapy

Whatever the reasons may be for choosing supportive therapy in a particular case, the strategy of maintaining repression and of not mobilizing unconscious conflict dictates that further regression should be avoided. Merely to bring unconscious material to consciousness through the process of regression is not in itself therapeutic, unless the patient is in a position effectively to deal with these conflicts and to find more satisfactory adaptations or solutions to them. To promote regression in a patient whose capacity to recover from it is limited or ineffective usually disrupts the patient's defences further. This is particularly important in patients who have already undergone a significant regression during the development of the neurotic illness.

This must also be kept in mind in situations where the spontaneous regressive process is still active and the level of psychic equilibrium has not yet stabilized. At such times of ongoing regression which is not readily reversible (as compared with regression in the service of ego), the patient needs all of the defences he can muster in order to maintain homeostatic equilibrium. Regressions which are induced in the absence of the ego's capacity to reverse them at will are more likely to be fixed. As a result, they tend to persist beyond the therapeutic situation itself, thus contaminating the patient's outside life and adjustment, and they may prove extremely difficult to reverse.

With these points of strategy in mind, the tactics of the management of regression in supportive treatment are different from those in an insight-directed approach. In attempting to reverse the regressive process, or at least to maintain the current level of regression without fostering it further, the therapist encourages the patient's attempt to 'think before you speak', rather than an uninhibited expression of ideas. There is an attempt to maintain the secondary process and more quickly to confront the patient with logic and reality, rather than to encourage the emergence of primary process thought-content. The therapist gives the patient more cues regarding his own personality and personal reactions, and by interacting with the patient in a more specific and overt fashion, he provides a realistic framework for the maintenance of the relationship between himself and the patient.

The therapist is also likely to intervene actively in a judgmental and directive fashion opposed to regression in the patient, particularly after the therapeutic relationship has been established and rapport is positive so that the suggestions are likely to be effective. At times this may be done by directly instructing the patient to give up the regressive behaviour, using a 'pull yourself together' approach. Such interventions are often made on the basis of an exhortation, the motivating force being the wish to please the therapist by being a 'good patient', and 'doing what you are told to do'. The emphasis is on the patient's needs consciously to control the overt manifestations of his regression, even at the expense of giving up his independence by requiring the reinforcing attitudes of the therapist to do this.

For example, in encouraging a clinging or dependent patient to return to work, the therapist might present this in the context of a request made on the patient with the expectation that the patient will do it to please him. With a patient in whom the defence of reaction formation against dependency is being encouraged, the therapist might present the same instruction to the patient, but on the basis 'You've got to get your pride back by showing yourself and everybody else that you can do this and not give in to your symptoms'. With a masochistic patient or a patient with an unconscious need for punishment, such interventions might be made in an aggressive, somewhat harsh and slightly punitive way, such as, 'This is ridiculous for you to behave that way. Stop it, and get yourself going. If you go on this way, you will alienate everybody, and they will be right, because you are acting like a spoiled child'.

When the patient makes a move, even if a minor one, in the direction of progress and reversing the regression, it is necessary that the therapist reinforce this with interventions appropriate to the patient's overall personality organization and pattern of defences, particularly those which he is attempting to strengthen.

The therapist must also use his ingenuity to help the patient find more socially acceptable outlets for expression of regressive fantasies or impulses. In suggesting such forms of expression, he must consider both the drives to be gratified, and the defences to be strengthened. For a patient with strong acquisitive impulses, a collecting hobby might serve this function, but in a patient with a reaction formation against such acquisitiveness, it may mobilize anxiety and an activity which involves collecting for others may be more appropriate. Finger painting and clay modelling may be appropriate outlets for derivatives of a wish to smear, but if fastidiousness and orderliness are important character defences, a more controlled and careful activity such as fancy sewing or detailed copying may be more appropriate. Exhibitionistic fantasies may be gratified by developing a talent or activity that can be performed or shown in front of others. But if the patient experiences anxiety over such wishes, a solitary pursuit will be more helpful. Aggressive and hostile impulses may be expressed through activities such as carpentry, sports or vigorous physical work. But in patients with reaction formations against such direct expression of aggressiveness, more passive and vicarious outlets must be found.

In situations where the therapist is unable to forestall or reverse the regression, it is frequently necessary that he enlist the aid of the patient's relatives or others in his external life, or at times that he arrange for hospitalization as a means of dealing with the disturbance.

Catharsis and Abreaction

The concept has previously been elaborated that when a drive or drive-derivative has been gratified, there is a temporary reduction of drive-tension, until drive intensity again reaches threshold proportions. In a general way, the same holds true for the discharge of certain affects. When there has been a conscious expression of feeling, there is often a decrease in its intensity, thereby reducing the necessity for the ego to ward off such affective experience through the use of unconscious defence mechanisms. Thus for the moment, the overall stress impinging on the ego is reduced, and a more stable dynamic equilibrium can be established in keeping with the temporarily lowered affective charge.

It is this phenomenon which forms the basis of the concepts of 'catharsis' and abreaction, in which the feelings associated with a particular event or conflict are expressed, ventilated and discharged consciously, thereby reducing their intensity. In commonsense terms, this is the basis of the ideas 'get it off your chest', or 'letting off steam'.

Patients may have a variety of secondary feelings related to the open display and expression of affect (i.e. shame over crying, or guilt over anger) and a further therapeutic effect may occur as a result of the acceptance of the patient by the therapist in spite of his expression of feeling. The patient often anticipates a negative and critical response from the therapist in this situation and prepared for this, he then meets a response different from the one anticipated. This experience may encourage the patient to set up a new ego expectation and perspective, and to identify himself with the therapist's unexpected response, thereby becoming better able to modify his own self-attitudes.

The tactics in supportive therapy therefore involve permitting or encouraging the patient to express those emotional reactions, attitudes and feelings *which are already conscious*. This permits a catharsis and ventilation of feeling, with the immediate tactical goal of helping the patient establish a more stable dynamic equilibrium. On the basis of an identification with the therapist after such an emotional experience, unconscious changes in ego or super-ego forces may occur. This may also occur at a preconscious level, as when a patient says: 'Ever since I told you about that problem, I have felt much better about it, although I don't know why.'

In supportive therapy, the focus is on those feelings and affective experiences which are currently conscious, and as in the general strategy of supportive treatment, no attempt is made to interpret unconscious affective experience. The emphasis is on lessening the current adaptive burden through temporary reduction of affective charge by catharsis and ventilation, thereby enhancing the ego's capacity to improve other defences against the unconscious conflictual components.

Initially in psychoanalytic therapy, catharsis and abreaction were thought to be curative, analogous to the draining of an abscess. However, this did not take account of the fact that the intensity of such feelings is derived from unconscious intra-psychic conflict, and there tends to be a recurrence of such an affective build-up as long as the conflict which produced it persists. Although dramatic changes in symptoms were observed to occur following such abreactions, these did not prove to be permanent unless the underlying conflict was likewise more effectively integrated or resolved.

Therefore, in insight-directed treatment, catharsis, ventilation, and abreaction are important, but chiefly as a first step towards ultimate development of insight and conflict resolution. The therapist continues to interpret the various resistances against affective experience, since after the affective component has been temporarily discharged, the ego is more capable of dealing with the conflict previously warded off.

These concepts are illustrated by the treatment approach to a traumatic neurosis, particularly where there has been a total repression of the traumatic experience. Various agents (i.e. sodium amytal, hypnosis, etc.) may be utilized to bring about the emotional discharge of the affects associated with the traumatic experience. Once the abreaction has occurred, the patient is better able to permit the memory of the experience itself to return to conscious recollection, and further working through can occur and the experience can then be integrated.

In the non-traumatic neurosis the same process occurs, but in a less dramatic form. Frequently it is only after the unpleasurable affect associated with a particular memory has been discharged, and the memory thereby 'detoxified', that a fuller exploration, understanding and integration of such a memory can occur.

Many of the therapeutic factors described as occurring in the supportive situation likewise occur with abreaction in insight-directed treatment. The major difference is that in the insight-directed approach, the therapist does not stop there, nor does he permit the patient indefinitely to ward off such affect through unconscious ego defence mechanisms.

Genetic Approach

Another important part of the therapeutic process involves the application of the genetic approach. This is particularly the case in insight-directed treatment where the concept of emotional insight involves the patient's increased awareness of the antecedents of his current behaviour, and of how the present behavioural patterns relate to those of the past. The therapist oscillates the focus of his attention between the present and the past, seeking for patterns, similarities and repetitions of conflict or experience, and when tactically appropriate, he calls the patient's attention to them through a confrontation or interpretation.

It must be emphasized that the strategy of the genetic approach is for the patient to develop an increasing awareness and insight into the nature of his *current* motivations and behaviour. The tactical goal of elaboration of earlier life experience is important only if this new understanding of past events and conflicts ultimately results in more effective interaction and adaptation to conflict and stress in the present. There may be intervals in which the patient elaborates extensively on past experiences, particularly during periods when repression is less and there may be a return of previously unconscious memories. At such times, both patient and therapist may focus almost exclusively on the past experiences, but eventually these should be connected with the patient's current life in a way which provides a deeper understanding of his present attitudes and conflicts. Although elaboration of childhood experience and conflict may provide some therapeutic assistance through catharsis and abreaction, the impact is significantly lessened if this material is not consciously associated to the current situation.

In supportive psychotherapy, the therapist's focus of interest is more likely to remain in the current material and situation, without attempting to establish meaningful connections to past conflicts, since to do so usually represents the reduction of defences, and remobilization of earlier conflicts and anxiety. If this occurs in patients with inadequate ego capacities for reintegration of such material, or if the ego capacity is adequate but for other reasons therapy was undertaken only for limited contact or goals, the patient may suffer an unnecessary and unproductive disruption of psychic equilibrium. In instances of severe failure of defences, there may be a spontaneous return of previously repressed memories and experiences. In such situations, the therapist listens and accepts the communications as they occur in the consciousness of the patient, but he makes no attempt at further exploration or undoing of defences. Instead, after the patient has recounted the memory in question, the therapist may attempt to focus the patient into something more current or reality-oriented, with the explanation that the emphasis should be on his immediately feeling better, and that in the long run it is best to avoid rumination over past experiences. This must not be presented to the patient as a prohibition or lack of interest, but rather in a positive fashion as being more pertinent to the patient's immediate needs.

SUGGESTED READING

ALEXANDER, FRANZ & FRENCH, THOMAS M. (1946) *Psychoanalytic Therapy*. The Ronald Press

BUHLER, CHARLOTTE (1954) The process-organization of psychotherapy. *Psychiat. Quart.* **28**, 287

FROMM-REICHMAN, FRIEDA (1950) *Principles of Intensive Psychotherapy*. The University of Chicago Press

MENNINGER, KARL (1958) *The Theory of Psychoanalytic Technique*. Basic Books Inc, New York

CHAPTER XIV

The Therapeutic Process: Insight and Working-Through

The ultimate aim of psychotherapy is an improvement in the patient's overall capacity for psychological adaptation. The differences between supportive and insight-directed psychotherapy have repeatedly been emphasized, in terms of the methods by which this aim is achieved, and the nature of psychological functioning which the respective goals represent.

Insight

To achieve the goals set for insight-directed therapy, the patient must first gain a degree of new insight regarding himself, and then make use of this awareness to achieve a more stable and mature level of adaptation. Insight involves an enhanced degree of self-awareness and recognition of elements in the individual's own mental and emotional life which previously had been preconscious or unconscious. Insight may occur at various levels and depths, from an intellectual understanding to a full emotional awareness.

At the more superficial end of this spectrum, the patient develops a more clear intellectual understanding and acceptance of an idea of which he had previously been only dimly aware; or of a new idea introduced by the therapist and accepted as valid by the patient on the basis of his confidence in the therapist's skill. At the other end of the spectrum, the patient has a subjective emotional sense of conviction and understanding of a new idea or concept resulting from his own personal experience. Patients describe this latter form of insight in various ways, such as: 'I suddenly see what you mean'; or, 'we have talked about this before, but it never made sense to me until now'; or, 'suddenly it is all so simple and clear'; or, 'that rings a bell'; etc. Another dimension of insight also occurs on a spectrum, and involves dynamic (cross-sectional) as opposed to genetic (longitudinal) awareness and understanding. The patient may develop emotional awareness and insight into current dynamic mental processes and thereby become aware of factors and forces which previously had escaped conscious recognition, but he may have no explanation or understanding of their origins. And a patient may have an awareness that certain events in early life were traumatic or significant, but have no insight into the delayed effects that these events have on his current life or personality.

The subjective experience of emotional insight is a highly meaningful one for the patient. It is usually the result of gradually lowered resistance against awareness of unconscious and preconscious conflicts, and increasing personal recognition and acceptance by the ego of the drive-derivatives and defences previously warded off. However, there are instances in which emotionally significant insight may occur rapidly with only a brief therapeutic contact, and result in significant intra-psychic change. In such cases, the patient usually has a pre-existing capacity for psychological awareness, the currently activated dynamic conflicts are close to consciousness, the therapist has been able promptly to grasp the essence of the current conflict, and for a variety of reasons the patient is rapidly able to establish a relationship of basic trust. Generally such a response occurs more readily for dynamic rather than genetic insights, but its effects can at times be dramatic.

Clinical examples of this include a 42-year-old factory worker who requested consultation for an intense work phobia of recent onset. In the first session, the therapist obtained a history of the present complaints, as well as background information to the effect that he had had a poor relationship with his father, had been a man of violent temper, had drunk excessively, and had been sexually promiscuous. After his marriage 6 years earlier he had undergone a major personality change, and the previous aggressive and unreliable behaviour had disappeared. In the second session several days later, the therapist concentrated on the onset of the phobia shortly after an incident with the supervisor in which the patient felt unjustly accused and criticized. The therapist suggested that the patient must have felt angry, and helpless, and probably had an impulse to hit the supervisor. The patient then recalled with feeling that he had a fantasy at the time of crushing the supervisor's skull with a piece of pipe lying nearby. He went on to express more of his hostility towards the supervisor. In the next session he reported that his anxiety had completely subsided and he was back at work without symptoms.

A 22-year-old college senior developed acute symptoms of inability to study, anxiety when attending classes, expectation of failure in spite of a good record, and depression. She had gone to school at great sacrifice by her parents, and had always worked hard. The therapist asked how she thought her parents would feel if she failed to graduate. She said they would be heartbroken, and with sudden awareness recognized that she wanted to hurt them and that for years she had felt angry at their pressure for her success. She immediately felt less anxious and depressed, and one week later reported a return of her ability to work.

A 20-year-old attractive but shy, inhibited, studious college student developed acute anxiety, fears of academic failure, obsessional doubts about his future, and difficulty in concentration. The symptoms occurred shortly after his first meaningful contact with an attractive girl who had taken the initiative to begin a sexual relationship with him. Throughout the interview the therapist made no interpretations at all, but as he talked the patient spoke of dividing people into those who worked and those who played, and thought he should belong to the former group. With a sudden feeling of recognition and relief he became spontaneously aware of the unreality of such stereotypes, and of the possibility of combining both activities. He left the session relieved and with a new sense of confidence.

A man sought consultation for marital discord which he blamed on his wife's emotional instability and neurotic disturbances. In between the two diagnostic sessions he suddenly recognized that he felt more comfortable and confident within himself when his wife was upset and troubled, and that he frequently behaved in ways to accentuate and intensify her difficulties, rather than to be helpful to her. He had no explanation of why he reacted this way or how it all began. When informed several weeks later that the therapist now had time available to begin regular treatment sessions, the patient stated that his marriage was much improved and he no longer felt the need for therapy.

In all these cases relatively superficial but meaningful dynamic insight extended the operations of the patient's conscious ego functions, thus permitting a new equilibrium to occur with dramatic symptom and behavioural response. Each of them also had further neurotic disturbances and character pathology which was untouched by these brief therapeutic contacts, and whether or not these would eventually produce other episodes of decompensation could not be definitely predicted.

It is the therapeutic importance of achieving this form of personal and emotional insight that makes insight-directed treatment so long and difficult with most patients. If intellectual insight alone were sufficient to produce a fundamental change, it would be possible much earlier in the course of treatment to explain to the patient his conflicts and disturbances or to encourage him to learn about himself through reading. Through study of the derivatives of unconscious conflicts, the therapist may quite accurately identify the general nature of the patient's disturbances early in the course of the treatment contact. However, in the time between the therapist's awareness and the patient's readiness to understand his conflicts in an emotional way, significant preparatory therapeutic work usually must occur. In general, the more emotional, immediate and personal is the experience of insight, the more effect will it have therapeutically.

Generally speaking, therapy is most effective if the development of insight proceeds from the conscious surface towards the unconscious depths of mental functioning, and from the current dynamic conflicts towards their genetically earlier editions. In the type of face-to-face psychotherapy discussed here, insight is generally not achieved (except for intellectual reconstructions) to ages more remote than the latency period. And often the most effective therapeutic work occurs in the exploration and elaboration of the conflicts, changes, and structuring of personality which occurred during that phase of development.

In other words, the therapist tries to help the patient unfold the patterns of conflict in an organized way, and does not attempt to 'jump ahead' to childhood when adolescent or adult conflicts are largely unexplored.

When setting the original goals, and when modifying them as necessary during the course of the treatment, the therapist must also keep in mind the level of insight which it is possible for the specific patient to achieve. In some instances, therapeutic strategy may dictate the focusing of insight on the various aspects of particular conflicts as they occur in the individual's current life, leaving unexplored the earlier determinants and manifestations of the same conflicts. In other instances, strategy may dictate the development of insight into some conflicts, while other conflicts or their derivatives are left unexplored. Such strategic limiting of insight requires consistent intervention by the therapist in ways which selectively encourage or discourage specific dynamic or genetic explorations.

Working-through: Insight Therapy

In earlier chapters, the tenacious and timeless nature of the unconscious drives and their derivatives have repeatedly been emphasized, as have been the functions of defence and their manifestation as resistance in the therapeutic process. As a result of these factors, and in contrast to the usual portrayal in movies and T.V., a single interpretation or conscious recovery of previously preconscious or unconscious material is not likely to produce the permanent change which is the goal of insight-directed treatment. (One possible exception to this is the acute traumatic neurosis, in which emotional abreaction of the traumatic experience may at times lead to rapid and lasting reintegration.)

The more usual pattern of treatment involves a step-wise and repetitive series of therapeutic interventions through which the patient is helped again and again to recognize and attempt to integrate psychic material previously warded-off. Resistances do not 'melt-away', and frequently the temporary reduction of a resistance may be followed by a more intense recurrence of the same resistance, or by the intensification of other patterns of defence in a compensatory fashion. In this way, after the patient has taken two steps forward, he frequently takes one or two steps backward, and this form of oscillation between progress and retreat is a common pattern during insight-directed treatment.

The working-through process involves this repetitive cycle of mobilization of conflict and anxiety, followed by a temporary symptomatic exacerbation, in turn followed by increasing conscious awareness of that which previously was warded off, and then by a partial resolution of conflict and reduction of anxiety as conscious ego processes of integration take control. Phrased differently, the process of working-through involves an oscillation in small increments between 'getting worse' and then 'getting better'.

The therapist, through his interventions and focusing, attempts to help the patient recognize the same conflict or constellation of mental processes in a variety of different current situations, as well as in genetically earlier forms. The therapist also attempts to vary the approach to the problems from the different perspectives of id, ego or super-ego functions.

The process of working-through thus involves the patient repeatedly extending his awareness of his problems in their different forms and from different points of view, until the desired degree of insight and understanding has been achieved. Sometimes this occurs in response to transference phenomena; at other times in relationship to conflict in the current life situation; and at other times in regard to conflicts in the past life of the patient. In this way, working-through results in a further elaboration and understanding of material which is increasingly conscious to the patient, but not yet fully integrated.

However, repeatedly bringing up the same material may represent a form of resistance in which the patient continues to stay on familiar and therefore 'safe' topics. The process of working-through is signified when each return of the material is accompanied by an affective component, or by changes in the material itself, particularly the elaboration of further details, or by new associations previously omitted.

During the working-through process, the therapist's job is to present his formulations in a form which will make the most sense to the patient, and permit the greatest degree of developing insight and expanding ego integration. It is important in this that the therapist avoid stereotyped interventions even though the material may be familiar to the patient. Repeating the same words or interpretations again and again tends to make the treatment dull and lifeless. One of the therapist's tasks is to find new and different ways of presenting his interventions. This includes such things as shifts in his point of view or perspective, changes in the language he uses, variations in the examples he chooses from the patient's material to illustrate concepts, or the use of varying and colourful analogies to illustrate his ideas. Sometimes an effective method of confrontation or interpretation may even be the telling of an appropriate joke.

The point has been made that insight alone has no magic qualities. It does not produce therapeutic change unless the patient is able to develop and integrate new patterns of behaviour, adaptation and ultimate internal modification on the basis of this new knowledge and understanding. Thus another important element in the process of working-through is the attempt which the patient makes to modify and change himself or his situation on the basis of his increasing insight. And the way in which the therapist intervenes in response to such attempts by the patient will significantly influence how effective they are.

When the patient begins to make changes in the direction of greater adaptation and more mature functioning on the basis of insight, working-through, or a change in intra-psychic organization, it becomes important that the therapist attempt to support such efforts or at least not oppose them.

In this way, the therapist helps to strengthen those elements in the patient's ego organization which are striving towards new and more effective modes of integration. Often first attempts at new adaptations or conflict solution will tend to be fumbling and awkward, or result in failure, or reflect other unconscious neurotic aspects in the total behaviour pattern.

For example, if a shy, inhibited and sexually anxious young man finally takes a girl out on a date, but the evening ends in discomfort and failure, the importance of the fact that the patient has made the effort to go out socially far outweighs the failure that resulted. At such a time, if the therapist focuses on the old neurotic and unconsciously self-defeating patterns, he will emphasize the patient's weaknesses, and not support the effort it required to make the attempt to change. In such a setting it would be more helpful explicitly to recognize the patient's positive movement, and to postpone consideration of the other neurotic components in the total experience until the time when such types of progressive movement are less difficult and more commonplace.

If an obsessional patient who has had intense neurotic anxiety about punctuality begins to come late to his therapeutic sessions, this in all likelihood represents the acting-out of a resistance. However, even more important, it also represents a sign of internal psychic change, and a beginning modification of the rigid character structure exemplified by neurotic punctuality. If the therapist immediately focuses on this behaviour, or emphasizes that the lateness represents a resistance, the likelihood is that the patient will interpret this as criticism for not following the rigid obsessional pattern, and the progress manifested by such behaviour will stop. In such a situation the therapist might instead accept the patient's lateness without comment, at least until the patient has had the helpful experience of being late without dire consequences or attack by the therapist. And when an intervention is made, it might be advisable to acknowledge the fact that giving up of the rigidity represents a step forward, but that none the less, the lateness represents some unverbalized aspect of the patient's reactions.

In other words, it is therapeutically important for the patient to realize that the therapist has recognized the efforts he is making, and changes which are occurring. At times this may become a form of transference resistance, in that the patient may then make further efforts as a direct attempt to please the therapist and thereby gain verbal or tacit approval. If this occurs, the therapist would then use the transference resistance itself as further material to be worked through.

Working-through: Supportive Therapy

In keeping with general strategy, concepts of insight and the working-through of conflict do not strictly apply to the supportive treatment situation, but a process similar to that of working-through does occur.

The strategy of supportive treatment may be summarized as calling for the gratification of drive-derivatives, the strengthening of a particular defence or group of ego defences, the modification of super-ego and ego functions chiefly by conscious or unconscious identification with the therapist, and/or the establishment of a less stressful or more supportive external environment.

As in the process of working-through during insight-directed treatment, a single tactical intervention in keeping with this basic strategy is seldom effective in producing the desired change. The patient in supportive therapy usually needs repetitive experiences with the same material, but as described in earlier chapters, from a different point of view than the patient in insight-directed treatment.

For example, several cathartic abreactions of the same material, or repeated gratification of drive-derivatives may be required before significant reduction in the intensity of conflict can occur. The strengthening of ego defences usually requires multiple interventions in connection with various situations of conflict. Unconscious identification with the therapist is a gradual process, and usually occurs only after repeated interactions, and seldom takes place on the basis of a single experience.

In a supportive therapeutic situation, the therapist actually uses appropriately repeated transference gratifications to reinforce any movements by the patient in the direction of more mature and stable levels of adaptation. Such reinforcements tend to perpetuate and entrench the new behavioural or feeling responses, and may thus result in modification of the patient's overall behaviour without his conscious awareness of the reasons for its occurrence. Once these new patterns of behaviour have been established with the help of the therapist's repeated reinforcement, the hope is that the satisfaction provided by the new modes of integration themselves, as well as the continuing transference gratification offered by the treatment relationship, will make such changes more ego-syntonic. It is on this basis that a lasting therapeutic change may at times occur in a supportive treatment relationship, although the more usual pattern requires a continuing or at least intermittent reinforcement of some type.

In applying such reinforcement supportively, one of the main therapeutic problems is for the therapist accurately to assess the psychodynamics and psychopathology in the specific patient. For many patients, particularly those with passive-dependent transference attitudes, or those in states of positive rapport, an overt sign of recognition, approval or pleasure from the therapist serves to provide such reinforcement. However, as previously emphasized, in patients with reaction-formations against dependency, or with needs to rebel against an authoritarian figure, or with intense guilt, or masochistic character disturbances, or with intense latent homosexual conflicts, etc., this type of intervention by the therapist may not only fail to reinforce the response in the patient, but may actually have the reverse effect. The therapist's task is to determine for each specific patient the types of intervention which are likely to be unconsciously reinforcing in a positive sense, and repeatedly to make use of them in achieving the supportive goals.

18

Rate of Improvement

The rate of the patient's progress in insight-directed therapy, as it is reflected in the process of working-through, may be seen as a geometric rather than a linear progression. Much of the early work in treatment is ego-preparation in which the interpretation of a defence or resistance, the mastery of the anxiety and conflict thus mobilized, and the resulting increased self-awareness produce an extension of conscious ego activity and a strengthening of the therapeutic alliance.

With the slightly greater awareness of previously unconscious conflict, the ego is strengthened. The patient is then in a position to tolerate further reduction of resistance, mobilization of anxiety and conflict and to seek further conflict resolution.

As the ego is strengthened in a step-wise fashion, the patient can tolerate greater increments of conscious awareness of conflict, and he becomes less anxious at the emergence of his own impulses, and has greater capacity for conscious ego control. The more the patient integrates and deals with these smaller increments of conflict, the greater is his capacity to integrate larger and deeper increments, and this produces the geometric rate of progress.

As a result, overall progress in insight-directed psychotherapy is often relatively slow or minimal in terms of subjective symptoms, behaviour, or integration during the early and middle phases of the treatment. However, as the ego functions become more conscious and effective, there may then occur rapid progress in all of these areas.

To some extent the same holds true in supportive therapy, where the therapist's interventions and the patient's interactions in the treatment situation also produce a strengthening of ego functions and defence, although not on the basis of insight or awareness. As defences become more effective, and conflicts are reduced in intensity, the dynamic equilibrium becomes more stable and there is a reduction of anxiety. This diminishes the needs for further unconscious defences and symptom formation, but in supportive therapy progress tends to be more linear in rate than is the case in insight-directed treatment.

However, in either form of treatment the patient's rate of progress may reach a plateau in which there is little or no further change over an extended period of time. This may be a function of the specific patient and his therapeutic capacity, or at times it may result from the particular therapist-patient combination. It is also often a function of the inherent limitations of the treatment method, and the patient may have already achieved as much success as is likely or possible.

If such a plateau occurs, it is important that the therapist evaluate the total therapeutic situation, and establish the reasons why progress has ceased. Appropriate overall management of this problem depends on the nature of the factors that produced it. Failure to make such an evaluation may at times result in treatment being automatically continued long beyond the point where it is serving a useful function for the patient.

SUGGESTED READING

FINESINGER, JACOB E. & REID, JOHN R. (1952) The role of insight in psychotherapy. *Am. J. Psychiat.* **108**, 726

GREENSON, RALPH R. (1965) The problem of working through. In: *Drives, Affects, Behavior.* Vol. 2, ed. Schur, Max. International Universities Press Inc, New York

GRINKER, ROY R. & SPIEGEL, JOHN (1945) *Men under Stress.* Blakiston Co, Philadelphia

LOEWALD, HANS W. (1955) Hypnoid state, repression, abreaction and recollection. *J. Am. Psychoanal. Ass.* **3**, 201

ROSEN, HAROLD & MYERS, HENRY (1947) Abreaction in the military setting. *Arch. Neurol. & Psychiat.* **57**, 161

THORNTON, NATHANIAL (1949) What is the therapeutic value of abreaction? *Psychoanal. Rev.* **36**, 411

CHAPTER XV

Counter-Transference

Introduction

In Chapter XII, the theory and manifestations of the patient's transference relationship during the course of a treatment experience were described. The counterpart of such reactions are those which the therapist may develop towards the patient during this process, and these are known as *counter-transference*.

Transference was defined as that part of the patient-therapist relationship which occurs at an unconscious level in the mind of the patient, and was distinguished from the more conscious elements of the patient's total reactions to the therapist. Counter-transference is based on unconscious forces within the therapist, whereby he reacts to the patient in ways which are to some degree inappropriate to the current reality of the therapeutic relationship, and are displaced from earlier relationships and experiences in his own life.

In Chapter II and III, the role of unconscious forces in normal mental life was developed. These factors also hold true for the psychotherapist. He has gone through the various vicissitudes of individual and species-specific development, and as in all human beings, there will remain residues of unconscious psychic conflict dating back to childhood and infancy.

Many psychotherapists are attracted to the field of psychiatry by virtue of their own interest in psychological and emotional phenomena, and they are more likely to be introspective and partially aware of their own emotional processes than is the individual whose interests lie in other spheres. Not infrequently, it is this awareness of his own unresolved internal emotional conflicts which stimulates a person to enter this field, at times in hopes of finding the solution to his own personal problems through work with patients. When properly integrated or resolved, such a personal experience with emotional conflict makes the psychotherapist more sensitive and respectful of the patient's illness and disturbances, and therefore, makes him a more skilful worker.

Although the resolution of personal conflicts may make the psychotherapist more sensitive and skilful, their unrecognized persistence may jeopardize or interfere with his successful therapeutic function. The therapist's ego also scans the environment seeking objects which can serve the gratification of unconscious drive-derivatives or defences, and the counter-transference may block or interfere with the therapeutic process if the therapist makes unconscious use of his patients as such objects. At other times, the patient may be consciously or unconsciously used by the therapist in his relationship to his professional colleagues. In such instances, the patient may become a source of pride and praise, or shame and criticism, and the therapist may react emotionally to the patient on this basis.

The differentiation must also be made between those elements in the therapist's reactions to the patient which are conscious, and those which are unconscious. A therapist interacting with a patient may at times experience such feelings as irritation, impatience, boredom, pleasure, satisfaction, curiosity, concern, uncertainty, confidence, sympathy, failure or success, etc. When such emotional responses are proportional and appropriate to the patient's material or behaviour, and they are conscious to the therapist, and do not directly motivate his therapeutic interactions, they are best considered *counter-reactions*. In fact, the therapist can make effective use of his own counter-reactions as a form of non-verbal data, indicating the impact which the patient produces on other people.

Using his observations of his conscious emotional reactions as a guide, the therapist can often detect the latent meanings behind the patient's communication or behaviour. For example, if he feels helpless and blocked in his therapeutic efforts, he can make other observations to determine whether the patient's latent wish is to defeat the therapy. If he feels pleased and satisfied, he may begin to wonder if the patient's transference wish is to ingratiate himself and gain approval from the therapist. If he feels irritated and annoyed, he may ask himself whether the patient is seeking to provoke an attack. As with all data from empathy and introspection, the therapist must consciously decide how to use such material in keeping with the overall strategy and the immediate tactical situation.

The term *counter-transference* is therefore generally reserved for the unconscious responses in the therapist towards the patient, resulting from the therapist using the patient as an object for transference. At times the existence and nature of the counter-transference reaction may be totally unconscious, while at other times only some of the elements in the reaction remain unconscious. But as in transference reactions, the counter-transference may involve elements of the drives and drive-derivatives, the super-ego, and/or the defensive or adaptive ego functions.

Manifestations

Analogous to transference reactions, the manifestations of counter-transference are variable and multiple, since any element or aspect of the therapist's mental processes may be cathected by counter-transference displacement. The manifestations themselves are limited only by the vicissitudes of the therapist's unconscious mental life and the various derivative ways in which it is integrated.

A. Generalized Reactions

The group of generalized counter-transference reactions involving a number of different patients may include such drive-derivatives as a therapist's need to be needed and to have others dependent upon him; or a need to feel himself to be omniscient; or a wish to control and manipulate people and their lives. They may chiefly involve certain groups of patients, as in a therapist who can function comfortably only with men, or only with women; or a therapist who is repeatedly unable to treat patients with particular types of conflicts, or specific disorders.

At times a therapist may use his patients to gratify such unconscious drives as voyeurism and curiosity, and be particularly energetic and eager to uncover the patient's innermost secrets, fantasies and details of behaviour; at other times a therapist may have a reaction-formation against such curiosity and be reluctant or unable to elicit such information. Some therapists may gratify unconscious aggressive impulses by inflicting unnecessary pain, discomfort or frustration on to patients; other therapists may experience anxiety in such circumstances, and thus be unable to maintain optimal therapeutic frustration of transference wishes. Some therapists may repeatedly be passively manipulated and controlled by their patients, and be drawn into undue or excessive activity.

At times therapists may have unconscious masochistic needs which lead them unconsciously to encourage their patients to make excessive demands, and then to try to meet these at the sacrifice of their own personal lives. Counter-transference reactions may cause some therapists always to become involved with the sickest patients who have the poorest prognosis, and then attempt 'to do the impossible'; while in other therapists, such patients may evoke a counter-transference response of hopelessness and avoidance. A therapist may unconsciously select the patients with whom he works on the basis of counter-transference reactions involving such things as certain diagnostic entities, the sex of the patient, specific age groups, physical attractiveness, intelligence, etc. Some therapists choose only to treat patients who will become intensely dependent, whereas other therapists may avoid such patients and choose only those who maintain distance and aloofness, and who remain independent of the therapeutic relationship. Some therapists may unconsciously respond in ways to evoke intense, and at times inappropriately regressive, transference reactions in all patients, while other therapists may respond in ways to suppress and avoid any development of transference reactions in their patients, both of which suggest the operation of counter-transference forces.

B. Specific Reactions

The other group of counter-transference reactions involves the therapist's unconscious responses to a particular patient, in which there are specific associations linking some element in the patient's material or behaviour to the unresolved conflicts within the therapist.

This might involve a patient who manifests conflicts very similar to those of the therapist, whereby the therapist's attitudes and interactions will be influenced by his attitudes towards his own unconscious disturbances. At times this may prevent the therapist from recognizing or fully understanding the conflicts presented by the patient, lest he also have to recognize the unconscious meaning of his own. At other times, it may lead him to project his own internal unconscious conflicts on to whatever material presented by the patient permits such a defence. For example, a therapist with unconscious conflicts over his own aggressions may emphasize the various manifestations of aggression in the patient to an undue extent and proportion; or a therapist with latent homosexual impulses may interpret homosexual conflicts in the particular patient out of proportion to their actual significance.

At times a patient may have had life experiences very similar to those of the therapist, which may thereby stimulate his unresolved conflicts; or a specific behaviour and attitude in the patient may evoke a moralistic response in the therapist, thereby impairing his ability to be effectively objective in his therapeutic role. At times characteristics of the patient or his behaviour may be specifically associated by the therapist to particular objects in his own past life, and thereby may evoke unconscious responses in the therapist more appropriate to the object from the past.

Some counter-transference reactions are covert and difficult for the therapist to recognize. For example, over-identification with a patient may be manifested by a relative loss of objectivity, or a tendency to take the patient's side against the objects in his environment, and a feeling they are hostile, unco-operative or frustrating. The opposite response of taking too great an emotional distance from the patient, and thus the therapist's inability to use himself as a perceptive instrument, may also be a manifestation of counter-transference. Failure to give the patient his full attention may at times be a reflection of the therapist's current problems, but may also be a manifestation of a counter-transference need to keep emotional distance from the patient.

The 'Pygmalion fantasy' in which the therapist attempts to mould the patient into an idealized image is usually the result of his using the patient for his own unconscious purposes. Therapeutic over-ambition and the setting of unrealistically high goals for the patient, as well as therapeutic under-ambition and the setting of inappropriately restricted and limited goals, may be influenced by counter-transference reactions. They may also influence the selection of the treatment modality in the choice between insight-directed or supportive psychotherapy, drug-treatment, hospitalization, electric-shock, hypnosis, etc.

Another manifestation of counter-transference may be a difficulty in understanding or integrating the material presented by the patient, particularly if such a difficulty is persistent. Some therapists have problems in permitting the patient to grow as an independent individual and to live his own life by standards or values different from those of the therapist himself. Often this is a particular issue at the time of termination. Analogous to the parent of an adolescent or a young adult, the therapist at times has difficulty in permitting the patient to grow and establish an independent existence, and may have unconscious needs continually to point out the persistent neurotic conflicts that have not been fully resolved, and thereby keep the patient in treatment for an unnecessarily long time.

These illustrations of possible generalized or specific counter-transference reactions could be elaborated indefinitely, but the emphasis here is to demonstrate the type of impact that unconscious counter-transference reactions may exert. The therapist's use of unconscious ego defences often results in repression, rationalization, displacement and other defence manoeuvres to explain or justify such reactions, and frequently the therapist's responses are not consciously recognized as manifestations of counter-transference.

Early in the history of psychoanalytic theory and therapy, it was thought that counter-transference reactions should be eliminated, and that they inevitably led to significant disturbances or disruptions in the therapeutic process. Further clinical experience and study, however, has indicated that it is probably never possible completely to eliminate all counter-transference reactions, and that they continue to occur even in seasoned and well-trained therapists.

Thus the problem for the therapist is the acceptance of counter-transference as a phenomenon which must be recognized in the therapeutic process and dealt with in ways to minimize its disruptive effects. It is therefore necessary that the psychotherapist be aware of himself and his own reactions and responses, in order that he may manage the inevitable counter-transference phenomena as they arise. The occurrence of counter-transference reactions is more frequent and prominent in inexperienced therapists, and the more familiarity that the therapist develops with his own preconscious and unconscious mental processes, the more can such reactions be minimized and controlled, if not eliminated.

Signals of Counter-Transference

Although the specific nature of a counter-transference reaction is highly variable and should be individually worked out in each instance, there are a number of non-specific manifestations which are relatively easy to recognize. Probably the most common signal of counter-transference is a persistent or recurrent significant block in understanding the patient and his conflicts. The therapist may also notice such things as the experience of anxiety during the therapeutic session or when considering the material after the treatment session is over. Such anxiety may at times be accompanied or replaced by the development of other neurotic symptoms, usually of a transient nature. Other signals may include a feeling of guilt, or the experience of intense emotional reactions towards the patient such as anger, jealousy, excessive concern and sympathy, sexual arousal, or love.

Such things as minor symptomatic acts, slips of the tongue, mistakes in appointments, errors in billing, etc., generally indicate a mobilization of unconscious conflict related to the patient. There may also be a conscious preoccupation with the patient beyond reasonable therapeutic interest. Such things as repetitively discussing or describing the patient to others, dreams or fantasies about the patient, and an eager or an unpleasurable anticipation of the patient's next visit, are useful indicators to suggest the existence of a counter-transference reaction. After the therapist has established a particular structure and routine of procedure for each patient, departures from them should be scrutinized as possibly related to counter-transference.

Management of Counter-Transference

In the management of counter-transference reactions, the first problem is for the therapist to recognize their existence and attempt to identify them as specifically as possible. This involves a continuing process of self-evaluation and introspection on the part of the therapist as he interacts with the patient, and a continuing alertness to the possible occurrence of counter-transference phenomena. It also requires an awareness of the various cues which may be used to indicate the existence of such a reaction, and a willingness in the therapist to accept the occurrence of such counter-transference reactions in himself without undue shame. In attempting to identify the details of a counter-transference conflict, it is essential that the therapist apply the same standards of honest and forthright self-appraisal to himself as he expects of his patient. Bringing a counter-transference conflict to conscious awareness can only occur after overcoming the therapist's own resistances.

In instances where the therapist, after reasonable efforts at introspection and self-evaluation, is still unable to recognize or identify counter-transference reactions, or in instances where there appears to be a persistent unresolved counter-transference response, it is often helpful to seek consultation with a colleague. By virtue of his greater distance from the immediate situation and greater objectivity, the consultant may be in a better position to help the therapist identify some of the counter-transference forces.

In situations where the counter-transference appears to be intractable, repetitive or a significantly generalized experience which interferes with the therapist's ability to carry out his functions, the therapist must consider personal psychotherapy in an attempt more clearly to deal with and resolve such counter-transferences.

In the meantime, when dealing with the patient in the face of an ongoing counter-transference reaction, it is wiser at such moments that the therapist attempt to minimize his activity and interventions until he has re-established his own emotional equilibrium and control, thereby reducing the extent of contamination of the therapeutic situation by the counter-transference. When the therapist is under the pressure of his own emotional responses to the patient, these will inevitably colour and influence his choice of words, tone of voice and the way in which he presents his interventions to the patient, possibly leading to subsequent complications or difficulties in the treatment situation.

If the therapist is aware of a persistent counter-transference attitude, it is sometimes possible to compensate for this by an offsetting conscious decision and control. For example, a therapist who tends to be overly ambitious for all of his patients may consciously be able to control this, and set more realistic limitations for himself as well as the patient. A therapist who is aware of an unneutralized sexual voyeuristic curiosity and who tends to intervene whenever sexual material is mentioned, may consciously be capable of offsetting this through control and through conscious efforts to intervene equally in other areas as well. Or a therapist who has an inhibition or a defensive need to avoid such explorations may likewise be able to compensate for this by conscious efforts in the opposite direction.

The emphasis must be on the therapist's willingness to accept the occurrence of counter-transference without undue guilt or shame, and on his honesty in self-appraisal in attempting to identify and understand such reactions. As with the patient in treatment, the therapist must then attempt to use such newly gained understanding and awareness to change his reactions and behaviour in the current situation. Unless the therapist is willing to face issues of psychological truth within himself, he is hardly in a position to request or require this of his patients.

Some schools of psychotherapy go so far as to encourage the therapist to express his counter-transference reactions and counter-feelings directly and openly to the patient on the assumption that this will encourage honesty in the patient, and will make communication between therapist and patient more effective and intimate. Some therapists believe that the therapist can and should use the therapeutic situation for his own treatment and further development as an individual.

At times such behaviour even reaches the proportions of the therapist significantly acting-out with the patient, as in the case of an overt sexual seduction, or of active personal participation in the patient's social and extra-therapeutic life. Those who hold to such positions often maintain that failure to do this is a function of inhibition or lack of openness and honesty in the therapist.

Opposed to this, however, is the argument that if the therapist is in need of treatment himself, he should make the necessary arrangements to place himself in the position of a patient with someone who can be therapeutically objective, rather than to use the patient for this purpose. Furthermore, when he uses the situation for himself, he departs from the position of a therapist to whom the patient comes for help. Instead, the therapist places himself in a position *vis-à-vis* a patient more akin to a non-therapeutic relationship between friends or acquaintances. Although in the latter there may at times be significant changes in both participants by virtue of the relationship and interactions between them, this is no longer a structured and stable therapeutic situation, and the dynamics of the relationship are thereby significantly altered.

This is different from the situation described earlier in a supportive relationship where, on the basis of a conscious decision based on the therapeutic needs of the patient, the therapist may reveal certain aspects of himself or his personality and reactions in an attempt to further the immediate tactical goals of the treatment. The chief distinction is that the tactical goal is the well-being of the patient rather than that of the therapist, and the intervention is designed to meet a particular need such as the fostering of identification, or the strengthening of a defence. In such a situation the therapist is not attempting to express and reveal emotional counter-transference responses, but is instead using himself as a model for the patient to emulate in the latter's struggle to establish a more comfortable dynamic equilibrium.

SUGGESTED READING

ABSE, DAVID W. & EWING, JOHN A. (1956) Transference and counter-transference in somatic therapies. *J. nerv. ment. Dis.* **123**, 32

BENEDEK, THERESA (1953) Dynamics of the counter transference. *Bull. Menninger Clin.* **17**, 201

GITELSON, MAXWELL (1952) The emotional position of the analyst in the psychoanalytic situation. *Int. J. Psycho-Anal.* **33**, 1

MONEY-KYRLE, R. E. (1956) Normal countertransference and some of its deviations. *Int. J. of Psycho-Anal.* **37**, 360

ORR, DOUGLASS W. (1954) Transference and counter transference: an historical survey. *J. Am. Psychoanal. Ass.* **2**, 621

REICH, ANNIE (1951) On Countertransference. *Int. J. Psycho-Anal.* **32**, 25

REICH, ANNIE (1960) On Countertransference. *Int. J. Psycho-Anal.* **41**, 389

CHAPTER XVI

The Therapeutic Process: The Use of Drugs

Introduction

The use of drugs is a traditional and important aspect of general medical practice. In recent years, advances in chemistry and pharmacology have led to the development of a large and increasingly complex group of drugs with specific psychotropic effects. The ready availability and relative safety of these drugs has led to an increasingly intensive and extensive use of such agents in the treatment of the various forms of psychiatric disturbances. With increasing frequency, this is being undertaken by the general medical physician as well as the psychiatrist.

Psychodynamically, the effect of many psychotropic drugs is to reduce the intensity of the specific unpleasant signal affects and affect states. The role of these affects in symptom formation has been discussed earlier. When the intensity of unpleasant affects is reduced by pharmacological methods, the needs for secondary elaboration and intensification of ego defence mechanisms is likewise decreased. As a result of this shift, symptom formation or maintenance is diminished.

The administration of any active substance or drug will produce a pharmacological response and will also have a psychological effect in the patient who receives it. The pharmacology and clinical indications for the use of the various specific drugs is a vast subject which will not be discussed here. The importance of the psychological effects is indicated by the fact that they produce undesirable and contaminating responses in the patient when such drugs are being pharmacologically evaluated. The frequency and intensity of this *placebo effect* has required the development of the double-blind method for clinical testing of new drugs.

In the primarily therapeutic situation, however, there is less need to distinguish between the pharmacological and psychological effects of a drug, since the chief aim in its administration is the well-being of the patient. In other words, the therapist should understand the dynamics of the placebo effect in order that this force may be harnessed and harmoniously used for its therapeutic value in keeping with the overall strategy and tactics of psychotherapy. While the placebo effect must be eliminated in the pharmacological testing of a particular drug, it can be used effectively when the drug is being given in a therapeutic situation.

Drugs and the Therapeutic Relationship

The psychological effects of drug administration can be understood in dynamic concepts as part of the overall patient-therapist relationship. As with other elements and phenomena of the patient-therapist relationship, interactions in connection with the giving and taking of drugs may be invested by the patient with a variety of conscious and unconscious reactions and responses.

For many patients the idea of treatment is consciously associated with the prescription and administration of medication in accordance with the general medical model. Where such expectations are fixed or intense, the patient may be consciously dissatisfied if drugs are not prescribed, and may experience doubts that 'merely talking' can be of therapeutic value. The use of drugs as a treatment adjunct may help to enhance the patient's feelings of positive rapport, and the conscious recognition of the therapist's concern for his immediate comfort. If the drug helps to relieve the patient's discomfort or conscious symptoms, the therapist's prestige and the patient's conscious confidence in him are strengthened. However, if the drug fails to produce the predicted relief, or if there are unpleasant side-effects from its use, the patient's conscious feelings of rapport and confidence may diminish.

The therapist's expectations of the drug, as revealed by his verbal and non-verbal attitudes in prescribing it, will be consciously perceived by the patient, and may influence the ultimate drug-effect in keeping with the overall dynamics of the relationship. The patient's conscious attitudes towards the taking of drugs may also significantly determine the final effects. These may include such things as fears of becoming addicted, shame over requiring their use, or specific previous experiences with the drug in question in himself or in others. At times patients may have conscious misconceptions or misinformation about the significance of a particular drug (i.e. 'Thorazine is only used in schizophrenia') and these may influence the ultimate response to it.

As in the other components of the patient-therapist relationship, the unconscious transference forces are far more significant than are the conscious ones, and in fact they frequently determine the nature of the latter. The same interrelationships of drives, drive-derivatives, prohibitions and defences occur in connection with the giving and taking of drugs, as in any of the previously described psychological experiences and inter-actions.

If the pharmacological effect of a drug produces a pleasurable experi-ence for the patient, or reduces the intensity of previous unpleasure, the drug itself and the person who provided it are unconsciously associated by the patient with the earlier need-gratifying objects. Both the drug and the therapist are thus endowed with transference derivatives from the earlier relationships. By virtue of these transference reactions, the immediate effects of the drug may be further enhanced. On the other hand, if the drug is ineffective, or if it produces an unpleasant pharmacological effect, or if there are significantly unpleasant side-effects, the transference responses may become mixed and related more to non-gratifying objects.

The use of drugs further lends itself to the projection and displacement of the patient's magical and omnipotent fantasies about the therapist and his powers of influence. The drug may also come to represent the therapist in a symbolic way, and as a tangible symbolic object it can provide for a variety of further transference displacements. These may include repeated reminders of such transference gratifications as the wish for love, control of the object, or the constant presence of the therapist. The fact that many of these drugs are taken by mouth may also symbolically serve the function of derivative gratification of unconscious incorporative drives. These in turn, particularly if accompanied by transference need satisfaction, may serve to enhance the process of identification with the therapist. One patient described this 'I feel more secure when I carry you around with me in this bottle of pills'.

In patients for whom a close relationship to the therapist provokes anxiety, or in patients who are reluctant to accept a psychological explana-tion for their symptoms, the administration of a drug may permit a rational-ization of the benefits of treatment by encouraging the patient to displace the explanation to the drug itself. In this way the defences against psycho-logical phenomena or the significance of a relationship to the therapist can be maintained.

Transference reactions may also help to explain instances where the patient fails to achieve the therapeutically desired effect from the drug, or may even develop unexpected adverse or negative responses to it. For example, when the transference is primarily negative, the patient may have an unconscious need to defeat the therapist and deny his strength or influence, all of which may be displaced to the drug he prescribes. If the unconscious transference fantasies are those of being poisoned, attacked or injured, the drug may serve as the displacement object for these fantasies and the defences against them, thus resulting in negative responses. In patients with intense conflict over oral incorporative or passive-dependent drive-derivatives, the taking of drugs may evoke greater anxiety with concomitant intensification of symptoms.

At such times, any drug which is tried may produce negative or unpleasant effects, and none of them produce the desired positive response. These negative effects may at times appear paradoxical in light of the expected pharmacological action. And if there are unpleasant pharmacological side-effects to the administration of a drug, the patient may exaggerate and elaborate these to the point that the drug can no longer be used.

The influence of the prevailing unconscious transference reactions is illustrated in the clinical phenomenon of a patient responding differently to the same drug when given by different therapists, or by the same therapist at different times. At times the patient may cease to respond favourably to a drug which previously had been used successfully, and at other times he may begin to respond to a drug which previously had failed, or had produced disturbing side-effects. Although factors of changes in tolerance must be considered on the basis of habituation and prolonged usage, the fact that such shifts in response to the drug may occur in either direction indicates that they do not provide the total explanation.

Recognition of such transference factors may also help in understanding the favourable responses to drugs taken in homeopathic dosage (i.e. the patient who takes only a fraction of the prescribed dose) or the lack of response in patients receiving large and sustained amounts of a drug. It may also be a factor in patients whose response to a drug is significantly delayed and occurs only after enough time has elapsed to permit the development of a meaningful and supportive transference relationship. The impact of transference forces may be so intense that in some instances the patient doesn't actually take the drug, and the mere possession of the pills, or even of the unfilled prescription, provides enough gratification and reassurance to permit a symptomatic response.

In other words, the prescription and administration of drugs by a therapist provides an object to which the patient may displace the various manifestations of unconscious transference reactions to the therapist. The final effects of the drug will reflect its specific pharmacological action, in combination with the specific nature of the transference and overall therapeutic relationship. These same principles on the use of medication hold true in general medical practice even though it is not specifically designed as psychotherapy. Many of the same transference components exist in the more traditional doctor-patient relationship, and much of the so-called 'art of medicine' revolves around their appropriate management and manipulation.

Insight-therapy

The use of drugs in insight-directed treatment entails a departure for the therapist from the neutral participant-observer role. Drug administration also involves an active manipulation by the therapist, and generally shifts the immediate emphasis in the direction of specific symptomatic relief. Furthermore, it may provide specific drive-derivative gratification, and it also involves the therapist in a continuous reality-oriented type of inter-action with the patient which may have later complications in the manage-ment of the transference. In addition, the use of drugs may mask the patient's symptoms, or obscure the understanding and elaboration of the specific psychic processes involved in their structure and exacerbation. This in turn may make it more difficult to mobilize the unconscious conflicts. Furthermore, the use of drugs to reduce or control symptoms or unpleasant effects may interfere with the strategic goal of increased tolerance towards such affects and symptoms.

In spite of these reservations, there may be times when the administra-tion of such drugs is indicated during the course of insight-directed treatment. Occasionally they may be used in situations where the patient's anxiety is so intense that it precludes his effective function in the thera-peutic process. The reduction in the degree of anxiety by pharmacological action may permit the patient to reduce the intensity of defences and resistance during the initial phase of access of a previously repressed conflict into consciousness. There may also be occasions when specific symptoms (i.e. insomnia) are so disabling that the patient needs sympto-matic relief more immediately than is generally possible with insight-directed treatment.

In such a situation the therapist may choose to prescribe the medication himself, and attempt to deal with the various transference manifestations and reactions to this as part of the overall therapeutic process. In other situations, however, the therapist may prefer to minimize the elements of transference gratification and manipulation and might arrange for someone other than himself (i.e. the family doctor, or an associate) to prescribe and regulate the medication, thus removing it from the immediate therapeutic interaction. This latter course, however, may make it difficult to bring the patient's reaction to the other physician into proper focus as a trans-ference manifestation.

19

Another situation in which drugs are sometimes used during insight-therapy is the treatment of a traumatic neurosis when the traumatic event itself has been fully repressed. The use of sodium-amytal or sodium-pentothal narcosynthesis in such a situation induces a controlled state of delirium, as a result of which there is a temporary interference in the patient's ability to maintain his ego defences. This may permit the return from repression of the traumatic event, accompanied by an emotional abreaction. After such abreaction the patient's anxiety at recall of the traumatic event may be sufficiently reduced to permit the recollection of this material when not under the influence of drugs. In such a situation, drugs are used temporarily to by-pass the patient's ego defences, with the ultimate aim of reducing the immediate impact of the material previously repressed and thus permitting its access to consciousness and ultimate resolution and integration.

Supportive Therapy

In supportive therapy, the use of drugs is extremely common, and the tactical interventions concerning them should be consistent with the overall therapeutic strategy. Drugs may be used to produce symptomatic relief based on the immediate pharmacological action of the drug itself. They may also be used as a means of helping the patient establish conscious rapport and unconscious transference displacement by virtue of the drive-derivative gratifications which they offer. After an appropriate transference relationship has already been established, the administration of drugs may be used in the specific transference manipulations called for by the overall strategy of the treatment approach.

The effects of the use of drugs on the transference relationship will be greater if the therapist spontaneously and willingly offers them, rather than doing so reluctantly or only after repeated demands or requests made by the patient. The way in which the drug is administered and the therapist's attitude towards it may also be significant in influencing the final effects of the drug. In passive-dependent patients who need to rely on an authoritarian figure, the administration of drugs should generally be accompanied by strong positive suggestion from the therapist. However, it is usually wise to phrase such a suggestion in the form of providing definite relief, the exact extent of which cannot be predicted in advance. If the therapist promises full relief from a symptom and this is not forthcoming, his authoritarian position and magical powers may be significantly reduced in the patient's mind. In patients with needs to rebel against an authoritarian figure, it is wiser that the therapist does not offer firm suggestions as to the efficacy of the drug, and possibly offers a somewhat uncertain prospect instead. The therapist might also leave the exact details of the administration of the drug more in the hands of such a patient, if pharmacologically feasible. On the other hand, in an obsessional patient with needs for precision and orderliness, the therapist's instructions should be detailed, precise and specific, and might even attempt to elaborate a minor ritual around the taking of the drug.

If the patient has strong and overt dependency needs, the therapist might prescribe the drug for regular and consistent usage, thereby repeatedly providing the patient with tangible evidence of interest and concern. In such a situation, the therapist might even consider giving the patient the actual pills, thereby enhancing the impact of the medication as a 'gift'. If a patient experiences anxiety when offered a gift, and utilizes reaction-formation against dependency wishes, the therapist would have the patient pay for his own medication, and thus reduce the transference significance of a gift.

The same considerations of drive and defence should enter into the decisions as to how frequently and for how long a time a patient takes the medication. For example, if there are no pharmacological contra-indications, more frequent administration of the drug in smaller individual dosage will tend to enhance the passive-dependent transference gratifications through repeated reminders of the therapist's concern, and symbolic incorporation of the therapist with each dose. Contrariwise, in patients for whom such drive-derivative gratification evokes anxiety, a smaller number of daily administrations of larger dosage or long-acting medication would be more in keeping with the patient's overall pattern of defence. The same concepts apply to the question of how long the patient is to take the medication, where the emphasis in some patients may be on the free and prolonged administration of the drug and in others on more restricted and brief use only at times of considerable distress.

The therapist must also be alert to the patient's own attitudes towards the taking of medication which at times may block his symptomatic response to the drug. Patients in whom reaction-formation against dependency is intense frequently manifest the attitude that the use of medication is a sign of weakness, and a cause for shame, as well as fears over the possibility of becoming habituated. When such attitudes are present, it is important that they be discussed prior to the prescription of the drug, and that the therapist attempt to intervene in ways designed to make it more acceptable to such a patient. It is frequently helpful in such cases if the therapist firmly insists that the patient take the medication, and emphasizes his own therapeutic responsibility and decision in the matter. In this way, the patient can rationalize and project the taking of drugs as a demand made on him by the therapist and therefore may feel less shame himself.

These illustrations of the way in which the therapist makes pharmacological and psychological use of drugs to achieve the specific tactical aim in supportive therapy could be elaborated in further detail. The general principal to be emphasized, however, is the same as in the management of other transference phenomena in supportive psychotherapy. Through the interaction of prescribing drugs in keeping with the realities of a therapeutic situation, the therapist provides the patient with another realistic intervention which is consciously appropriate to a therapist-patient relationship. This permits the therapist to use such interventions in ways to gratify specific drive-derivatives or strengthen defences in his attempt to help the patient reduce psychic conflict and stabilize the dynamic equilibrium. The fact that these interventions are realistically appropriate and are focused at the level of therapeutic interaction permits the patient to concentrate on the current reality of the relationship, and hence emphasizes the elements of conscious rapport. In this way, the unconscious transference components of the patient's response (i.e. wishes for tangible evidence of love, gratification of oral incorporative drives, symbolic internalization of the therapist, etc.) remain repressed, and the therapist permits or encourages the patient to maintain his defences against awareness of them. On the other hand, if drugs are used during insight-directed treatment, such unconscious transference manifestations and derivatives might be ultimately brought to the patient's conscious awareness.

These same issues regarding the use of drugs in supportive therapy are manifested even in the instance of treating a patient who is a professional colleague. At times the therapist's impulse may be to permit the colleague to prescribe or regulate his own medication. However, this ignores the fact that the professional colleague has the same unconscious drives and defences as the patient who is not a colleague. The transference components in the use of medication will not be utilized to the fullest if the colleague's professional knowledge of drugs is overemphasized.

Use of a Placebo

At times when the therapist wishes to induce a purely psychological response in the patient, he may be tempted to use a true placebo for this purpose. In the usual therapeutic situation this is unwise for a number of reasons. It places the therapist in the active role of 'fooling' the patient, and as such may at times stimulate counter-transference responses of 'victory' or contempt for the psychological forces and reactions within the patient. Furthermore, the therapist himself, the pharmacist who fills the prescription, or the associate (i.e. nurse) who administers the substance may give subtle non-verbal cues to the patient that administration of this medication is in some way different from others. If the patient begins to suspect that he has been fooled, his reaction is likely to be one of humiliation, anger and an inability subsequently to trust the therapist. This in turn will result in a breaking off of the useful therapeutic relationship and usually a loss of whatever symptomatic improvement has occurred. The patient will need to 'save face' by further proof that he is ill, and may develop symptoms recalcitrant to any form of therapeutic intervention.

The therapist should always use a chemically active substance in such a situation, even if given only in very small doses, since this will permit him to make effective use of the medication for the desired therapeutic purposes, while not harming the patient, or running the risk of an adverse psychological effect.

Hazards of Drug Therapy

A number of psychological hazards exist in the use of drugs during psychotherapy. Where possible, the therapist should anticipate their occurrence on the basis of his dynamic understanding of the patient's conflicts, and he should respond accordingly.

One such problem is the occurrence of psychological habituation or chemical addiction to the drug being prescribed. In patients prone to develop such a response (i.e. alcoholism, compulsive eating, overt passive-dependent yearnings, etc.) the therapist must keep this in mind when deciding such things as the amount of the drug to prescribe, who should control the administration of the substance, whether or not to permit the prescription to be refilled, etc.

Another hazard in regard to drugs is their use in patients who are potentially suicidal, or are likely to act-out suicidal gestures. In such instances, the therapist must weight the risk of a suicidal attempt in which the patient may use the drug that has been prescribed. However, he must also recognize that the patient may have a variety of transference responses to the implied concern or lack of trust if he sharply limits the amount of the drug which is prescribed, or arranges for someone other than the patient to control its use. The resolution of such a dilemma may often pose a very difficult clinical problem.

For a variety of reasons, some patients may take drugs in larger amounts than prescribed (but not with suicidal intent) while others may refuse or forget to take the necessary medication. In such situations the therapist must intervene to regulate the drug usage more appropriately, but his interventions should be in keeping with the individual's basic dynamic personality organization.

The therapist must also remain alert to the possibility that any drug may at times induce a low-grade chronic delirium in the patient. Such a delirium, although not blatantly obvious, may interfere with ego function and thus disturb the psychic equilibrium, thereby evoking increased signal anxiety. The tendency at such times may be for the patient or the therapist to increase the dosage, thus producing a vicious circle. Other patients on long-term drug therapy complain of dulled emotional or intellectual responsiveness, and describe feeling 'like a zombie'. This in turn may increase such affects as anxiety, depression, or hopelessness, and may indirectly stimulate further symptom formation. The same is true when a side-effect of a drug interferes with an important function in the patient (i.e. producing insomnia or drowsiness, interfering with sexual potency or response, etc.). Unfortunately, a not uncommon impulse is to then prescribe another drug to counteract the side-effects of the first, and the problems are then often compounded.

Another hazard in using drugs in the treatment of patients with psychiatric illness involves the therapist placing excessive reliance on the pharmacological efficacy of the substance itself. The risk is in minimizing the importance of the patient's other therapeutic needs. The use of drugs in psychotherapy is best understood as an adjunct to the therapist's armamentarium, and they should not be considered a substitute for his other therapeutic activities.

SUGGESTED READING

BRACELAND, FRANCIS J., GRINKER, ROY R. & MEDUNA, L.J. (1957) Use of drugs in the treatment of neuroses, and in the office management of psychosis. *Mod. Med. (Minneap.)* **25**, 190

KUBIE, LAWRENCE S. & MARGOLIN, SYDNEY (1945) The therapeutic role of drugs in the process of depression, dissociation, and synthesis. *Psychosom. Med.* **7**, 147

MANDELL, ARNOLD J. (1968) Psychoanalysis and psychopharmacology. In: *Modern Psychoanalysis*, ed. Marmor, Judd. Basic Books Inc, New York

MASSERMAN, JULES H. & MORENO, J.L. ed. (1958) *Progress in Psychotherapy*. Vol. 3, Part IV, Psychopharmacology. Grune & Stratton, New York

OSTOW, MORTIMER (1962) *Drugs in Psychoanalysis and Psychotherapy*. Basic Books Inc, New York

CHAPTER XVII

The Therapeutic Process: Termination

The importance of the termination phase in psychotherapy and the impact that the handling of termination can have on the final results of treatment are often insufficiently recognized or appreciated.

A number of different types of termination may be described. It may occur when therapy has been successful as well as when it has been unsuccessful. Termination may be elective on the part of the patient, the therapist, or both, but it may also at times be forced by external circumstances in the life either of the patient or of the therapist. Termination may have been set from the beginning of treatment (i.e. where treatment is planned for a specific number of contacts; in instances of crisis intervention; or where the patient or therapist has only a limited time available for treatment). But termination may also occur in an indeterminate fashion and may be dependent on the nature and outcome of the therapeutic process. The type of treatment will influence the type of termination that occurs, and the management of this phase should be consistent with the form and strategy of therapy that has been undertaken.

Dynamics of Termination

The dynamics of the termination phase and of the patient's reactions to it are variable and are dependent on the nature of the treatment that has occurred, as well as the nature of the patient's personality, problems, and previous experiences. However, the reactions can be classified as relating to conscious reality factors, and to neurotic factors in the total situation.

Realistically, the patient may have a response to the degree of improvement which has occurred, manifesting pleasure and satisfaction at termination where improvement has been significant, or disappointment and dissatisfaction where improvement has been limited or non-existent. In the latter instance, the patient may have a variety of responses expressing discouragement or depression at having to accept in himself the continuing presence of neurotic symptoms or disability, or a recognition of his own

273

limitations. Even in instances where there has been significant improvement, there may be partially realistic concerns over the possibility of a recurrence of symptoms after treatment is over.

Another realistic factor may be a response to the loss of the therapist, who has in some ways been a real person in the patient's life. This is particularly likely if the treatment has been meaningful and effective, in which case the therapist and his skills will have played a significant role for the patient, and there may be attendant feelings of gratitude, as well as regret at not seeing an important figure again. In many ways, the relationship between the therapist and patient in psychotherapy is a unique one, bringing with it a number of realistic satisfactions which the patient may find difficult to give up. Furthermore, even though the patient while in psychotherapy may have made a more effective and mature adjustment and adaptation, he none the less will also experience partially realistic uncertainties about functioning on his own and anxiety about the future and what it may hold for him.

In addition, there may be reactions in the patient to no longer having to undergo the expense and inconvenience in terms of time and money which the ongoing therapy involved. There may also be reactions in terms of the patient's increased independence after termination, as well as a realistic anticipation of his opportunities in the future.

However, termination also involves a number of responses on a neurotic or unconscious basis and it is these reactions which must be clearly understood in order that an optimal therapeutic result can be obtained. The chief of these factors is the nature of the transference relationship and the way in which it has been dealt with during the ongoing therapeutic process. The greater the degree of transference involvement and conscious awareness in the patient, the more intense will be the neurotic components of the reaction to termination.

For such patients, the termination of treatment and the separation from the highly cathected object (the therapist) implies a frustration of the patient's persistent neurotic transference wishes. Such a frustration tends to evoke a conflict between the patient's wish for health, maturity, independence and realistic life satisfactions, as opposed to his continuing wish for dependency, gratification of neurotic childhood wishes and, hence, continuing illness and disability as a means of maintaining the ties to the transference object (the therapist). This final frustration tends to provoke disappointment and pain in the patient, and in response to this, may further stimulate the development and intensification of negative transference reactions. These negative transference reactions may, in fact, reach a peak of intensity greater than those occurring earlier in the treatment. Prior to the termination phase, patients frequently maintain the fantasy that by being a 'good patient' there is the possibility ultimately of obtaining the love of the therapist. The setting of the termination dashes this hope, and hence, there is often less reason for the continuing suppression of negative transference feelings.

In addition, the end of treatment may involve the patient in an experience of loss of what had been a significant and meaningful object in his life. This is particularly likely in patients who have sustained earlier losses of key figures in their lives, and for them termination often represents a re-experiencing of affects and conflicts from the earlier experience. Such a loss, with the awareness that termination means the end of the relationship, is frequently unconsciously experienced by the patient as equivalent to the death of a loved object, and hence will be accompanied by sadness and grief.

During the termination phase, patients will try to avoid the frustration, pain, grief, negative transference, and need for the work of mourning in a variety of ways. Some patients will want to terminate immediately, rather than experience or express such conflicts. Others will attempt to maintain such defences as repression, denial, displacement, reaction, formation, etc., to ward them off. Frequently patients will manifest a recurrence of symptoms or regressive behaviour as a means of expressing the feeling they are not ready to terminate, or of expressing the wish to begin therapy again. Some patients may bring up new problems, again as a means of expressing the wish to prolong the therapeutic contact. Others may try to displace these conflicts and act-out with people outside of treatment. At times there is a search for a substitute object to take the place of the therapist and provide the hoped-for gratification of neurotic strivings. This may also occur in the fantasy of some form of continuing contact with the therapist, frequently on a social basis. Another reaction may be a depreciation of the therapy and its results, as a means of reassurance to the patient that he is not losing anything of value. During this phase, there may be very precise repetitions of reactions and behaviour patterns in response to previous separations from key objects earlier in the patient's life.

Generally speaking, the deeper that the transference involvement has been during the course of treatment prior to the setting of the termination date, the more intense will be the termination reaction. And in some instances, the setting of a termination date may stimulate previously latent transference wishes which had been successfully defended against earlier.

These dynamic conflicts are operative in all patients who have experienced significant transference reactions, whether or not they were consciously interpreted. In some instances they are entirely unconscious, whereas in others the derivatives of these conflicts may be conscious to the patient. Regardless of the type of therapy, the more significantly the patient has involved himself emotionally to the therapist, the more intense will be the termination conflicts. Contrariwise, the more the patient has avoided or minimized an emotional investment in the therapist, the less conscious and intense will such reactions to termination be.

Termination of Unsuccessful Treatment

Therapy may be unsuccessful or only partially successful for a variety of reasons. These may include factors within the patient or his overall situation; or factors within the therapist and his particular skill; or the particular combination of patient and therapist who, for specific transference or counter-transference reasons, are unable to work together effectively. In such an eventuality, either the patient, the therapist, or both, may consider terminating the treatment arrangement.

A. By the Patient

When the patient's decision to terminate treatment results from a realistic appraisal of the current situation, he will usually have brought the matter up for discussion with the therapist, and the decision will have been made in an objective fashion. The pros and cons of the decision will have been consciously considered for a reasonable period before the termination occurs.

Frequently, however, the patient's decision to terminate treatment is significantly influenced by current transference factors in the therapeutic relationship. These may be the result of transference frustration and the patient's refusal to tolerate it or the fantasy of finding the gratification he is seeking in a relationship with someone else. At times, it may represent the patient's wish to use termination as a threat to the therapist in an attempt to manipulate or control the therapeutic situation. At other times, it may be a defence against the intensification of transference wishes, and analogous to a phobic reaction, may dynamically represent the patient's wish to avoid the situation in which unacceptable unconscious drive-derivatives are stimulated.

In such instances, the termination itself is often impulsive and sudden and the patient may merely not come for further treatment sessions, or may announce during a session that he is not returning. The nature of the final decision, and the patient's reluctance to discuss it openly with the therapist in advance, as well as accompanying anxiety, intense affect, or neurotic uncertainty all may indicate the existence of unconscious components in the termination.

The therapist must accept and recognize the patient's privilege of terminating the therapeutic arrangement at any time, and in the counter-transference reaction to such a termination, the therapist must be prepared that some of his cases will turn out this way. However, an impulsive and neurotically determined decision in this regard is not in the patient's overall best interest. It is important that the therapist encourage the patient to discuss the decision for termination in the treatment setting. If this can be done, the therapist is frequently in a position to help the patient recognize some of the components in the decision, in which case the patient may elect to continue the treatment. However, in situations where the patient refuses to discuss the matter further, or does not keep subsequent appointments, the therapist can only accept the patient's decision. He may indicate directly or by a letter to the patient his willingness to discuss the matter further if the patient elects to do so.

In such a situation, the therapist must also keep in mind the possibility of a conflict between the maintenance of confidentiality, and his implicit obligation to the patient's responsible relatives. If the patient is psychotic or seriously disturbed, or if there is a significant suicidal risk or possibility of seriously self-destructive behaviour, the therapist's obligation generally would be to inform the patient's family of the termination, in order that they may make other appropriate arrangements. If treatment has been oriented from the outset that the therapist will have contact only with the patient, or if none of these potentially serious consequences are likely, the therapist would be prone to maintain the confidentiality of the patient's decision.

B. By the Therapist

At times the decision to interrupt or terminate the therapy may be made by the therapist, even if the patient does not concur. Therapy may have ended in a stalemate, in which progress appears to have been halted for an extended period of time, and little further change is occurring. In such a setting, it is sometimes useful to suggest interruption in the treatment for

6 months or a year. This gives the patient an opportunity to see how he functions alone, to test his motivation and improvement and to test the intensity of his continuing symptoms and disturbances. Then if the patient returns for further treatment, he is frequently motivated to do more than merely continue the current stalemate indefinitely.

It is important that the therapist accept the fact that there will always be some patients with whom he will fail, or in whom therapeutic progress will cease. In such a situation, to continue work indefinitely may not be in the patient's best interest in the long run. The therapist must keep in mind the possibility of sending the patient for consultation with another therapist to try to assess the nature of the process which is blocking the treatment. Another possibility is to consider referring the patient to another therapist who may approach the problem from a different perspective, or with whom transference or counter-transference reactions may be sufficiently different to permit more effective therapeutic utilization.

Another indication for such a transfer is the situation in which treatment is instituted initially at the level of immediate and active support with the strategy of stabilization, symptom relief, and reduction of anxiety. Not infrequently, however, an assessment of the situation after stabilization of the acute regressive process may reveal that the patient has a potential for more intensive insight-directed psychotherapy with the goal of a more basic and lasting change. Frequently in such a situation, the original therapist, by virtue of his extensive interactions with the patient during the supportive phase, is so involved in a reality relationship to the patient that it would be extremely difficult to revert to the type of neutrality required for transference development in insight-directed treatment.

Another factor at times may be the occurrence of an unresolved counter-transference reaction, which only the therapist may be in a position to recognize, and thus only he may be aware of his inability effectively to help the patient further.

In all such situations, it is important that the therapist bring the matter up for discussion with the patient directly and openly, and that he give the patient sufficient warning prior to the time of actual interruption or termination to prepare for it, and to make any other arrangements that may be indicated. If a therapist suddenly imposes a termination of treatment on the patient against the latter's desires, the patient will have difficulty in establishing future effective therapeutic relationships, since he may anticipate a repetition of the sudden termination and hence be reluctant to invest emotionally in a new relationship.

Not infrequently the decision that the treatment has not been successful may be a mutual one between the therapist and the patient. In such a case there should be reasonable and objective discussion prior to any changes being made in the therapeutic agreement. This permits both patient and therapist to consider the reasons for the therapeutic failure and to assess whether or not transfer to another therapist is indicated, or whether the patient would be better off to stop treatment altogether. At times it may be indicated for the therapist to offer his help in arranging for subsequent treatment with someone else. However, if there are significant negative transference factors in the current treatment failure, these may be displaced to the next therapist if he is chosen by the present one.

For External Reasons

In other instances, treatment may be terminated prior to its successful conclusion because of factors unrelated to the immediate therapeutic interaction and situation. These would include such things as geographical moves by the patient or therapist which preclude further treatment, intercurrent and prolonged physical illness, the patient's inability to maintain the financial agreement, etc. Not infrequently such non-therapeutic factors can be anticipated in advance and they should be taken account of in setting treatment goals from the outset. For example, if a patient is aware at the time of initial referral that he will be leaving the community 6 months hence, it may be wiser not to begin intensive insight-directed treatment, recognizing that it is unlikely to be successful in the relatively short time available. The same would hold if financial limitations are apparent from the outset.

The most common form of this type of forced termination is that which occurs in institutional settings or in training programmes where the completion of the therapist's training or shift in his assignment within the institution makes is impossible for him to continue the treatment. Such terminations will involve all of the previously mentioned dynamic forces, but in addition they include the introduction of another major factor into the transference relationship. This is the fact of a unilateral decision by the transference object, without regard for its effect or impact on the patient, which recreates the arbitrary nature of some parental relationships. Such a circumstance will add both realistic and transference components to the patient's reactions, and the therapist needs to be alert to the various disguised and derivative ways in which such responses may be expressed by the patient. Whether or not they are interpreted and worked over is a function of the nature of the treatment contact and experience.

Where such factors have not been anticipated and occur unexpectedly, it is important that the therapist be alert to the possibility that the patient may use an apparently reality oriented event or decision for transference displacement. For example, the timing of a decision to make a geographical move may be determined by unconscious forces within the patient.

However, where such factors force the termination of the treatment arrangement, it is important that the therapist and patient discuss this matter in advance, and that the therapist attempt to help the patient make whatever further treatment arrangements are necessary.

Termination of Successful Treatment

When the issue of termination arises in the course of a treatment relationship which has been successful, its significance and the tactics of the management of the termination phase are a function of overall therapeutic strategy.

Strategy in Insight-directed Therapy

In insight-directed treatment, the strategic goal of maximal self-development and independent psychological functioning requires that there be a resolution of the transference relationship as the final step in the treatment process, and to a great extent this occurs during the phase of termination. Not infrequently there is a persistence of the fantasy of ultimate gratification in the transference up to the time that the termination is announced and planned. Dynamically, the termination of treatment may have the unconscious significance to the patient of ultimate frustration of transference wishes.

The dynamics of the termination conflicts were previously described. For all these reasons, the patient who approaches the termination of successful insight-directed psychotherapy is being asked to give up an extremely meaningful object and object-relationship. This experience of loss of the object may be accompanied by sadness, grief and anger at the object over the felt rejection. In a non-therapeutic situation of loss of an important object, the individual must go through the process of grief and mourning to a varying degree, depending on the significance of the object. But the anticipation is that when there has been an elaboration and resolution of the grief-work, there will again be a readiness and capacity to invest in new objects. In the usual situation of loss, the absence of grief and mourning is frequently an indication of their repression, and they may then persist indefinitely or serve as the source of subsequent neurotic disturbance.

The patient in the termination phase of psychotherapy who is experiencing sadness or grief over the loss of the therapist must similarly go through the process of mourning and grief-work to resolve this loss. The more that the patient consciously experiences and elaborates the sadness, depression, anger and helplessness at the loss, the greater is the possibility of his working through to a resolution of his transference relationship. The more that the patient avoids the experience of grief, the greater is the potentiality for an unresolved and persistent transference relationship, and thus a failure to achieve the full benefit of insight-directed therapy as well as the possibility of subsequent neurotic disturbance in the future.

The more intense the patient's transference reaction has been during the course of the therapy, and the greater the degree of regression in the service of the ego, the more intense will be the experience of loss and grief, and therefore the need for mourning and grief-work. The more that the patient during treatment has avoided the development of a transference relationship, and the more that the transference has been denatured or weak, the less intense will be the experience of loss and the accompanying grief. However, as described earlier, the patient's resolution of his conflicts will also be less effective and less meaningful.

Therefore, in the termination phase, the strategy of management requires that the therapist provide the patient with an opportunity to elaborate and work through the grief and mourning reaction in whatever intensity the patient has experienced it.

Strategy in Supportive Therapy

In accordance with the overall plan of supportive treatment, strategy during the termination phase calls for the continuing attempt at reduction of conflict and stress, and the avoidance of mobilization of the negative transference.

To this end, the emphasis in the termination phase of supportive therapy is on the continuing positive rapport, and the attempt at maintenance of a positive state of transference. If feelings of anxiety, rejection, sadness or anger are conscious to the patient, he should have an opportunity to ventilate these in conscious expression, as described earlier for other phenomena during supportive treatment. However, no attempt is made to undo resistances against such reactions as long as they remain repressed and unconscious. The emphasis is on a continuing relationship, even if at a reduced level of intensity and, as described earlier, no attempt is made to resolve the transference components. Instead, such residual components are used to continue the reinforcements and identifications previously described.

Therefore, instead of emphasizing the termination of the relationship, the therapist would be more inclined to emphasize his continuing interest and his continuing availability should the patient require it. In supportive treatment, some patients may never be in a position formally to terminate therapy, and a continuing therapeutic relationship may be essential for their support and maintenance of equilibrium. In other types of patients, however, the therapist may allow the patient to use interruption or termination of contact as a defence against further involvement or awareness of the transference. Termination may also at times fit the defensive need of reaction-formation against dependency.

Indications for Termination

The general criteria for the termination of treatment are the accomplishment (or near accomplishment) of the goals which were set when therapy was undertaken. Another criterion may be the partial accomplishment of the goal which has been set, but the recognition by the therapist that, for one reason or another, full accomplishment of the previously set goal is not feasible, and there must be an acceptance of more limited benefits. If possible, termination of treatment should not coincide temporally with other situations of crisis, or major change in the patient's life. The termination of treatment itself may consciously or unconsciously represent a loss and stress for the patient. If this is superimposed on other major stresses in the individual's life, it may further precipitate neurotic disequilibrium. Furthermore, if the patient faces changes in his life such as marriage, divorce, change in job, death of a loved person or the birth of a child, etc., he may need the ongoing therapeutic relationship to sustain and help him to adapt to whatever the change may be, at least during the immediate adjustment period.

A. Insight-therapy

In insight-directed therapy, some of the specific indications for termination include such things as evidence that there has been a significant structural change in the personality. The definition of such structural change is a complex issue, but it includes a shift in the drives and drive-derivatives toward genital primacy, with a relative decrease in the importance of pre-phallic drive-derivatives. It also includes a modification of super-ego functions, with a decrease in primitive or authoritarian moral precepts, and an increase in conscious personal decisions by the patient regarding his own moral value system. There should also be an extension of conscious ego functions with decreased need for unconscious defences, partial conflict resolution, and an increase in conscious control of residual conflicts. There should also be evidence that the patient has developed some degree of awareness and personal insight into the nature and derivative manifesta-tions of his conflicts, and some degree of understanding of their origins. All of these points must be judged in relationship to the goals originally set for the particular patient and how closely they have been approached.

Another criterion is the significant improvement or elimination of presenting symptoms, or at least evidence that there is improvement in the patient's capacity to tolerate those symptoms or conflicts which remain. Other criteria include such things as improvement in the patient's capacity for mature object-relationships and for work in whatever form or field the individual has chosen. Finally, there should be evidence that the patient has developed some capacity to recognize and explore his conflicts by himself, and thus to carry on the therapeutic process alone. Since stress and conflict are ubiquitous throughout human life, the criterion for termination is not their complete elimination, but rather the improvement in the individual's ability to identify, and then to adapt to the conflicts he must face. In other words, insight-directed treatment should prepare the patient to carry on some of the therapeutic work himself after the termina-tion of the formal treatment agreement.

In any specific instance, these criteria will not be met to the same degree, and at times termination is indicated even if one or more of them are not yet fulfilled. As mentioned above, the emphasis in this connection is on how closely the patient has approximated the goals that were initially set, and also there may be occasions when termination is indicated in spite of partial failure to achieve the pre-set goals.

B. Supportive Therapy

The chief criteria for termination in supportive therapy are the state of the patient's symptoms, the stability of the dynamic steady state, and the reversal of the active regression. Included in this is an improvement in the patient's ego capacity for defence. These various criteria must be assessed against the background of the importance of an ongoing transference or

20

therapeutic relationship in the maintenance of the remission which has occurred. In other words, in situations where the maintenance of an ongoing therapeutic relationship is required to achieve and maintain the supportive goals that have been set, termination may never occur, and the therapist may continue seeing the patient indefinitely. In other situations, if the patient can maintain the symptomatic improvement without necessity for an ongoing treatment relationship, termination may occur in a more definite fashion.

The concept of a transference cure was elaborated in Chapter XII, and if such a transference improvement is occurring, this in itself may be an indication to consider and plan for termination. The strategy here is to attempt to reduce the intensity of this response so that it may continue at a plateau of relatively dilute positive transference and conscious confidence, rapport and satisfaction. If the patient develops too intense a relationship, the unconscious transference wishes will be likewise intensified, and may then become conscious to the patient. At that point, their frustration may lead to a negative transference response, with loss of the symptomatic remission previously gained. In other words, to avoid the mobilization of a negative transference, the time to consider the reduction of frequency and intensity of the therapeutic relationship is when symptomatic improvement begins and appears to be well established as an ongoing process.

Tactics in Insight-therapy

The termination phase in insight-directed treatment begins after the patient or the therapist first raises the issue of when termination should occur. Initially this may be done in a tentative way, and discussion may be indefinite while the possible reactions to such an event are explored. Not infrequently it is the therapist who must initiate this since the patient may be reluctant to do so, if he is now comfortable by virtue of the transference resistances described earlier. Eventually, the patient and therapist should come to an agreement and set a definite date for termination.

In setting this date, it is important that the therapist keep in mind the strategic necessity for the patient to have sufficient time in which to develop and experience his reactions to termination, and ultimately to work them through and resolve them in a therapeutically effective way. This requires that the therapist anticipate how intense the termination reaction is likely to be, and as mentioned earlier, it tends to be proportional to the intensity of the transference relationship that has previously been established. In some patients, several weeks may be sufficient time for this, and in other cases, several months or more may be required.

If the patient has had significant separations from key objects early in life, the likelihood is that in the transference relationship during termination there will be a greater intensification of conflict over separation from the therapist. Not infrequently during the termination phase, the transference reaction may involve a precise repetition of the conflicts and affects which occurred in response to the earlier object loss.

During the termination phase the mobilization of conflict related to separation and object-loss, the negative transference, and the uncertainties of the future and independence will be accompanied by the intensification of anxiety. Such mobilization of conflict and anxiety may result in a variety of defensive or integrative attempts, and may be manifested by a variety of resistances to the therapeutic tasks imposed by the termination phase.

One major source of resistance is the wish to avoid the sadness and grief, and to avoid the work of mourning in the therapeutic relationship. Patients may wish to terminate immediately, rationalizing this in various ways. However, such a plan usually represents the wish to avoid the experience of grief and the mobilization of conflict. The patient may attempt the denial of the importance and meaning that the relationship has had for him, thereby depreciating the idea that termination represents any type of significant loss. Another frequent manifestation of resistance is the attempt to find a substitute object who will replace the therapist and thereby permit the patient to ward off the impact of the loss as well as to perpetuate the regressive transference wishes. This may involve such things as seeking out another therapist or physician, or falling in love, or making use of the spouse or a friend to serve as a therapist.

Other manifestations of resistance may include expressions of concern whether the illness is resolved, or whether the patient will be able to manage on his own. Another frequent resistance is the verbalization of feelings of disappointment in the therapy, and feelings that little or nothing of significance has been accomplished. This frequently represents an attempt to emphasize that the loss is not a significant one, and thereby to avoid the experience of grief. The patient may try in various ways to have the therapist feel guilty for the termination, and possibly try to postpone its occurrence. At times this includes the development of a recurrence of symptoms, often the same symptoms that caused the patient to seek therapy in the first place. The latent meaning behind this is the wish not to terminate, and instead to 'start over', or to make the therapist feel that the termination is premature and that it is essential for the patient to continue in active treatment. It may also represent an indirect expression of hostility and aggression against the therapist and a way of saying 'you haven't done anything to help me'. At other times, hostility over termination may be expressed directly, or there may be a displacement of anger away from the transference and on to other objects in the environment.

In other words, a wide variety of responses may occur at the prospect of terminating treatment. It becomes essential that the therapist recognize such manifestations as related to the transference, and that his role be one of repetitively interpreting the resistances in the light of the termination dynamics, and that he attempt to help the patient consciously complete the task of separation and termination. During this phase it is also important that the therapist not permit himself to be manipulated into repetitive postponement or withdrawal of the termination date, and that he maintain the therapeutic attitude and help the patient resolve the conflicts mobilized by the termination.

In instances where the transference relationship has been a significantly affective and regressive one, it is advisable to maintain the constancy of the therapist's activity as well as the basic frequency and duration of sessions up to the very end of the treatment. In this way, there may be the optimal maintenance of the transference relationship for mobilization of conflict and ultimately for conflict resolution. In less intensive treatment experiences, or in situations where the transference relationship has not developed to the same extent, or where the patient has a more limited ego capacity, it may be advisable gradually to reduce the frequency of interviews during the final phases of the termination in order to minimize the acuteness of the loss, and to help the patient more gradually resolve and accept the transference frustration. Such a gradual giving up of the object may make the final phase less stressful, and less anxiety-provoking.

Another aspect of the therapist's task during termination is repeatedly to interpret the patient's anxiety over emancipation and the development of independence and self-fulfilment and his oscillation and conflict between progress and regression. Through his interpretations and interventions the therapist attempts to help the patient's movement in the direction of progress, and by avoiding gratification of regressive transference wishes during the termination phase, he helps to promote the patient's ultimate level of adaptation and health, and to discourage regression back to symptoms and illness.

In other words, in insight-directed therapy when the time comes for the fledgling to fly by himself, it is essential that the therapist respond with kind but firm insistence that the patient make the necessary efforts to sustain himself and then fly alone. As in nature generally, this at times means 'pushing the baby out of the nest' although standing by in case further help should be necessary. At times the therapist must accept the possibility that some of the patient's neurotic complaints or symptoms may not have been fully resolved at the time of termination. However, if significant structural change has resulted from the treatment, major further symptomatic and behavioural improvement may take place after the termination has actually occurred.

Tactics in Supportive Therapy

The tactics in the management of termination in supportive psychotherapy follow from the strategy outlined earlier.

Since the strategy is to maintain repression of the negative transference, and to avoid having the patient experience the termination as a significant loss, the tactics are designed to permit the patient to maintain his unconscious resistances. The therapist emphasizes the termination as an interruption of the relationship, and as a further sign of progress. The therapist must reinforce this through appropriate unconscious gratification.

Interventions are also designed to permit the patient to maintain an ongoing and unresolved relationship with the therapist, based on positive conscious rapport, and encompassing the unconscious positive trans-ference components. The intensity of the actual relationship which is necessary for the patient to sustain the support offered by the therapist varies greatly and is a function of all the various factors which contribute to his disturbances. For some patients, the knowledge that the therapist is available to them, should they ever need him again, is sufficient and in this way many patients can be carried supportively for indefinite periods of time with only occasional visits or clusters of visits at times of acute stress or crisis. Another tactical way to maintain the relationship is to ask the patient to send the therapist a card (i.e. at Christmas) letting him know how the patient is faring. Other patients who may need somewhat stronger reinforcement of the relationship might be told to call the therapist after a particular elapsed time (i.e. 6 months or 1 year), with the indication that this will result in a follow-up appointment. When a slightly stronger intensity of relationship is desirable, the therapist may actually make a specific appointment even if it be 6 months away, since the knowledge of having the appointment can frequently be sustaining of the trans-ference relationship. Other patients may need a regular, albeit infrequent, appointment (i.e. once every 3 months), as a means of fostering a relationship of ongoing rapport and unconscious transference, but one which is not so intense that it threatens the patient's defences.

For example, a young woman with a severe schizo-affective disorder was seen for weekly sessions during the first year of treatment, and made significant symptomatic improvement. Sessions were gradually spaced out, and reduced to regular half-hour appointments once every 3 months, the total duration of treatment being 9 years. During this time she was able to marry, make friends for the first time, make a stable decision not to have children, find new interests and activities, and continue her symptomatic and behavioural remission. Rapport was consistently positive, and although the patient had exacerbations of anxiety and symptoms from time to time, she was capable of waiting for her regular appointment to discuss them. Treatment was terminated only because the therapist left the community, and the patient underwent a significant but normal grief reaction at the time of his departure.

In situations where a patient is seen in a clinic or in an institutional setting, the attempt may be made to displace the transference away from the individual therapist, who may not be permanently available, to the institution itself by emphasizing that the clinic or hospital will always be interested in the patient's welfare.

For example, a chronic schizophrenic woman was seen for a 15-minute interview once every 3 months by interns who rotated through the clinic service every 6 months. She would be passed from one intern to the next, and as long as this arrangement was maintained, she continued to function at home. If one of the interns felt he was not accomplishing anything for this patient and suggested that since so little was being done she might discontinue coming entirely, the patient would have an almost immediate recurrence of her florid psychosis and would require several weeks of inpatient hospital care to restabilize. As long as she could be seen at this frequency by someone in the clinic, the patient could maintain herself outside a hospital setting.

As mentioned earlier, the patient treated in supportive therapy may also have consciously mixed or negative reactions to the suggestion of termination, or of reducing the frequency of sessions. When such reactions are already conscious to the patient, it is essential that the therapist intervene in ways to permit the patient to express them, but not to elaborate and develop the unconscious components of such reactions.

Another tactical manoeuvre during termination in supportive therapy is to point out to the patient that there may be symptomatic recurrences from time to time, and that he cannot expect to remain completely symptom-free. However, the emphasis is on the probability that the patient will tolerate such symptoms effectively. If the patient has already been fore-warned about the recurrence of a symptom, it will not take him by surprise and, therefore, will not jeopardize his rapport and confidence in the therapist. Such anticipation is also likely to help the patient to control the intensity of a recurrence if it occurs. If the therapist had essentially sug-gested that the patient's illness is completely over, and then recurrence of a symptom should occur, the patient may lose confidence, and may also experience increasing concern that all of his disturbances are returning.

Contact after Termination

In the months immediately after the termination, the patient may again contact the therapist with the request to resume treatment. If the previous therapy has been supportive and particularly if the therapist had emphasized to the patient his availability in the future if needed, it is essential that the therapist see the patient as promptly as possible, even at the expense of personal inconvenience. The immediate availability of the therapist in times of need or crisis is an extremely important aspect of the continuing transference, and permits the patient to maintain a sense of continuity and the security that such a relationship brings. This also frequently permits the patient to make immediate and brief use of the relationship, at times being seen only for a few sessions. After the immediate crisis has subsided, the patient can again interrupt his treatment. If there are difficulties or long delays in resuming active contact with the therapist, the patient may be reluctant to again interrupt treatment, lest he again have trouble in returning at another time.

A number of patients may also test the therapist and his promise to see them again if needed, so that if there are long delays, the therapist will have 'failed' the test. Furthermore, if the patient verbalizes a need or wish to see the therapist again and this is frustrated, there is a strong possibility that the previously positive rapport and transference will become more ambiva-lent or negative, and the previous gains from treatment may be jeopardized.

In insight-directed treatment however, the therapist must be more cautious if the patient should call requesting a resumption of therapy. The therapist's position should be that he is available to the patient to re-evaluate the current situation, but that any decision to resume regular therapeutic contacts must await the outcome of such an evaluation. The therapist must be aware that the patient may still be experiencing a reaction to the termination. The patient's request to resume therapy may represent a manifestation of regressive transference wishes, and may represent the patient's initial reactions to the inevitable frustrations of adult and independent living.

If the therapist immediately agrees to resume regular therapy, this may foster such regression and may be interpreted by the patient as an indication that the therapist agrees he is still immature and unable to handle his own problems. It is often wiser after evaluation to suggest that the patient continue his efforts to function independently and to consolidate the previous therapeutic gains, at least for a number of months. Not infrequently during this interval a patient may make significant progress in consolidating his awareness and the new patterns of adaptation and integration which he had evolved.

Furthermore, if the patient has such an interval of time to struggle with his residual problems on his own, the issue of motivation will become more clarified and crystallized should it eventually prove necessary to resume regular therapy. If the patient immediately returns for further therapy, and if his anxiety or symptoms subside with the return to the transference object, the patient's motivation will be difficult to assess and will perhaps be aimed more at immediate relief of symptoms than basic awareness and understanding. On the other hand, if the patient has had a 6- or 9-month interval during which there has been persistent symptomatology and difficulty, his motivation may be further enhanced to work out the basic conflicts in a definitive way. Not infrequently in such a situation, the patient may resume therapy and make more effective use of it than the first time, since his own experience has demonstrated the impermanence of improvements based chiefly on a transference relationship.

In such a situation the therapist's position is analogous to that of a parent whose child has grown up and has recently left home to establish himself. If the child immediately 'gives up' and wants to return home when faced by the inevitable frustrations and difficulties of independent and adult life, it may be in his ultimate best interest that the parent not permit this. The parent may more effectively encourage him to return and face the problems, knowing of the parent's concern for his welfare, but recognizing that it is now appropriate for him to be independent and to mature.

Counter-transference

In this connection, the therapist must be alert to the possibility that counter-transference responses may influence his decisions and interventions around the issues of termination, and these may make it difficult effectively to exploit and deal with the special problems involved. The therapist must relinquish his ties to the patient and be willing to experience and resolve whatever feelings he has in this regard. He must be able to tolerate the various transference phenomena described earlier, and not permit the patient to evade the grief and work of mourning. Such counter-transference reactions as overly intense attachment to the patient, or fear of provoking frustration for the patient, or therapeutic over-ambition, or over-identification with the patient may lead the therapist to prolong the treatment relationship and have difficulty in establishing and carrying through an effective termination.

Probably the most common effect of the counter-transference is in the creation of 'blind spots' so that the therapist does not recognize the patient's termination responses. Many therapists evade the entire issue by letting the treatment gradually fade out without a definite termination phase, or by announcing or permitting a quick termination without time to explore the patient's reactions to it. In instances of forced termination by the therapist, the issues are often evaded by automatically transferring the patient to another therapist and thus minimizing the problem.

In the opposite direction, forcing a premature termination of treatment may also be a reflection of counter-transference factors. These include such things as therapeutic underambition, or unconscious wishes to prove that effective therapy can be brief, or dislike of the patient, or reluctance to become involved in a long-term relationship, or a feeling that continuing supportive therapy is not worth while, etc. As with counter-transference generally, such unrecognized reactions in the therapist tend to have an adverse effect on the final outcome of the treatment.

Summary

The termination of psychotherapy is in many ways dynamically similar to the normal developmental stage of late adolescence. The adolescent is much involved in the problems of dependence and independence, self and identity, and the conflicts between the challenges of the real world ahead as compared with the regressive satisfactions of the childhood which has been left behind. This is a developmental stage for the normal individual through which he must pass in order fully to achieve adult maturity. To the degree that these adolescent conflicts and issues are not resolved during development, the individual may suffer later disturbance and inhibition of optimal adult functioning, with a continuation of conflicts or attachments that belonged to an earlier era in his life.

So too the patient in psychotherapy needs to pass through this phase of termination and, to whatever degree possible, express and resolve the conflicts that it entails, in order that in his final level of adjustment he may achieve whatever degree of maturity and self development he is capable of reaching. It is the therapist's task (analogous to the task of the good parent) to help the patient cope with the various conflicts and anxieties involved in termination, and in spite of the patient's wish to avoid the discomfort or pain they produce, to help him pass through this 'developmental stage' and thence out into the world beyond.

SUGGESTED READING

COLBY, KENNETH M. (1951) *A Primer for Psychotherapists.* The Ronald Press

DEWALD, PAUL A. (1965) Reactions to the forced termination of therapy *Psychiat. Q.* **39**, 102

DEWALD, PAUL A. (1966) Forced termination of psychoanalysis: Transference, Countertransference and reality responses in five patients *Bull. Menninger Clin*, **30**, 98

FREUD, SIGMUND (1938) *Analysis Terminable and Interminable.* Collected Papers, Vol. 5, 316. The Hogarth Press, London

GREENBERG, RAMON (1963) Manifestations and management of patient's reactions to disruptions of psychotherapy. *Compr. Psychiat.* **4**, 330

KEITH, CHARLES (1966) Multiple transfers of psychotherapy patients: a report of problems and management. *A.M.A. Arch. Gen. Psychiat.* **14**, 185

RANGELL, LEO (1966) An overview of the ending of an analysis. In: *Psychoanalysis in the Americas*, ed. Litman, Robert E. International Universities Press Inc, New York

ORENS, MARTIN (1955) Setting a termination date. *J. Am. Psychoanal. Ass.* **3**, 651

PUMPIAN-MINDLIN, EUGENE (1958) Comments on technique of termination and transfer in a clinic setting. *Am. J. Psychother.* **12**, 455

Series of Papers on Termination of Analysis (1950) *Int. J. Psycho-Anal.* **31**, 179–205

CHAPTER XVIII

Psychoanalysis and Insight-Directed Psychotherapy

Introduction

In Chapter VII, a spectrum of psychotherapy was described running from supportive treatment at one end, to formal psychoanalysis at the other, with insight-directed psychotherapy between them. In the subsequent discussion on the theory and technique of psychotherapy, consideration has been directed chiefly to that portion of the spectrum ranging from supportive treatment to insight-directed psychotherapy, and to a comparison and contrast between these two treatment approaches.

In the Introduction to this book, the distinction was made between psychoanalysis as a specific method of therapy applicable to a relatively small number of patients, and psychoanalysis as a general theory of behaviour, personality and psychopathology. The applications of psychoanalytic theory to the situation of psychotherapy and the extrapolations from psychoanalysis as a method of treatment has meant for many therapists a considerable confusion and a failure to distinguish clearly between analysis and insight-directed treatment. For a variety of motives, many other workers have a more active wish to deny that a significant difference exists between these treatment modalities. Furthermore, the applications of psychoanalytic theory and technique to the treatment of different and broader categories of mental illness, and the introduction therewith of a variety of parameters, has further obscured for some individuals the unique identity of classical psychoanalysis as a treatment and research method. To highlight these differences, it is now necessary to delineate psychoanalysis as a method of treatment and to distinguish it from insight-directed psychotherapy based on psychoanalytic principles.

The point has been emphasized earlier that supportive and insight-directed therapy are easily distinguishable from one another in their pure forms, but that these distinctions tend to become somewhat obscured in the mid-portion of the spectrum. The same concept holds for the distinction between dynamically oriented insight-directed psychotherapy, as opposed to formal psychoanalysis. These are readily distinguishable from one another in their usual forms, although they likewise exist on something of a spectrum.

Not infrequently, however, the therapeutic process for some patients in whom an attempt is being made at formal analysis may be more akin to that seen in psychotherapy. This is particularly the case in patients with extremely rigid character structure, or in patients who have major inhibitions in psychological mindedness or in their capacity for communication. On the other hand, there are patients seen in briefer forms of psychotherapy whose therapeutic attitude, progress and communication resemble and partially approach the behaviour and responses of patients seen in formal analytic treatment. In the discussion to follow, therefore, the contrast between analysis and insight-directed psychotherapy will be made on the polar basis of the ends of this spectrum, as was done earlier in the distinction between insight-directed and supportive psychotherapy.

Strategy of Psychoanalysis

The strategy of psychoanalysis is to re-establish the nuclear infantile and earliest childhood conflicts through the development in the patient of a full-blown regressive transference neurosis. By experiencing this regressive transference neurosis, the patient has an opportunity for the undoing of the infantile and childhood amnesia, and for exploration and developing awareness of the primary process. The development, exploration and ultimate resolution of the transference neurosis becomes the central theme of the analysis and becomes the vehicle by which, in successful cases, there is a resolution of the nuclear infantile and early childhood conflicts. When such nuclear unconscious conflicts have been resolved, their symptomatic and characterological derivative expressions will likewise be modified. Accompanying such resolution will be a decrease in the psychic energy involved in unconscious defence against such conflicts, and as a result such energy becomes available for use in reality-oriented activity and behaviour.

The goals of analysis are the general reorganization and reintegration of personality structure and function, and the fullest possible maturation of the individual, with development and utilization of whatever innate talent and ability he has for productive activity and mature object relatedness. In successful cases there is not only a relief of the presenting symptoms and neurotic character patterns, but there is also an increase in such things as general sensitivity and responsiveness, creativity, effective adaptation, mature forms of drive discharge, and improved capacity to adapt to stress.

Such patients indicate that compared to their pre-treatment status they now lead fuller and richer lives.

Strategy of Psychotherapy

The strategy of psychotherapy, on the other hand, involves the establishment of a transference relationship (as opposed to a regressive transference neurosis) in which there is an emotionally meaningful experience of the *derivatives* of the infantile and early childhood conflicts, with an attempt to resolve or modify patterns of integration, structural organization, and behaviour at the level of these derivative conflicts. A deeply regressive transference neurosis is not only unnecessary in the psychotherapy situation, but is actually unwise, and if it does occur, it frequently complicates and disrupts the treatment effort. As has been mentioned in other connections, regression for its own sake has little therapeutic value. And a transference relationship in insight-directed treatment must ultimately be resolved for optimal therapeutic benefit. By virtue of the other inherent limitations in insight-directed therapy as compared with analysis, the resolution of a regressive transference neurosis in psychotherapy is extremely difficult and most frequently is unsatisfactory.

In this framework, the extent and depth of insight is significantly less than in analysis, and is chiefly related to the deeper preconscious derivatives of the nuclear unconscious conflicts. The patient's awareness is chiefly of the secondary process derivatives of primary process thought. The transference relationship is chiefly used to help the patient become increasingly aware of the nature of his current interpersonal attitudes and reactions as mirrored in his transferences to the therapist. The goals of treatment, therefore, are less ambitious in terms of the degree of insight and structural change that can be achieved. The lifting of infantile amnesia is not a goal of insight-directed therapy, and the recall of genetic conflictual material is focused chiefly from latency and adolescence forward towards adult life.

Quantitative versus Qualitative Differences

In one sense, these distinctions in strategy are related to sharp *quantitative* differences in the depth of regression, and in the intensity of the transference neurosis. However, these quantitative differences in turn produce major *qualitative* effects on the overall nature of the treatment process. During the course of original psychosexual development, there occurs a gradual evolution from primary process to secondary process thinking. At the beginning of the latency period, with the usual generalized repression of infantile and childhood conflict, awareness of primary process thought is sharply diminished and most conscious thinking and fantasy occurs in secondary process form. Those earlier memories that are retained in consciousness are usually screen memories organized in accordance with the secondary process.

If the therapeutic regression and transference relationship is focused at the latency or adolescent levels of development (as in psychotherapy) the patient's conflicts, fantasies and communications will be structured and expressed in accordance with the secondary process. Only if the regression and transference neurosis re-establish the infantile and early childhood situation (as in successful analysis) can there be a significant exploration of fantasy and conflict in terms of the primary process.

Thus the qualitative distinctions are a reflection of the extent to which there is an uncovering and exploration of the primary process in analysis, as compared with the elaboration of secondary process derivatives in psychotherapy.

Tactics in Psychoanalysis

The differences in tactics between the two treatment methods is a function of the basic differences in overall strategy. A number of factors and forces in the analytic situation favour the establishment of a regressive transference neurosis. Generally speaking, the frequency of analytic sessions is greater (usually 4 or 5 sessions per week), thus permitting more continuity of material from session to session and intensifying the exposure of the patient to the analyst and the analytic situation. This tends to enhance whatever potentiality the patient has for the development of an intense relationship to the analyst.

The use of the reclining position on a couch with the analyst sitting behind and out of the patient's visual field further fosters the regressive trend. In this situation, the patient is less aware of the reality of the analyst's behaviour, and reality cues such as movement, posture or facial expression are eliminated. The appearance and secondary sexual characteristics of the analyst likewise are eliminated from the patient's immediate visual awareness, thereby further permitting a more free projection of the patient's fantasies in the transference neurosis. For example, if the patient is sitting face-to-face with a male therapist, it becomes far more difficult to develop and express maternal transference fantasies of an immediate and psychically real nature. When the analyst is out of view, such fantasies can be more readily developed by the patient who may at those moments experience the male analyst in a female form with all of the accompanying secondary female sexual characteristics. (The same types of transference distortions of gender may occur in the instance of a female analyst.)

In the analytic situation, the basic rule is that of free association, with a greater communication of the details of the immediate thoughts, fantasies, sensations and other subjective experiences. In this connection, the analyst makes a freer and more specific use of silence in the analytic situation than can usually occur in psychotherapy. The emphasis in psychoanalysis is on the intra-psychic life of the patient, and the entire analytic situation is designed to facilitate its emergence into conscious awareness. Often in psychotherapy attempts are made directly to apply these analytic techniques of free association and prolonged silence, but the other elements in the treatment situation make this of doubtful value to the patient.

In the analytic situation, there is usually a greater emphasis on the use of dreams as a means towards the exploration of the patient's unconscious emotional life through detailed associations to the various component parts of the dream. This same detailed approach is emphasized in the exploration of unconscious fantasies, and in specific reconstruction or recovery of early repressed memories and experiences. In analysis there is generally less focusing of material by the analyst who instead tends to follow the line and pattern of the patient's associations wherever they may lead, seeking always to deepen and broaden the patient's awareness of his own unconscious mental life.

It is often mistakenly assumed that the analyst is not interested in the current reality of the patient's life experience. The analyst, however, emphasizes in his interpretations to the patient the ways in which the current reactions to the reality that he faces are repetitive derivatives of the basic unconscious infantile conflicts and disturbances.

As compared with psychotherapy, analysis generally involves a longer duration of therapeutic work. In the earlier history of analytic therapy, particularly when the topographical hypothesis served as the basis for the theory of treatment, analysis tended to be relatively brief (sometimes as short as a few months). However, with the increasing awareness of the complexities of human mental life, and with the reorganization of the basic theory of treatment in accordance with the structural hypothesis, and with awareness of the nature and extent of unconscious resistances, the total duration of analysis has tended to become longer. In the context of present-day analytic theory, a complete analysis can seldom occur in less than approximately 2 years, and often the total duration of treatment is considerably longer.

Tactics in Psychotherapy

The tactics of insight-directed psychotherapy show significant differences from those applicable to analysis, although they are derived from general psychoanalytic theory and from general experience in analytic treatment. To achieve the strategic goal of a transference relationship which does not develop into a full-blown regressive transference neurosis, the interviews in psychotherapy are generally conducted in a face-to-face situation. Interviews are frequent enough to permit some continuity and carry-over from one session to the next, but generally speaking, are at a lesser frequency than in the case of analysis (i.e. one or two sessions per week).

In an insight-directed treatment situation, the patient is encouraged to express himself with a minimum of conscious withholding and editing, and resistances and defences against this are interpreted and dealt with as part of the therapeutic process. However, free association as it occurs in analysis is usually not a treatment tool in psychotherapy. Compared with psychoanalysis, the therapist in insight-directed treatment does not use silence as much, and he tends to be more active and frequent in his interventions, confrontations and interpretations.

The type of material which is fostered by the therapist's interventions tends to be of the deeper preconscious and more superficial unconscious varieties, and there is a lessened emphasis on dreams and on the elaboration of unconscious fantasies. Dreams will occur in the communications of the patient in insight-directed treatment and they are often of great use to the therapist as a means of assessing the current dynamic problems and the state of the transference relationship. However, a detailed inquiry and associational analysis of dreams usually goes beyond the limitations of this form of treatment, and the same is true for the detailed exploration of unconscious fantasies. Instead, the therapist tends to emphasize apparent generalized patterns of behaviour, reactions or relationships, and he tends to summarize and co-ordinate the material communicated by the patient and actively to relate it to the patient's current life and experience.

In psychotherapy, the therapist also tends to focus the material in accordance with his dynamic diagnostic formulations and in keeping with the limitations of the treatment method. This type of sector or segmental approach may mean that the therapist helps the patient to gain insight and understanding in the resolution of certain conflicts while leaving others deliberately untouched or unexplored. In other words, the therapist in insight-directed treatment actively sets a limit on the extent and depth of the insight and awareness towards which the patient is working.

The duration of this form of treatment is usually less than that of an analysis, in keeping with the differences in overall goals of the two approaches. Not infrequently in some particularly sensitive or psychologically 'ready' patients, significant insight into focal conflicts can be developed in a relatively short therapeutic contact and can have lasting therapeutic effect. Oftentimes this may occur in patients who might have derived greater benefits from a prolonged and formal psychoanalysis, but in whom for various reasons analysis has not been undertaken.

From the foregoing, it might be summarized that insight-directed psychotherapy stands roughly midway on a spectrum between supportive psychotherapy and psychoanalysis. And furthermore, the distinctions in the strategy and tactics of insight-directed therapy as compared with analysis are of a similar magnitude to those distinguishing insight-directed treatment from supportive psychotherapy.

Therapeutic Complications

Some of the major therapeutic complications arising in the course of insight-directed treatment come at times from a failure to distinguish this therapeutic approach from psychoanalysis. Many therapists are reluctant for various reasons to accept the inherent limitations of this treatment method, and at times attempt in an inappropriate fashion to apply the techniques and goals of analysis to psychotherapy. To this end, patients are frequently seen in the reclining position, or use is made of the 'method of free-association', or there is a heavy emphasis on dreams and fantasies. Implied behind this misuse of the therapeutic situation is the attempt by the therapist to achieve the benefits and goals of an analysis but using the methods of psychotherapy. It is such attempts as these which frequently result in therapeutic stalemates, or in regression which has little therapeutic usefulness, or in major and at times disruptive acting-out of transference or other neurotic manifestations.

When properly applied and carried out, insight-directed psychotherapy can result in significant and lasting therapeutic and constructive change for the patient, and as such it is a treatment approach of major importance. However, even though it is based on analytic principles and even though it makes use of certain analytic techniques in a modified fashion, it is not and should not be confused with analysis itself. It is important for the

21

psychotherapist to keep these distinctions clearly in mind, so that he may operate to the utmost efficiency within the framework and limitations of his chosen treatment method.

SUGGESTED READING

ALEXANDER, FRANZ (1954) Psychoanalysis and psychotherapy. *J. Am. Psychoanal. Ass.* **2**, 722

ARLOW, JACOB A. & BRENNER, CHARLES (1966) The psychoanalytic situation. In: *Psychoanalysis in the Americas*, ed. Litman, Robert E. International Universities Press Inc, New York

BIBRING, EDWARD (1954) Psychoanalysis and the dynamic psychotherapies. *J. Am. Psychoanal. Ass.* **2**, 745

FROMM-REICHMANN, FRIEDA (1954) Psychoanalytic and general dynamic conceptions of theory and of therapy. *J. Am. Psychoanal. Ass.* **2**, 711

GILL, MERTON M. (1954) Psychoanalysis and psychotherapy. *J. Am. Psychoanal. Ass.*, **2**, 771

GITELSON, MAXWELL (1951) Psychoanalysis and dynamic psychiatry. *Arch. Neurol. & Psychiat.* **66**, 280

GITELSON, MAXWELL (1964) On the identity crisis in American psychoanalysis. *J. Am. Psychoanal. Ass.* **12**, 451

HAMMETT, VAN BUREN O. (1965) A consideration of psychoanalysis in relation to psychiatry generally. *Am. J. Psychiat.* **122**, 42

Panel Reports—Annual Meeting (1953) (1954) Psychoanalysis and dynamic psychotherapy—similarities and differences. *J. Am. Psychoanal. Ass.* **2**, 152

RANGELL, LEO (1954) Similarities and differences between psychoanalysis and dynamic psychotherapy. *J. Am. Psychoanal. Ass.* **2**, 734

STONE, LEO (1951) Psychoanalysis and brief psychotherapy. *Psychoanal. Quart.* **20**, 215

WALLERSTEIN, ROBERT S. (1965) The goals of psychoanalysis: A survey of analytic viewpoints. *J. Am. Psychoanal. Ass.* **13**, 748

CHAPTER XIX

Implications for Community Psychiatry

The systems and programmes for delivery of health care are currently under enormous social pressures for change. The problems are how to provide medical care for those segments of the population who, for one reason or another, were not effectively included in the previously existing systems of health care delivery. The basic principle that adequate and effective health care is no longer a privilege but is to be considered a right for every person regardless of social or economic class, makes it necessary to re-assess and re-evaluate the methods previously used in providing health care, particularly for the underprivileged. The old pattern of the individual physician making his own direct arrangements with his patient on a fee-for-service basis is an inadequate model to meet current social pressures. Health care needs of the future will require innovative changes of clinic organization, group practice, prepaid insurance, convenient availability of health services, organized preventive programmes, etc. And the dehumanizing of the patient which has unfortunately accompanied some of the advances in medical science will require the development of new approaches regarding the organization of medical care.

The recent development of community psychiatry and the concept of the community health centre illustrate these issues. While still unclear in many of their specific functions, areas of interest, and roles, these developments represent the first steps in the evolution towards a new form of care for the psychiatrically ill.

However, there is a hazard that the increasing social pressures to treat larger numbers of patients by briefer techniques may lead to an overlooking of the valuable contributions which painfully learned past lessons about psychotherapy can offer, even though in a new setting. The techniques to be evolved will be more rational and effective if they are consistent with the cumulatively acquired general theory of motivation, mental functioning, and behaviour. Even in this setting, psychoanalysis and psychoanalytic theory can contribute significantly to the rationale for the development of these techniques.

The population of patients seen in the usual community mental health centre tends to be different in a number of characteristics from those seen in the more traditional psychiatric agency or those seen in the usual private practice of psychiatry.

Although these individuals share the same basic human drives and pass through the same stages and levels of psychosexual development as have been described earlier, the environmental, social, and cultural forces impinging upon them have exerted a significant influence on the form and pattern of adaptation and resolution of conflict that is achieved. In other words, the 'average expectable environment' is quite different from that which is expectable in middle-class society. Although generalizations are hazardous and possibly inaccurate in the individual instance, certain generalized patterns and effects on the mental apparatus become discernible.

From the standpoint of the id, there is often a relative lack of gratification of oral libidinal strivings and need satisfactions, with frustration of dependency demands, and a resulting problem in establishing basic trust. Deprived, depleted, insecure, or hopeless parents will tend to have greater difficulty providing for the psychological needs of their children. And where the mother, for various reasons, must leave the care of the young child to older siblings or to others, these problems tend to be compounded. Such experiences tend to be reinforced subsequently if hunger, malnutrition, lack of adequate heat or shelter, etc., are regular or commonplace. The normal reaction-formations against pre-phallic drives tend to be less effectively established, and as a result such drives are often more directly discharged. Overcrowding, lack of privacy, multiple sharing of beds, early and frequent exposure to various aspects of sexuality, etc., will all exert an influence on the intensity and form of expression of phallic and oedipal strivings. The discharge of hostility and aggression (arising from conflict at all psychosexual levels) tends to be more immediate, direct, and physical in its expression. And the sub-culture provides both stimulation and acceptance of such overt aggressive drive-discharge.

From the super-ego standpoint, a variety of developmental distortions are prone to occur. Most likely is a failure of effective internalization, so that morality and value systems remain dependent on external sources of control and internal guilt feelings are lessened. The models for identification in establishing super-ego functions also tend to be externally oriented, or they may be individuals who characteristically use primitive physical violence as a means of expressing prohibitions. Super-ego function may often be paraphrased as 'it's all right as long as you don't get caught', rather than an internally controlling sense of guilt for wrong-doing. And the ego-ideal will frequently involve values and attributes very different from those of the traditional middle-class ideals.

However, the most significant and disabling effects of these forces is their impact on the development of component ego functions. A relative lack of appropriate and meaningful stimulation at key stages tends to produce severe (and at times irreversible) arrests in the development of such ego functions as intelligence, judgment, abilities for verbalization, reading, capacity for conceptual or abstract thinking, etc. Absence or repeated separations from parents, unpredictable or erratic parental behaviour, uncertainty regarding drive satisfaction, transient relationships with large numbers of people, etc., all tend to contribute to difficulty in the establishment of object constancy. Premature expectations for self-care and independence make it more difficult to establish a stable self-concept with a sense of basic security and confidence. The models available for identification are often ineffective in their capacity for mature adaptation and problem-solving. Stimulation of verbal communication skills is often deficient, and as a result the development of empathic understanding of others is hampered. This tends to make the use of control mechanisms such as verbalization or elaborate fantasy less effective or gratifying, and also tends to promote narcissistic fixations. Coping with overt violence and aggression from parents and/or peers promotes the use of identification with the aggressor as a mechanism of defence, with subsequent continuation of the same behaviour patterns.

In later developmental stages, stress and lack of opportunity in such areas as education, economic security, social mobility, occupational limitation, etc., contribute further to ego handicaps by blocking opportunities to develop effective and satisfying displacements or sublimations. Issues of racial or social discrimination significantly influence the basic identifications and images of the self. The greater intensity of realistic danger situations tends to promote more extensive use of projection as a characteristic defence, and awareness of 'out-group' status and depreciation by the rest of society further reinforces the use of such projective mechanisms.

Problems of psychopathology in lower-class populations include the full gamut of disturbances seen in other groups. But as a result of the issues described above, they tend to be even more complex, multi-determined, and difficult to modify.

The focus of effort in the field of community psychiatry may be on the provision of therapeutic facilities and services to the individual patient, or to the family group of which he is a member. It may also, however, be

21§

focused at the level of the community at large, including attempts to modify the underlying social, economic, and educational deprivations and stresses; attempts at prevention of social disability and psychological illness; programmes for early recognition and treatment of psychopathology, or programmes for improving or enriching life in the community. In some of these latter programmes, the consulting psychiatrist may find himself in roles far removed from the traditionally therapeutic physician-patient relationship, and he may be involved in the development of community programmes for mental health education, in work with schools and teachers, in advising courts and probation officers, in work with governmental, social, or legal agencies, etc. However, a consideration of these elements is beyond the scope of this presentation.

In regard to providing therapeutic services for lower-class patients, however, a number of additional characteristic problems must be recognized, with appropriate technical innovations introduced.

Problems for Patients

Given the previously described limitations of self-observation, psychological awareness, and capacity for verbal communication, these patients tend to be psychologically unsophisticated. It is likely that they will have many misconceptions regarding the role and functions of a psychotherapist, and they are not likely to have confidence in the effectiveness of verbal interaction. Their perception of their own problems and the priorities they develop are likely to be quite different from those of the middle-class therapist. Their goals and motivations tend to be more exclusively symptom-oriented, and immediate, and they are often in need of active help in solving current or practical problems. The motivation for treatment is frequently the result of pressures or requirement by a legal or social agency as a consequence of maladaptive behaviour that has come to the agency's attention.

The therapist and the clinic may represent to the patient the personification of 'the establishment' and the power structure from which he feels excluded, and his conscious expectations concerning available help will be influenced by his previous experiences with other analogous agencies. In addition, the less conscious transference reactions are often negative, suspicious, or mistrustful, based not only on previous specific personal relationships to key figures, but also on the projections resulting from the social and environmental issues described previously.

For this group of patients, the various reality problems relating to the therapy itself tend to assume considerable significance. Issues such as the cost of transportation, prescribed drugs, and the therapy itself, or of geographic convenience, or the risk to employment, or loss of income from time taken out of a working day, or provision of care for children while attending the clinic, etc., will influence the patient's motivations and response.

Problems for Therapists

The usual middle-class therapist has had a life experience and system of values so different from those of the lower-class patient that his capacity for empathy and understanding may be severely taxed. He must also be sure that the heirarchy of priorities he establishes for the therapy is consistent with the patient's priorities, since the possibility of discrepancy is considerable. His mode and style of communication, both verbal and non-verbal, must be adjusted to the patient's limitations, and his choices of idiom must be understandable by the patient.

The therapist must be capable of tolerating the at times unstable or exaggerated transference reactions which may not be offset by self-observing ego function. And he must recognize that in many cases basic trust will be established only slowly and after repeated 'proofs' of his interest and therapeutic intentions.

The central importance of identification in supportive therapy was previously described. But with this patient population the therapist must recognize that the major differences in background, race, experience, education, value systems, ego capacities, etc., between himself and the patient may make it difficult to promote such identifications.

And in view of these marked differences between himself and his patient, the therapist should be particularly alert to the possible development of significant counter-transference responses.

Implications for Treatment

The procedural organization of services should be simplified for the patient in order to provide prompt and direct access to help. Patients whose personality organization and life style is towards immediate or short-range goals generally cannot tolerate significant delays when they finally apply for treatment, often at times of crisis. A waiting period for initial evaluation, or a long waiting list for definitive treatment tend to reinforce negative transference expectations. Walk-in clinics where patients do not need an advance appointment are helpful, even if the initial contact or evaluation can only be very brief. The availability of emergency services on a 24-hour basis fills an important need and can promote a sense of confident expectation of help and interest. Operation of clinics at hours convenient for the working population (i.e. evenings) will tend to enhance shaky motivation and reduce the stress or sacrifice that therapy might otherwise demand.

Given the difficulties in empathy, interpersonal relationships, and negative transference expectations described earlier, it is helpful if the patient can have immediate contact with the person who will be his ultimate therapist, regardless of that person's professional identity (i.e. psychiatrist, psychologist, social worker, psychiatric technician, etc.). When a patient in acute distress is seen promptly by a therapist who can then continue the treatment contacts, the rapid development of any positive transferences or rapport can be capitalized upon, and the effectiveness of brief treatment procedures tends to be enhanced. The more traditional clinic intake procedure of a series of screening interviews by one or more individuals before the patient is assigned a regular therapist forces the patient to make but then break therapeutic relationships, and places an additional series of obstacles and stress between the patient and the help he is seeking. It interferes with the development of any immediate positive transferences or rapport, and makes positive identification with the source of gratification or help more difficult.

For the majority of patients seen in such settings, brief, supportive, crisis-oriented therapy with limited goals will be the treatment of choice. However, those patients who can effectively benefit from longer, definitive, or insight-directed approaches will be recognizable during the initial brief therapeutic efforts. They may then be selected for further or more extensive evaluation, placed on a waiting list, or transferred to a different therapist. But if they are appropriate cases for insight-directed or long-term therapy, presumably they will be capable of tolerating the necessary delays or changes.

The central importance of identification with the therapist in supportive treatment has been described earlier, as have the difficulties and problems in this process when the patient and therapist have widely differing social class origins, experiences, value systems, and styles of communication. These issues make it necessary to consider methods by which this process of identification can be enhanced. One possibility is the recruitment and training of therapeutic personnel whose origins and experiences are closer to those of the patients to be served. Even if such individuals lack other important professional qualifications, they may provide more easily reachable models for identification, may more readily experience empathy for the patient, may be capable of more direct communication, and may be able to provide more appropriate concrete solutions to immediate problems. Where such personnel are to be used, the professional therapist would serve as an educator, consultant, and supervisor.

The activities of the therapist in supportive treatment have been described in earlier sections. In work with patients from lower socio-economic groups the *real* elements of the therapist–patient relationship are of particular importance. Such a relationship frequently represents the first sustained experience the patient has ever had with a consistently accepting, helpful, emotionally stable, and effective person who is himself capable of adapting to life's stresses. By his active interest, concern, participation, and if necessary, environmental interventions in the problems the patient faces, the therapist presents himself as a model for problem-solving. Since such patients tend to be limited in their capacity for abstract or conceptual thinking, it is generally more effective to focus on concrete, specific, current issues or problems which are high on the patient's priority list, and to offer practical (but dynamically appropriate) suggestions and solutions. By actively demonstrating his concern and respect for the patient as a person, the therapist also promotes the patient's own sense of self-esteem and pride. Such an approach requires a prompt recognition of the dynamically important forces, an assessment as to which of these forces can be modified, and then an actively maintained focus upon them with exclusion of irrelevant or unmodifiable factors.

There are instances of unmodifiable psychopathology and/or social disability, where the patient nevertheless needs an on-going therapeutic contact. If there is dynamic evidence that an excessively dependent or demanding transference relationship will gradually develop towards an individual therapist, it is sometimes helpful to have such transferences diluted and experienced towards the clinic itself. This can be done by having a team of therapists who take turns in seeing the particular patient.

In addition to the practical values of increasing the number of patients being treated, and of saving therapists' time, there are a number of dynamically significant reasons for using various types of group therapy with underprivileged patients. In a group setting, the individual patient is supported by his peers, and group identification may be more firm and effective than identification with the therapist alone. The group offers a setting for the sharing of common problems and of attempted practical solutions, which are often outside the personal experience of a middle-class therapist. The group also offers an opportunity for role-playing as a means of developing empathy, awareness, and new behaviour patterns. The group situation also reduces the demands or expectations for verbal communication by the individual patient, and the observations of other patients can help to make up for difficulties in introspection and self-observation.

In family groups the therapist can actively and concretely demonstrate the problems and reactions between family members, and illustrate new specific methods for coping with them. Role-playing with family members interchanging parts can serve to increase mutual awareness and open paths of communication between family members.

Activity groups may be useful in offsetting attitudes of isolation and helplessness among the individual members. They are particularly appropriate for adolescents and delinquents where the activity fosters a relationship to the group leader which can then serve as a bridge for more stable identifications and the establishment of new value systems. Such project-oriented activities may also be helpful in providing outlets for displacement of unacceptable impulses and the eventual development of effective sublimations. The proverb 'actions speak louder than words' is particularly appropriate for people in whom verbal communication is limited.

Summary

The provision of effective psychiatric services for the underprivileged represents a major challenge from many points of view. It will require the development of bold and new approaches to the prevention and treatment of psychiatric illness. However, the application of dynamic understanding to the particular problems faced by this social group will permit a rational evolution of programmes and services to meet their needs.

SUGGESTED READING

BAUM, EUGENE (1966) Psychotherapy drop-outs and lower socio-economic patients. *Am. J. Orthopsychiat.* **36**, 629

DORN, ROBERT M. (1966) The role of the psychoanalyst in community mental health. *Comm. Ment. Health J.* **2**, 5

DUHL, LEONARD J. & LEOPOLD, ROBERT L. (1968) Relationship of psychoanalysis with social agencies: Community implications. In: *Modern Psychoanalysis,* ed. Marmor, Judd. Basic Books Inc, New York

EWALT, JACK R. (1966) Projections for community mental health services. *Am. J. Psychiat.* (Suppl.) **122**, 51

G.A.P. Report 69 (1968) The Dimensions of Community Psychiatry

MINUCHIN, SALVADOR (1968) Psychoanalytic therapies and the low socio-economic population. In: *Modern Psychoanalysis*, ed. Marmor, Judd. Basic Books Inc, New York

Special Section (1967) Innovative approaches to therapy. *Am. J. Psychiat.* **123**, 1388–1438

SUTHERLAND, JOHN (1966) The psychotherapeutic clinic and community psychiatry. *Bull. Menninger Clin.* **30**, 338

CHAPTER XX

Evaluation of Therapy

The evaluation of the results of psychotherapy is an extremely difficult and complex problem in terms of the general therapeutic effectiveness of a particular form or type of psychotherapy, and also for the individual therapist assessing the treatment of a particular patient. A number of different studies have been done, or are in process, in the attempt to provide answers to the questions of what actually occurred in the therapeutic process, what was the eventual result, and what factors were responsible for the final outcome, whether successful or unsuccessful.

The problems of evaluation arise in part from the extremely large number of variables within the patient, within the therapist, within the therapeutic situation and in the vicissitudes of the patient's current life during the treatment. Most of these variables cannot be experimentally controlled in the natural therapeutic setting, and hence their impact is difficult to establish in a definitive way. On the other hand, when attempts are made experimentally to control or manipulate particular variables in advance, this has a contaminating impact on the therapist and the therapeutic process, and changes the total situation.

Another group of problems in evaluating the results of treatment revolves around the issue of who is best able to make such an assessment. In many ways the therapist himself is in a position to know more than anyone else concerning the nature of the patient's conflicts and disturbances, the changes that have occurred, the course of the therapy, and the various events or turning points in the treatment. By virtue of his clinical and theoretical knowledge, the therapist is also in a position to know significantly more than the patient regarding the degree to which underlying change or conflict resolution has occurred. He is also able to compare the nature and degree of change in the particular patient with the general experience in the therapy of other patients manifesting similar as well as differing conflicts and disturbances.

However, the therapist will have access to information chiefly (if not exclusively) from the patient, and therefore, some of the data on which to base an assessment of the total impact of treatment may be missing. For example, the patient's overt behaviour in his interactions with the environment may be quite at variance with what the patient himself describes, and hence the therapist may not be aware of the discrepancy. Furthermore, the therapist has the problem of his own bias in evaluating the results of his therapeutic efforts. Such biases may influence the therapist in either direction when making his overall assessment of the outcome, and they may also influence his understanding of the factors which account for the particular success or failure. Such biases may be personal and involve the therapist's own self-image as a therapist, or they may be theoretical and reflect his adherence to a particular system of thought or understanding of the process of therapy.

Likewise, the patient himself is often an unreliable judge regarding the outcome of treatment. If the therapy did not completely fulfil the patient's magical expectations of what should happen, he may be led to underestimate those changes which actually did occur. If the patient has had a recurrence of symptoms as a manifestation of transference resistance during the terminal phases of the treatment, he likewise may underestimate the internal structural changes which took place and think that the therapy was a failure. If the therapy ended with a symptomatic remission, the patient may equate this with a cure even though there may have been no resolution of the underlying conflicts and no evidence of structural reorganization. At times the patient may judge certain results to have been positive, whereas the therapist or others in his environment may see them as manifestations of continuing disturbance. Some patients may have a need to feel that there has been major benefit from treatment, thereby to justify the investment of time, effort and money, when in actuality there may have been little or no change. At other times, the patient may have an incomplete understanding of the factors in the therapeutic process which led to the success or failure, and his understanding is frequently distorted, or influenced by persisting unconscious transference forces or other conflicts. Frequently the patient's assessment is influenced by the passage of time, so that his evaluation of treatment might be very different (in either direction) at the time of actual termination as compared with 1 or 2 years later.

Other people in the patient's reality environment may likewise be unreliable as judges of change, since they can make direct observations only of the patient's objective behaviour but will have no direct access to any subjective changes. And even some of the behavioural changes which the patient or therapist might recognize as signs of improvement, may be considered by his relatives to be a lack of improvement or regression in the patient's condition.

For example, a patient after therapy became significantly less masochistically submissive, and instead, was more assertive and outspoken at home. Her husband felt that 'She is much harder to live with, and is much worse'. A 28-year-old man, whose conflicts involved an intense passive-dependent relationship to his mother, began to emancipate himself, to find interests outside the parental home, established a meaningful relationship with a girl, and ultimately moved into his own apartment. The mother's reaction to therapy was that it was successful when it had initially helped the patient to feel more comfortable and less phobic, but the final outcome had taken her son away from her, and therefore therapy had made him much worse. A 35-year-old man's presenting symptoms included a compulsive need repetitively to consort with prostitutes. During the course of treatment, this symptom improved greatly. The wife's appraisal was that the therapy had done him no good at all. She was unaware of the change regarding the prostitutes since she had never known about it in the first place.

Such examples could be multiplied indefinitely, but they would only indicate that the other people in the patient's environment may likewise be biased and unreliable as judges of the outcome of a treatment experience.

Another possible judge of the outcome of treatment would be some other therapist who might examine the patient and assess the results. On the one hand, this person would be more neutral regarding the outcome and less biased than the original therapist. However, there would be inherent limitations in the material he could obtain from the patient in a few sessions, particularly regarding inner subjective experience. In such an interview situation, the patient's motivation to reveal himself would be very different than it had been with his own therapist, and the problems of establishing a relationship with the new examiner would likewise influence the data which the examiner might get. Furthermore, the examiner would have less direct knowledge of the goals that had been established for the therapy, and might have difficulty in evaluating what the significant therapeutic factors had been in producing success or failure. Furthermore, seeing the patient only at one particular point in time, the examiner might have difficulty in assessing whether the patient's current level of function represents a significant change from his earlier patterns. Another issue in regard to a neutral examiner is his theoretical orientation, and whether or not it should be the same as that of the original therapist. This question has particular significance in comparing the effectiveness of differing therapeutic methods (i.e. analytically oriented vs. behavioural therapies).

Ideally, in the evaluation of therapy, attempts should also be made to determine the nature and basis of any observed changes, and to specify the factors or forces that led to them. Is the change genuine and lasting, or is it transitory? Is it based on insight and working through, or on the transference relationship? Is it based on identification, denial, displacement or some other unconscious ego mechanism? Is it the result of a change in the patient's reality situation which occurred independently of the therapeutic work?

Implicit in these questions is the issue of whether, particularly in insight-directed therapy, evaluations are more accurate at the time of termination of the treatment, or at some time in the more remote future (i.e. after a few years). In view of the strategy to help the patient towards a full and productive development of himself and a greater capacity to deal with the inevitable vicissitudes and conflicts of life, the full evaluation of the degree to which these goals have been reached must wait until the future has become the past. However, if the therapist arranges for such an evaluation of the patient after a considerable lapse of time, there is frequently a risk that such a contact may remobilize latent and unresolved transference reactions, and therefore it may not be in the patient's best therapeutic interests.

In patients whose therapy was not successful, a search should also be made to delineate the possible reasons for the failure. In this connection, occasionally therapeutic benefits from insight treatment are delayed, and although change may seem minimal at the time of termination, there may be considerable progress in the subsequent period.

Another problem is the evaluation of the situation in which the patient broke off treatment after just a short time. Added to all of the other complexities is the issue of whether or not the patient was properly evaluated at the beginning, and whether the treatment undertaken was appropriate. Was the failure a result of factors within the patient alone, or might a different therapist or different therapeutic approach have produced a different outcome? Such questions are particularly difficult to answer precisely, since even a subsequent attempt at treatment with another therapist may be influenced in one direction or the other by the previous therapeutic experience.

This discussion is meant primarily to emphasize the tremendous number of variables in the therapeutic situation which cannot be controlled experimentally, but must nevertheless be considered in the appraisal of results of a treatment undertaking. A full evaluation would include study of the data available from all of the different sources and points of view described above, and in some of the current research projects on the results of psychotherapy, this is being done. However, as is apparent from the methodological problems described in these studies, the difficulties, complexities and investments of time and manpower are considerable.

However, in spite of the difficulties, inaccuracies and limitations, ultimate growth and development of the individual therapist requires that he make an honest, self-searching and critical appraisal of his therapeutic results in every patient. This should include not only the gross judgment as to the degree of success or failure, but also the possible factors and reasons for it. Furthermore, if a patient's treatment was unsuccessful, the therapist should evaluate and try to consider what other things might have been done to avoid such a therapeutic failure. If the result was partially successful, the therapist should consider whether there were other ways by which he could have helped to make the treatment even more effective. If therapy was judged as successful, the therapist should try to delineate the factors which led to the success, so that these may be readily available to him for use in subsequent treatment situations.

The results of therapy must always be evaluated on the basis of how closely the final outcome of the treatment for the particular patient approximated the goals which had been set initially, or modified as the treatment progressed. Therefore, no single yardstick can be used to evaluate the results of various forms and approaches to psychotherapy. Even among cases treated supportively, 'success' of treatment may have different implications. For one patient, it might involve full remission of presenting symptoms; for another it might be merely the recovery from an acute psychotic regression and stabilization at the level of chronic neurosis outside of a hospital.

The major emphasis in evaluating the results of supportive treatment is the status of the patient's overt symptoms and behaviour. This includes the degree to which there has been remission of the presenting complaints, as well as the stability of the level of dynamic equilibrium which was established as a result of the treatment. Unconscious structural personality change may have occurred on the basis of identification with the therapist, and may be reflected in modifications of ego and super-ego function. The degree to which this has taken place, and the effects which it may have on the stability of the dynamic equilibrium are further criteria regarding the success of treatment.

However, such things as the persistence of unexplored or unresolved conflicts, the continuing use of unconscious ego defences or the persistence of ego-syntonic neurotic character traits and symptoms cannot be judged as manifestations of therapeutic failure. The strategy of supportive treatment does not involve attempts to modify these processes.

In insight-directed treatment on the other hand, the main criterion for evaluation of results is the degree of structural change which has occurred in the individual's personality, and the nature and depth of understanding and insight into his own mental functions and conflicts which the individual has achieved. The possibility that the patient will experience a recurrence of symptoms or anxiety during the termination phase was described in Chapter XVII. Hence, the status of the patient's symptoms at the time of the termination of treatment is a less significant factor in evaluating therapeutic change, although it is one that must still be considered. The presence of symptoms at the end of treatment is not itself an indication of therapeutic failure, as it might be in supportive treatment. And vice versa, if a patient in insight-directed treatment shows no evidence of structural change, or of insight into the origins and nature of his conflicts, but has had a remission of symptoms, such a result would have to be assessed as relatively unsuccessful in light of the original goals.

The type of structural change that must be evaluated is the degree of ego modification and conscious extension of function into previously unconscious aspects of mental life. Also included would be such things as modification of object relationships, capacity to tolerate frustration or anxiety and ability effectively to interact with the environment in the maintenance of adaptation. The degree of super-ego change away from the primitive and automatic unconscious responses and towards conscious ego integration is another manifestation of structural change which must be evaluated. There should also be an assessment of changes in the relative intensity of the unconscious drives and drive-derivatives, and of the progress the patient has made towards the achievement of genital primacy.

In other words, in insight-directed treatment the evaluation of results is based on the degree to which lasting structural change has occurred in the direction of emotional maturity as these concepts were defined in Chapter III. However, as described in Chapter XIV, therapeutic strategy may be aimed at achieving varying depths and degrees of insight and structural change. Therefore, the extent of the changes which took place must be evaluated on the scale of the degree of modification which was the goal of treatment. For example, if the goal of therapy was a major reorganization and reconstruction of the personality, the degree of change necessary to permit a successful evaluation of treatment would be significantly greater than if the initial goal had been a superficial insight-directed attempt to modify only the more immediate or focal elements of the patient's unconscious conflicts.

For example, a 37-year-old professional man entered intensive insight-directed treatment with the conscious goal of definitively resolving major personality problems, narcotic addiction and depression. The disturbances had destroyed his marriage, ruined his career, involved him in an intensely disturbed second marriage and alienated him from friends and family. He underwent a progressive symptomatic improvement to the point that after 6 months of treatment he had begun professional work for the first time in 4 years, and there was relief from the intense anxiety and depression. However, he became increasingly resistant to further therapeutic work, emphasized his symptomatic remission and partial achievement of pre-morbid function, and after a year of treatment he terminated contact. From the standpoint of the patient's subjective symptoms, there had been marked improvement. However, his conflicts over aggression, his sexual disturbances, his masochistic and ungratifying marital situation, his narcissistic withdrawal and his neurotic inhibition of his potential persisted unchanged. From the standpoint of the goals initially set and maintained for this patient, treatment was a relative failure in spite of the positive symptomatic response. And contrariwise, if the goals had been those of supportive treatment, the outcome would have been considered successful.

Each therapist must develop his own body of experience and clinical sophistication in order to improve his therapeutic abilities. An important aspect of this is the necessity for constant appraisal of himself, his interactions with patients and the tactics and vicissitudes of the treatment process. These must finally be judged in the light of their impact on the outcome of treatment. It is in this way that the therapist accumulates his personal collection of clinical experiences. And it is on this basis that he gradually evolves his own personal therapeutic style.

SUGGESTED READING

BRONNER, AUGUSTA F. (Chairman) (1949) Round Table: the objective evaluation of psychotherapy. *Am. J. Orthopsychiat.* **19**, 463

G.A.P. Report 63 (1966) Psychiatric Research and the Assessment of Change

KNIGHT, ROBERT P. (1952) An evaluation of psychotherapeutic techniques. *Bull. Menninger Clin.* **16**, 113

MILES, HENRY H.W., BARRABEE, EDNA L. & FINESINGER, JACOB E. (1951) Evaluation of psychotherapy with follow-up study of 62 cases of anxiety neurosis. *Psychosom. Med.* **13**, 83

PFEFFER, ARNOLD Z. (1961) Follow-up study of a satisfactory analysis. *J. Am. Psychoanal. Ass.* **9**, 698

PFEFFER, ARNOLD Z. (1962) The meaning of the analyst after analysis (Abstract), *Psychoanal. Quart.* **31**, 441

VOTH, HAROLD M. *et al.* (1962) Situational variables in the assessment of psychotherapeutic results. *Bull. Menninger Clin.* **26**, 73

WALLERSTEIN, ROBERT S., ROBBINS, LEWIS L. *et al.* (1956, 1958, 1960) The Psychotherapy Research Project of the Menninger Foundation. 1st Report, *Bull. Menninger Clin.* **20**, 221–280; 2nd Report, *Bull. Menninger Clin.* **22**, 115–166; 3rd Report, *Bull. Menninger Clin.* **24**, 157–216

WALLERSTEIN, ROBERT S. (1963) The problem of the assessment of change in psychotherapy. *Int. J. Psycho-Anal.* **44**, 31

Index